History and Modern Nursing

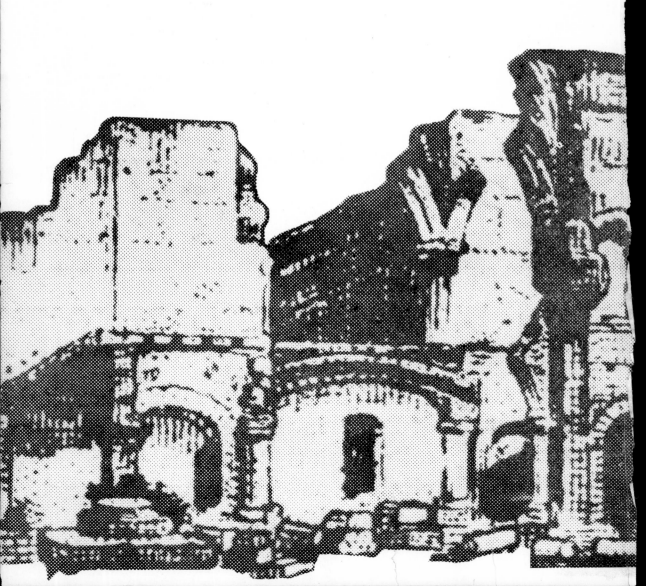

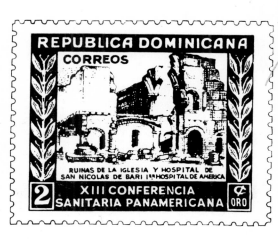

REPUBLICA DOMINICANA
CORREOS
RUINAS DE LA IGLESIA Y HOSPITAL DE
SAN NICOLAS DE BARI 1ᵉʳ HOSPITAL DE AMERICA
2 ¢ ORO
XIII CONFERENCIA
SANITARIA PANAMERICANA

by Lena Dixon Dietz, R.N.

Graduate of the University of Iowa Hospital School
of Nursing; awarded the Certificate of Merit by the
State University of Iowa, 1947. Formerly Science
Instructor, Hospital Latino-Americano, Puebla, Mex-
ico; Science Instructor, Aultman Hospital, Canton,
Ohio; Director of Nurses, Passavant Hospital,
Jacksonville, Illinois; Clinical Instructor in Medical
and Surgical Nursing, Michael Reese Hospital School
of Nursing, Chicago; Editor-in-Chief of The Nursing
Survey.

F. A. DAVIS CO.

Philadelphia

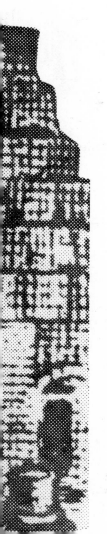

Printed in the United States of America

This book is dedicated to my daughters, Charlotte Dietz Horton and
Helena Dietz Laurent

Preface

Although nursing is as old as the human race, it is only during the past century that it has struck out boldly toward professional status. One of the characteristics of a profession is the interest in its history as a means of appreciatng the accomplishments of the past and as an instrument in planning further developments.

In this history no attempt has been made to separate nursing from medicine. These subjects have been closely interwoven since early times, even as they are today. For example, as late as 1890, nurses could not legally give hypodermics; only a doctor could pierce the human skin. The present controversy: "Shall nurses do venipunctures?" clearly indicates that there can be no historical separation of nursing and medicine. Because of this, nursing and medicine have been combined to show the development of both as they have been influenced by great historical events.

Since sociology is a part of the curriculum, nursing among primitive peoples has been omitted. Instead, the prevention of disease and the care of the sick is given as described in recorded history.

Also, since this history has been written for American nurses, the author has purposely given considerable space to the events in American history that have directly influenced nursing and medicine. These in turn have made possible the prestige accorded nursing in the United States.

Modern nursing is the day-by-day development of all fields of nursing as they are influenced by education, legislation, economics, and organizations.

Increased education for women in all fields of nursing has increased educational standards for schools of nursing. Modern nursing, therefore, to keep pace with modern medicine, requires women and men with broad educational backgrounds. Nurses are no longer ''the keeper of the keys'' and ''the handmaiden of the physician.'' Nursing is a service profession which carries with it all the implications of social and scientific advancement in the prevention of illness, the actual care of the sick, and rehabilitation.

The subjects in Units II, III, IV, and V are guides for the nurse-student and later for the graduate nurse to insure continued professional growth. With this background the nurse will understand nursing organizations, the Economic Security Program, legislative procedures, legal hazards in nursing, and many more subjects that will arise as nursing expands.

Through professional reading and organizational activities the nurse can keep abreast with the constantly changing pattern of modern nursing.

MRS. LENA DIXON DIETZ

Acknowledgments

No one can write a book alone. For this reason the author wishes to express sincere appreciation to those who have given directly of their knowledge, time, experience, and effort to help in the preparation of a book which the author hopes will be useful to the nurse-student in making her aware of the history of her profession and to help her make a satisfactory adjustment to modern nursing.

Appreciation is expressed to the following: Dorothy E. Anderson, Director of Nursing Service, Chicago Chapter of the American Red Cross, for assistance with the chapter, "The Red Cross."

The American Red Cross, Washington, D. C., for a careful review of the history of the Red Cross, both national and international.

Sister M. John Francis, Order of the Holy Cross, for bibliography and use of the archives on the life of Mother Angela Gillespie.

Amy Frances Brown, author, who shared her research on early collegiate schools of nursing.

Russell J. Burt, attorney, Canton, Ohio, for the review of the chapter, "Legal Problems."

Viola A. Callan, Director of Nursing Service, Children's Hospital, San Francisco, for quotations from the early files of the first hospital west of the Rocky Mountains.

Sisters of Columbus Hospital, Chicago, for information about the founder, Mother Cabrini.

M. Cordelia Cowan, author, who shared her accumulation of books, calendars, and scrapbooks on nursing history.

Alice Distad, Librarian, Michael Reese Hospital School of Nursing, who contributed many references for Unit I.

Frank J. Isherwood, photographer for the Hall of Fame of the International College of Surgeons, Chicago, for the use of illustrations.

W. F. James (MC), U.S.N. (Ret.), Executive Director of the Hall of Fame of the International College of Surgeons, Chicago, for many of the pictures used in this book.

Sister Justina, Administrator, DePaul Hospital, St. Louis, for an historical summary of the Sisters of Charity in founding the first hospital west of the Mississippi River.

Katrina Johnstone, Librarian, Michael Reese Hospital School of Nursing, who contributed greatly to the bibliographies of Unit I.

MacKinlay Kantor, author, for information on the prison camps of the Civil War.

Stanley Kaval, photographer, for assistance and advice in the preparation of illustrations.

Thomas E. Keyes, Chief Librarian, Mayo Clinic, Rochester, Minnesota, for his historic investigation of the *Prayer of Maimonides*.

Harriet T. Lane, author, who provided a bibliography on the work of the Ursulines in Charity Hospital, New Orleans.

James E. Laurent, business analyst, for helpful suggestions in review and arrangement.

Aurelia Lehozki, member of the Illinois Board of Nurse Examiners, for a careful review of the chapter, ''Registration and Interstate Licensure.''

Bertram Levin, roentgenologist, Michael Reese Hospital and Medical Center, for a review of the life of William Conrad Roentgen.

Myrtle Lewis, Director of Nurses, Mary Thompson Hospital, Chicago, who provided information on the first school of nursing in the Middle West.

Brother Maurice, Director of Nursing, Alexian Brothers Hospital School of Nursing, Chicago, for information and pictures of the origin and development of the Alexian Brothers and their hospitals.

Elma A. Medearis, Senior Professional Assistant, Museum of New Mexico, for information on the early Spanish explorers.

Timity J. O'Connor, member of the Civil War Round Table, for information on the prison camps of the North during the Civil War.

The Community Relations Department of Passavant Hospital, Pittsburgh, for information and pictures of the first Protestant hospital in the Western Hemisphere.

The Public Relations Department of Pennsylvania Hospital, Philadelphia, for the picture of the Great Court of the Hospital.

George A. Bender, Director of Institutional Advertising, Parke, Davis and Company, Detroit, for the pictures: A History of Medicine in Pictures. These are reproduced by special permission of Parke, Davis and Company, who commissioned the original oil paintings and by whom they were copyrighted. These pictures are painted by Robert A. Thom.

Edith D. Payne, Director of Nurses, St. Luke's Hospital, Chicago, for information concerning the early history of St. Luke's Hospital.

The Chamber of Commerce, Danville, Kentucky, for information and pictures of the Ephraim McDowell Shrine.

William Arthur Rodgers of the *South Town Economist*, for pictures of the Confederate Cemetery, Chicago.

Will Ross, Inc., Milwaukee, for the picture of the Augustinian nun from the series, "They Caught the Torch."

Dunbar Smith, Battle Creek Sanatorium, Battle Creek, Michigan, for information and pictures of early nursing in the Middle West.

Gordon Snider, Consultant in Tuberculosis, Michael Reese Hospital and Research Center, Chicago, for information on Dr. Edward Trudeau.

Kenneth Starr, Curator of Asiatic Archeology, Chicago Museum of Natural History, for his help and interest in finding authentic material on China.

Friedrich Sternthal, Historian, Hall of Fame of the International College of Surgeons, for information on early medicine in China and India.

Reed and Margaret Teitsworth, West Reading, Pennsylvania, for history and pictures of the Revolutionary War in eastern Pennsylvania.

Margaret C. Tibbits, Director of the School of Nursing, McLean Hospital, Waverley, Massachusetts, for information on early schools of nursing offering instruction in care of the mentally ill.

Audrey E. Toft, Director of Nurses, St. Luke's Hospital, Jacksonville, Florida, for information and pictures of the first hospital in Florida.

Charles LeTourneau, Editor-in-Chief, *Hospital Management*, for the use of illustrations from that publication.

Virginia A. Turner, former editor of *Nursing World*, for information on the early organization of American nurses.

Major Hubert J. Van Kan, Audio Visual Branch of the Public Information Division of the U. S. Signal Corps, for pictures of American wars.

Mary Jane Venger, Director of Nurses, Mount Sinai Hospital, New York (formerly Director of Nurses, Louisville General Hospital), for historical data and pictures of the first hospital west of the Allegheny Mountains.

Carol V. Webster, member of the Legislative Committee of the Illinois Nurses' Association, for the revision of the chapter, "Nursing Legislation."

Paula C. Weins, Psychiatric and Psychosomatic Institute, Chicago, for information on psychiatric nursing.

Stella Wuerffel, who provided information on the Saxon immigration and the later founding of the Lutheran Hospital, St. Louis.

Gladys B. Yost, Educational Director, Woman's Hospital, Philadelphia, for information on the early history of that hospital.

Anne Zimmerman, Executive Director, Illinois Nurses' Association, for assistance with the chapter, "American Nurses' Association."

Those students whose interest in nursing history provided a stimulus for continued historical investigation.

Both students and graduates who, by bringing their professional problems to the author, have furnished the basis and incentive for Units II, III, IV, and V of this book.

Table of Contents

UNIT II. ORIENTATION OF THE GRADUATE NURSE

UNIT III. OPPORTUNITIES AND PREPARATION

UNIT IV. ORGANIZATIONS: NATIONAL AND INTERNATIONAL

UNIT V. PROFESSIONAL RELATIONSHIPS

UNIT I

History of Nursing

CHAPTER 1

Introduction

What is the meaning of history? Why is it important for nursing students to study the history of their profession? Further, do the victories and defeats of the past have a real meaning for all nurses today?

There are a number of interlocking definitions of history. The most common definition of the word *history* is "the past of mankind." Even a superficial glance tells us that the meaning of the word in this sense is incomplete because the past of mankind, for the most part, is beyond recall. Louis Gottschalk says " . . . history becomes only that part of the human past which can be meaningfully reconstructed from the available records and from influences regarding their setting."[1] But when we look back through the years, the meaning goes deeper than that of a logical inquiry into the past.

Perhaps the meaning of history can best be summed up in three short lines from the first of *The Four Quartets* by T. S. Eliot:

> *Time present and time past*
> *Are both perhaps in time future,*
> *And time future contained in time past.*[2]

From these interpretations, we see that history is an endless cycle; there-fore, says Herbert J. Muller, "it cannot have a final meaning. We are

---

[1] Louis Gottschalk, *Understanding History* (New York, Alfred A. Knopf, 1956), p. 48.

[2] T. S. Eliot, "Burnt Norton," *Collected Poems* (New York, Harcourt, Brace and Company, 1936), p. 213.

constantly drawing upon the past. It constitutes all the experience by which we have learned: it is the source of our major interests, our claims, our rights, and other duties. It is the very essence of our identity."[3]

Why study nursing history? Like everyone else, nurses must turn to the past for clarification of the present—for a fuller comprehension of what has happened, and how, and why. And in this whole process of interpreting and evaluating the facts, attempting to answer the questions of how, why, and what of it, nurses are inevitably committed to certain assumptions about the nature of nursing and its place in society and about the role he or she, as a nurse, must play in this society.

Unfortunately, nursing history-as-happening seems to have preference over nursing history-as-record. But it is to both that nurses must turn for wisdom and understanding. There is always a need for students to know concurrent events in general history in order to orient themselves in any particular period of nursing which they are studying.

In writing to an outstanding leader in many aspects of American life, the President of the American Association of University Professors asked the late Judge Learned Hand to express his thoughts on the subject: What should be the basic objectives of higher education viewed in its relation to the welfare of America in contemporary life, its short-term and long-term future? Judge Learned Hand, one of the nation's greatest jurists, voiced the need for students to have a wider knowledge of history:

I think that the prime purpose of "higher education" is to establish the right habit of thinking, by which I mean thinking that holds its conclusions open to revision and is ready to consider only new evidence that is apparently reliable. That habit I believe is better acquired by a wide acquaintance with history, letters, and the arts than by specialized but limited disciplines. . . . The main thing is what will be the student's temper of approach to his problem when he gets through.[4]

The findings of a significant study conducted by Frances Cooke MacGregor indicate that the cultural approach is of great benefit to the student nurse because it helps her to solve patient problems arising out of cultural differences in attitudes, feelings, and reactions. In discussing with student nurses the need of a scientific attitude and an appreciation of scientific methods, MacGregor reports some interesting questions asked by students: "Is it (scientific attitude) not likely to get in the way of tender loving care treatment that is stressed in our classes? Is it not apt to make a nurse detached or perhaps even cold in her relationships with patients? Is not the scientific attitude incompatible with compassion?"[5]

As MacGregor indicates, a scientific attitude and compassion are not identical but neither are they mutually exclusive.

[3] Herbert J. Muller, *The Uses of the Past* (New York, The New American Library, 1954), p. 36.

[4] AAUP *Bulletin*, Summer, 1956, p. 264.

[5] Frances Cooke MacGregor, *Social Science in Nursing* (New York, Russell Sage Foundation, 1960), pp. 63-64.

Sometimes people conform to patterns of behavior because they are expected to conform to certain standards, but usually they are taught to do so by formal or informal education, perhaps both. Historians and sociologists assign the name "culture group" to those persons who follow the same general pattern of behavior.

According to Margaret Mead, culture is not biologically inherited; instead, it is a "body of learned behavior which a group of people, who share the same tradition, transmit entire to their children, and, in part, to adult immigrants who become members of the society. It covers not only the arts and sciences, religions and philosophies to which the word culture has been historically applied, but also the system of technology, the political practices, the small intimate battles of daily life, such as the way of preparing or eating food, or electing a prime minister or changing the Constitution."[6] For example, we all need food, but we have different ways of conveying it to our mouths. In America, we use forks; in China, chop sticks; and Hawaiians use their fingers to eat certain foods.

When the group becomes very large and its organization complex, says Joseph Ward Swain, "a culture is called a civilization."[7] Reference is made frequently to both terms in this volume.

But what bearing do cultural differences have on nursing and patient care in American hospitals? Why should the nurse know about the magical and superstitious beliefs and practices of other peoples, especially when she functions in a highly scientific medical environment? Of what use is it for her to know that among some primitive peoples mothers insist upon burying the umbilical cord in the ground? What good will it do for the nurse to know that the sickroom of a Guatemalan Indian must be crowded with visitors to keep the evil spirits away? And what difference does it make if the attitude of the Chinese toward food is different from that of the student nurse? Of what benefit is it for the student to know that the primitive natives of Africa and Australia believe that sickness is caused by a disease devil who enters the human body?

One answer to these questions is that we are living in a fast-changing world; physical distances are shrinking, and American nurses are currently serving in more than thirty-one countries. Today's student may choose a similar assignment after she graduates. To come closer to home, while the student's patient population may be homogeneous today, tomorrow she may be assigned to a ward whose patient population is heterogeneous. If the student recognizes the cultural differences among her patients, it will help her to have a better understanding of her own attitudes as well as those of her patients.

MacGregor cites a good example of how recognition of and respect for cultural differences can promote better patient care:

---

[6] Margaret Mead, *Cultural Patterns and Technical Change* (Paris, United Nations Educational, Scientific and Cultural Organization, 1953), pp. 9-10.

[7] Joseph Ward Swain, *The Harper History of Civilization* (New York, Harper & Brothers, 1958), p. 4.

A public health nurse in a well-baby clinic was trying to stop Mexican mothers from feeding their babies so many beans, and start them using more milk. Month after month she inveighed against the beans. Finally, in despair, she said, "Well, then, at least feed them the water in which the beans are cooked [in which some of the nutrients would have been preserved]." The babies began to show signs of better nourishment. When she said, "You see, the bean water helps," the mothers answered: "Oh! It's not just the bean water. When you stopped talking against our beans we started following your advice and began giving them more milk."[8]

So we see that while differences in cultural patterns may seem insignificant at times—as in the case of using chop sticks instead of forks, and feeding the babies beans instead of milk—it is most important that the student understand that each civilization, culture, and subculture has its own distinctive way of life—that its members' ways of doing things are normal to them. Therefore students, as well as graduates, can no longer afford to ignore the cultural differences related to ethnic backgrounds.

Some cultures change rapidly, others slowly. But even the most progressive civilizations retain much of their legacy from the past. The purpose here is to study historically the stream of influence on nursing that has flowed from ancient times to the present. The two criteria which have helped to shape the author's point of view are: What kind of people have nurses been and how did they respond to the conditions in their environment; what measures were necessary to promote the growth and cohesion of nursing? In short, the dominant themes of this book are evolution and growth of nursing. As we shall see in the following pages, nursing has followed a course that is strange and somewhat obscure.

Although the art of nursing is of great antiquity—as ancient as humanity itself—nursing history does not stand out as distinctly as political, religious, or even medical history. Nursing history is interwoven with general history.

To understand more fully the development of nursing we must trace the evolution of medical beliefs and practices to find any remnants of nursing history. We shall begin by examining the medical concepts of ancient civilizations in order to detect the first threads of nursing history; the chapters thereafter will deal with the many social forces that have charted nursing's course from the most remote past to the present. While it is not the purpose here to make predictions, any book about the past inevitably contains some reference to the future.

REFERENCES

DOLAN, JOSEPHINE A.: *Using Postage Stamps to Teach History of Nursing.* *Nursing Outlook* 9:164-165, 1961.

EVANS, JESSIE C.: *The Modern Point of View in the Teaching of History.* Amer. J. Nurs. 17:952-957 (from the Proceedings of the 20th Annual Convention of the American Nurses' Association, April 26-May 2, 1917).

FABRICANT, NOAH: *Stamps that Mark Milestones of Medicine.* *Today's Health* 35:26-27, 1957.

---

[8] MacGregor, *op. cit.,* p. 79.

CHAPTER 2

Early Medicine and Nursing

Nursing history is an episode in the history of woman and, according to Victor Robinson, M.D., the entire history of nursing may be summed up in sixteen words: "the nurse is the mirror in which is reflected the position of woman through the ages."[1]

There are other historians who assume that early nursing was united with medicine, but these historians have failed to provide any concrete evidence that medicine and nursing followed parallel courses of development. There is an occasional reference to the word "nurse" in ancient literature, but no details as to the kind of preparation she had or how she functioned.

Whatever be the truth regarding the source of nursing history, the nurse reader will observe throughout nursing's course many twistings and turnings—perhaps partial breaks but never any complete breaks.

Where shall we begin the long but fascinating journey of looking backward, yet keeping an eye on the present so that the future may come into view?

Any division in the fields of history is always quite arbitrary, because historians rarely agree as to what should be included in each division. For convenience, however, we may divide human history into three periods: *ancient,* from the first written records to the fall of Rome in 476 A.D.;

[1] Victor Robinson, *White Caps* (Philadelphia, J. B. Lippincott Company, 1946), p. vii.

medieval, from the fall of the Roman Empire to the great period of exploration which began with the discovery of the West Indies by Columbus in 1492;
modern, from 1492 to the present.

If the nurse of today is curious about how her counterpart ministered to
the sick in ancient Babylonia (*ca.* 2000 B.C.), she will find that the ancient
nurse, though not referred to as such, was probably a domestic servant who
gave instinctive care to the sick and needy. If we use the present-day concept
of the nurse, we can find no counterpart for the twentieth century nurse in
ancient civilizations.

It will be necessary to first follow the development of medical science, not
so much for the purpose of trying to detect relationships between medicine
and nursing, but to emphasize the social forces shaping and reshaping the
conditions of a changing world.

The earliest civilizations settled along the Indus, Euphrates, Tigris, and
Nile Rivers. The first people we meet among the ancient civilizations are
the Sumerians, who established themselves in Babylonia.

Babylonia. The practice of medicine in ancient Babylonia was far advanced
with respect to legal and penal concepts. The Code of Hammurabi contained
statements of great historical significance both to physicians and nurses,
because it established for the first time legal and civil measures, thereby
regulating the practice of physicians and providing greater safety for the
patient. For example, the Code stated:

*If a physician shall produce on anyone a severe wound with a bronze operating
knife and cure him, or if he shall open an abscess with the operating knife and
preserve the eye of the patient, he usually shall receive ten shekels of silver;
if it is a slave, his master shall usually pay two shekels of silver to the
physician.*

*If a physician shall make a severe wound with an operating knife and kill
him, or shall open an abscess with an operating knife and destroy the eye, his
hands shall be cut off.*

*If a physician shall cure a diseased bone or a diseased organ, he shall receive
five shekels of silver; if it is a matter of a freed slave, he shall pay three
shekels of silver; but if a slave, then the master of the slave shall give to the
physician two shekels of silver.*[2]

The medical world must give much credit to Babylonian medicine for its
enrichment of drug therapy, for its concepts of hygiene and social medicine,
and for codifying the responsibilities of the physician.

Whatever the duties of the Babylonian nurse—slave or domestic—he or
she lived in a civilization of people skilled in calculation and observation,
though perhaps less objective in their treatment of data than were their
neighbors across the valley.

[2] Arturo Castiglioni, *A History of Medicine* (New York, Alfred A. Knopf, 1958), p. 40.

Egypt. Across the valley from Babylonia was Egypt, where the people lived an entirely different kind of social and political life, even though the two civilizations developed about the same time (*ca.* 4000 B.C.).

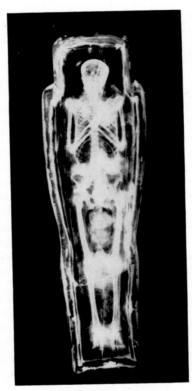

X-ray of a mummy in a case, 2000 years B.C. Note the pathologic process in the joints. (Courtesy of the Chicago Natural History Museum, from the Pollock-Bridgeman Collection.)

If we regard Egypt as "the gift of the Nile," the striking differences between the two civilizations become apparent. The whole subject of Egyptian civilization viewed in relation to the political, social, economic, and social life of the nation has captured the attention of peoples throughout the ages.

In the peace and quiet of their valley, the Egyptians worked out their own cultural pattern—without regard for time. Yet one of their most important inventions was the solar calendar of 365 days, with twelve months of thirty days each and five extra days added at the end of the year.

The Egyptians were advanced mathematicians. As skilled architects, they designed their buildings with a colossal style, the most famous of their monuments being the pyramids. The most reliable source of information on Egyptian culture are the inscriptions on the papyrus.

The development of medicine in Egypt did not follow an orderly course with respect to time and form. Influenced by the orient, Egyptian medicine was chiefly mystic and priestly; but it was empirical and realistic where contact with nature persisted longer and where the influence of African civilization was felt strongly.

In Egyptian mythology the control of health was in the hands of gods. Imhotep (He who cometh in Peace) was the most important of these gods, and was the first acknowledged physician. He is thought to have lived about 2980 B.C., although some Egyptologists place the date much earlier—about 4900 B.C. Although Imhotep was worshipped as a god, there is evidence that he was a historic person. The medical library dedicated to him in Memphis, Egypt, contained papyrus scrolls from which the Greeks later derived much of their medical knowledge.

Egypt is credited as being the healthiest of all ancient countries. The Egyptians made great progress in the field of hygiene and in sanitation, which is an important aspect of preventive medicine. Today we think of preventive medicine as being a modern concept, yet the Holy Scriptures show clearly that the Egyptians, under the leadership of Moses, practiced principles of good hygiene.

Moses, the adopted son of Pharaoh's daughter, undoubtedly had been educated at the University of Heliopolis (now Cairo) and had become learned "in all of the wisdom of the Egyptians." Some of the hygienic principles followed by the Egyptians concerned restrictions on eating meat, care in the choice of edible foods found in the desert, methods taken to curtail the spread of leprosy, and means of disposing of human excreta.

Because of the warm climate and lack of any form of refrigeration, meat was forbidden to be eaten after the third day as described in Leviticus 7:16-19 and 19:5-8. The Jews, in bondage for generations, were suddenly thrown into a desert country and forced to live off the land. The detailed list of foods that could be eaten is found in the eleventh chapter of Leviticus. It is evident that all forms of skin eruptions were automatically considered to be due to leprosy. Elaborate precautions were taken to prevent its spread and the person having a cutaneous lesion was isolated at once by the priest-physician. Chapter 14 of Leviticus describes the thorough terminal disinfection for leprosy; Chapter 15 the method for gonorrhea. The disposal of human excreta is described in Deuteronomy 23:12-15. If modern civilizations would use the same method where flush toilets are unavailable, hookworm might be eradicated.

Diagnosis achieved an advanced position in the Egyptian civilization, with each physician a specialist. As for therapeutics the Ebers papyrus lists approximately 1000 prescriptions. Some of the remedies used by the Egyptians are known to us today: honey, beer, yeast, oil, dates, figs, onions, garlic, flaxseed, and fennel. Some of the medicines prescribed were myrrh, aloes, crocus, opium, and lead prescriptions. Medicines were supplied in pills and suppositories, forms still used today.

It is now known that there was a college for physicians in Egypt in 1100 B.C., and perhaps long before that. The physicians of this college were employed by the state and were required to treat indigent patients without cost. Were there any hospitals connected with the early seats of learning? Studies to date reveal no trace of buildings identifiable as hospitals, but it is believed, however, that there were sanitoria connected with the temples and that they may have been used for the sick. Who cared for these patients? Certainly not the physicians. Undoubtedly some form of instinctive nursing care must have existed at this time, but there is no conclusive evidence that such was the case.

Palestine. Of all the ancient peoples, the Hebrews seem to have been the most democratic in sharing their knowledge with succeeding civilizations. Although much of this knowledge was borrowed from their neighbors, the Egyptians and Assyro-Babylonians, the Jews carefully evaluated it and adapted it to their own system of values.

From the standpoint of the care of the sick, the Jews, in contrast to the tenets of their neighbors, believed that the ordinary man was entitled to the same medical treatment as the aristocrat.

M. Adelaide Nutting and Lavinia L. Dock give an interesting example of the Jews' concern for the sick:

To visit the sick in order to show them sympathy, to cheer and aid and relieve them in their suffering, is declared by the Rabbis to be a duty incumbent upon every Jew even if the sick person be a Gentile . . . [3]

The ancient Jews provided an *xenodochium or pandok* for travelers and the destitute; the *ptochotropheum* or Sick House was attached to the *pandok*. Reference is made to the fact that "if anyone be sick, he is cured by medicine from the common stock . . . " But we do not know who administered this medicine, since no mention is made of nurses.

The practice of medicine by the Jews differed from that of all other ancient peoples in that it recognized one God as the source both of health and of all diseases. It was to this one God that the people of Israel turned for the cure of their ills. This concept, which has been referred to as unitarian, tended to dispel from among the Jews the magic practices and superstitious beliefs common among other ancient civilizations.

Since one God had the power to cure or inflict illness, it is easy to see why the Jews felt compelled to follow the divine precepts and also to carry out all of the religious practices that contained an element of hygiene and sanitation.

In the Biblical concept of medicine the priests were the supervisors of all religious practices and also the only ones to whom medical functions were assigned. This concept made physical purity equivalent to moral purity, thus the Jewish people attained high levels of hygiene and sanitation.

Whenever a person became impure, either by contracting some contagious disease or by committing an evil deed, he could become pure again by par-

---

[3] M. Adelaide Nutting and Lavinia L. Dock, *A History of Nursing* (New York, G. P. Putnam's Sons, 1935), p. 64.

taking in certain ceremonies. Bathing was an important part of the purification process, and held an important place in religious rituals. For example, no Jew could enter the temple without taking a bath if he had had contact with impure persons or things. Any person who had entered a house in which there was a dead person was considered impure for seven days and had to be washed on the third and seventh day with the water of *purification*. Any person affected by a urethral "issue," the issue most likely being gonorrhea, was said to be impure, and whoever had any contact with him had to wash his clothing, take a bath, and remain impure until evening. After the flow was stopped, the victim with the issue was required to wait seven days before he was regarded as pure. A woman was considered impure during menstruation according to Biblical law.

Soldiers going to camp were supposed to take with them an instrument to dig a hole in the ground to bury the feces. In the light of current sanitary measures, this is a primitive idea, but for that age it was an advanced concept of sanitation.

In the Talmud is found the later medical concepts of the Jews. The Talmudic laws indicate that the people of Israel regarded diphtheria as the most infectious of diseases. Tumors of the lung and cirrhosis are also identified in these laws. Some surgery, such as that for correction of anal fistula, the reduction of dislocations, and Caesarean section, was performed. A sleeping potion was given as preoperative preparation.

Jewish medicine made an important contribution to all other civilizations, it provided the basis of all social hygiene. For the first time in history the people were given legislative protection, and at the same time there arose the concept of sanitary legislation, which imposed restrictions upon them.

China. Respect for deep-rooted traditions, the veneration of sayings of ancestors, and rigid emphasis on insignificant details brought to a halt what

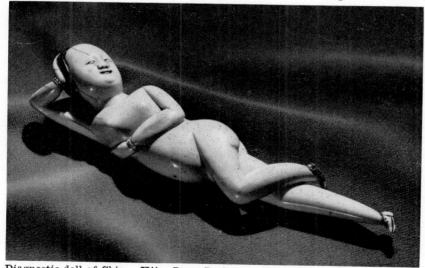

Diagnostic doll of China. K'ien-Lung Period (1736-1795). (Courtesy of Chicago Natural History Museum.)

had been a brilliant Chinese civilization. Chinese medicine first flourished and then regressed in much the same way as did the arts and natural sciences.

The original concept of Chinese medicine, unlike that of other ancient civilizations, is of great interest to doctors and nurses. In China the physicians were accorded exalted positions and frequently were found presiding among the gods. Chief among these gods were Pan Ku, the most ancient, who formed the universe; Hua To, an exponent of acupuncture and credited as being a great surgeon who practiced operations on the brain and abdomen; the Emperor Shen Nung, one of the chief medical gods and said to be the father of Chinese medicine; and Chang Chung Ching, known as the Chinese Hippocrates, who flourished about 170 A.D.

Emperor Shen Nung was the first to compile an herbal, which listed more than 100 remedies. He is also the inventor of the acupuncture technic.

Diagnosis was made on the basis of a complicated pulse theory—the human body was compared with a chord instrument; the different pulses represented

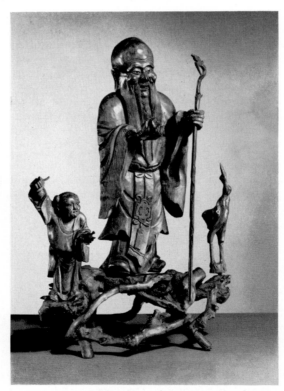

The god of Longevity, the most popular household deity of China, with dragon staff and peach of immortality, accompanied by a youth and a crane; the crane is an emblem of long life. Ming Period. (Courtesy of Chicago Natural History Museum.)

the chords. The well-being of the body was determined by examining the pulse, of which there were 200 types. It took seven hours to perform this procedure.

The Chinese physician placed no faith in the patient's history as a diagnostic aid, preferring instead to rely on observation. Our chief interest in Chinese medicine is found in its materia medica consisting of fifty-two volumes. Many of the drugs used in ancient China are still used in modern medicine. Seaweed, rich in iodine, was used many centuries ago in China for the treatment of goiter. Today iodine is still used in goiter therapy. The Chinese gave liver for anemia; we have liver preparations today that are administered intramuscularly. From the white poppy the Chinese extracted opium and gave it for the relief of pain. Leprosy was recognized as a specific disease and was treated with chaulmoogra.[4] The Chinese long employed ephedrine, prepared from the mahung tree, for asthma and upper respiratory diseases; in the early 1920's this drug was brought to the United States and carefully refined. It is now a standard drug.

The Chinese used inoculation in the treatment of smallpox before Edward Jenner successfully used cowpox vaccine in 1789. The ancient Chinese tradition of tea-drinking, which requires boiled water, has long been a most effective measure against a grossly contaminated water supply. Other than this, the Chinese contributed little to our concepts of sanitation and public health. Essentially Chinese medicine was characterized by a rigid, closed system which has remained practically unchanged throughout the centuries. No reference is made to nurses in ancient Chinese literature.

We have now reached the point in history where, for the first time in the unfolding of medical science, we find specific duties outlined for the nurse.

India. The most important sources of information on the practice of medicine in India are *vedas,* the sacred books of the Hindus, some of which date back to 1200 B.C.

In lesson *ix* of the *Charaka-Samhita* an interesting account of the team concept is presented. The team concept, as practiced by the Hindus, consisted of the physician, the drugs, the nurse, and the patient. The *Charaka-Samhita* outlined the specific duties of the team members:

Physician. *Thorough mastery of the scriptures, large experience, cleverness, purity (of body and mind) are the principal duties of the physician.*

Drugs. *Abundance of virtue, adaptability to the disease under treatment, the capacity of being used in diverse ways, and undeterioration are attributes of drugs.*

Nurse *(always male, or in rare cases only females). Knowledge of the manner in which drugs should be prepared or compounded for administration, cleverness, devotedness to the patient waited upon and purity (both of mind and body) are the four qualifications of the attending nurse.*

---

[4] Chaulmoogra oil was used extensively by leperologists in this country for many years. However, the present treatment with the sulfonamides gives better results.

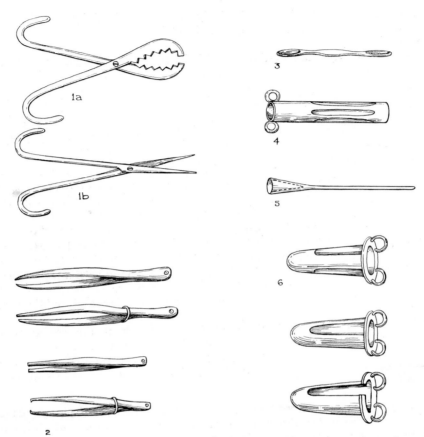

Instruments used in India in the year 100 **A.D.** Instruments such as these are still in use in India. 1a, plier; 1b, scissors; 2, tissue forceps with and without teeth; 3, orthopedic plate; 4, syringe; 5, catheter; 6, proctoscope.

Patient.   *Memory obedience to direction, fearfulness, and communicativeness (with respect to all that is experienced internally and done by him during the intervals between visits) are qualities of the patient.*

As in the task of cooking, a vessel, fuel, and fire are the means in the hands of the cook; as field, army, and weapons are means in the victor's hands for achieving victory in battles; even the patient, the nurse, and drugs are the objects that are regarded as the physician's means in the matter of achieving a cure.

Like clay, stick, wheel, threads, in the absence of the potter, failing to produce anything by their combination, the three others, viz., drugs, nurse, and patient, cannot work out a cure in the absence of the physician.[5]

[5] Nutting and Dock, *op. cit.*, pp. 32-33.

The knowledge of medicine portrayed in the *vedas* included major and minor surgery, as well as diseases of the nervous and urinary systems. The insistence that the nails of the physician and the midwife be kept short and that sweet-smelling drugs be burned in the operating room to prevent devils from getting into the wound hints of modern microbiology.

Hindu culture was then at its zenith and India was in touch with such foreign countries as Greece. Some of the implements used by the Hindus have come down to us and appear to have been the models for the design of later models. There are numerous practitioners in India who still employ these implements in their daily work.

Following this period of activity there was apparently a reaction in the life of the nation caused by the advent of Buddhism and Jainism, with the attending widespread cult of nonviolence. All manipulative effort and infliction of pain, even for the alleviation of pain, was suppressed.[6]

Three centuries before the Christian era, King Asoka, a Buddhist, published an edict to establish hospitals throughout India. These hospitals were still maintained some 900 years later when a Chinese traveler, Fa-Hiam, wrote in 599: "physicians inspect their diseases and according to their cases, order them food and drink, decoctions or medicines everything in fact that may contribute to their ease. When cured they depart at their own convenience."[7]

Nurses were employed in these hospitals. Records show that the qualifications for nurses (male attendants) were markedly similar to those we expect of our present-day practical nurses and attendants. A description of the duties required of nurse attendants, as translated from the old books, reads as follows:

After this should be secured a body of attendants of good behavior, distinguished for purity or cleanliness of habits, attached to the person whose service they are engaged, possessed of cleverness and skill, embued with kindness, skilled in every kind of service that a patient may require, embued with general cleverness, competent to cook food and curries, clever in bathing or washing a patient, well conversant in rubbing or pressing the limbs, or raising the patient or assisting him in walking or moving about, well-skilled in making or cleaning beds, competent to pound drugs, or ready patient, and skillful in waiting upon one that is ailing, and never unwilling to do any act that they may be commanded (by the physician or the patient) to do.[8]

The public hospitals in India were schools of medicine, and reportedly the senior physicians took the students into their homes. When Buddhism fell, public hospitals were abolished (*ca.* 750-1000 A.D.). Nursing and medicine were doomed with the conquest by the Mohammedans, since the Brahmins believe that it is unsanitary to touch blood or morbid matter.

[6] K. G. Pandalai, *Surgery in Ancient India.*

[7] Charles U. Letourneau, A History of Hospitals. *Hospital Management* 87:59, 1959.

[8] Nutting and Dock, *op. cit.,* p. 34.

Greece. In Greece, as in most ancient civilizations, treatment of disease was primarily in the hands of the priests who combined empirical medicine with impressive rituals and charms to work their cures. Aesculapius, the god of medicine, had as his symbol the single serpent staff, a carry-over from snake worship in prehistoric times when man attached the powers of wisdom, rejuvenation, and long life to the serpent. Even today the image of the snake remains the emblem of the wisdom of the physician. But later a secular group of medical practitioners appeared who, like the priests, ascribed their origin to Aesculapius. The secular group, however, rejected religious aids, made few claims to miraculous cures, and through a combination of observation and empirical knowledge gradually placed medicine on a rational basis.

The creative period of Greek medicine produced Hippocrates, who was born in approximately 460 B.C. and was thus a contemporary of Pericles, Sophocles, and Socrates. Hippocrates, the second of seven sons of a physician, has been known for over 2000 years as the father of medicine. Although the period was far from the beginning of modern general history, modern, rational medicine dates from the time of Hippocrates. Some sixty pieces of medical writing known as the Hippocratic Collection are available to us. These emphasize the value of observation rather than the cause of disease. One of the greatest contributions made by Hippocrates was his insistence that magic and philosophical theories had no place in medicine. Equally important was his contribution to medical ethics.

An illustration of the rational and superstition-free approach of Hippocrates is found in the opening paragraph *On the Sacred Disease* (Epilepsy) in which he says: "It is thus with regard to the disease called Sacred: It appears to me to be nowise more divine, no more sacred, than other diseases but has a natural cause from which it originates like other affections. Men regard its nature and cause divine from ignorance and wonder because it is not at all like other diseases."

Today's medical and nursing students are admonished to treat the whole person as though this were a modern concept. Hippocrates, however, in 400 B.C. advised his students that in order "to care for so much as an eye one must treat the whole body."

Pupils of Hippocrates were required to take a pledge, known as the Hippocratic Oath, which is well known to modern physicians. (The Nightingale Pledge for Nurses[9] is patterned after this ancient oath.)

It is regrettable that the great teacher Hippocrates made no direct reference to nurses in his writings. It may be inferred, however, that some of his teaching was directed along the lines most nearly related to the present-day concept of practical nursing. For example, his instructions were that fluid diet only should be given in fevers, and he advised cold sponging for high temperatures. For acute tonsillitis he requested hot fomentations and hot gargles, cathartics, and cool drinks. For colic he recommended warm enemata and warm baths, hot fomentations, purgatives, and anodynes.

---

[9] Formulated in 1892 by a committee of nurses of the Farrand Training School of Harper Hospital, Detroit. Mrs. Lystra Gretter was chairman of the committee which dedicated the pledge to Florence Nightingale.

In classical Greece the work of women was restricted to the household, where the mistress of the mansion gave nursing care to the sick slaves.

Rome. "According to Pliny, the younger, the Romans got along well without physicians for a period of 600 years, relying on superstitions, religious rites, dietetics and household remedies."[10] Although the physician came late to Rome the population was fundamentally healthy. Rome had a pure water supply brought by aqueducts from distant sources; the personal hygiene was good; and devotion to physical exercise and athletics was unusually well sustained.

The practice of medicine reached Rome by way of Greece. After the conquest of Corinth by the Romans in 146 B.C., many Greek physicians were brought to Rome as war prisoners. From them the Romans acquired a knowledge of medicine, and in time there were skilled Roman physicians and surgeons. Though the Romans adopted Greek medicine there is evidence that they were not entirely happy with it, for Pliny repeated Cato's imprecations upon Greek physicians who "seduce our wives, grow rich by feeding us poisons, learn by our suffering, and experiment by putting us to death."

Will Durant, in his book, *Caesar and Christ,* tells us that under Emperor Vespasian schools were opened to teach medicine and the state paid recognized professors to teach in them. Greek was the language of instruction, as Latin is now the language of prescription, and for a like reason—its intelligibility to persons of diverse tongues. Graduates of the medical schools were given a title, and after Vespasian, they alone could legally practice medicine in Rome. While the laws against the nonlicensed and the quack were stern, there continued to be quacks, but sound medical practice did increase.

The Romans, engaged in war as they often were, did much to develop military medicine; first-aid, field-ambulance service, and hospitals were available to wounded legionnaires. Private hospitals (valetudinaria) were opened by physicians and from these evolved the public hospitals of the Middle Ages.

The state appointed and paid doctors to look after the poor, and families sometimes contracted with a doctor to attend their health and illnesses for a period of time. Roman medicine eventually reached a high degree of specialization—there were urologists, gynecologists, eye and ear specialists, and dental practitioners. Wealthy Romans could have gold teeth, wired teeth, false teeth, bridgework, and plates. There were many women physicians, some of whom wrote manuals on abortion, which were popular among great ladies and prostitutes.

Surgeons also specialized and used in their practices surgical instruments not unlike those used today.[11] The surgeons performed plastic surgery (first

---

[10] Maurice B. Gordon, *The Romance of Medicine* (Philadelphia, F. A. Davis Company, 1949), p. 534.

[11] Many of these surgical instruments may be seen at the Hall of Fame of the International College of Surgeons in Chicago. In this museum, individual nations are assigned rooms where precious and antique articles pertaining to surgery are preserved. A visit to this museum would be of interest to all nurses.

developed by the Hindus), tonsillectomies, cataract operations, and many other surgical procedures.

The Romans, however, contributed little or nothing to drug therapy. They borrowed from the Greeks the use of sulfur[12] for the treatment of skin diseases and for fumigating the rooms of those with infectious disease. They also used mandragora juice or atropine as an anesthetic, but beyond these there is little to say for their drugs. Whereas Hippocrates had made sparse use of drugs, depending instead on fresh air, massage, hydrotherapy, bloodletting, enemas,[13] and purgatives, the Romans took a step backward and recommended such repulsive substances as human entrails and the excreta of dogs. Even Galen applied a boy's dung to swellings of the throat.

One lasting contribution of the Romans was their translation of Greek medical terminology into Latin terms which have been used in medicine ever since.

The Americas. An interesting example of ancient sanitation can be seen today in the sky-city of Ácoma, near Albuquerque, New Mexico. The superb mesa of Ácoma is one vast rock rising abruptly from the plain to become a perpendicular air-island 357 feet high with a practically level top. The peculiar erosion of the beautful sandstone has formed many deep chasms, and the visitor will see that one of these chasms is used for the storage of drinking water, while another, at a considerable distance away, is used for refuse and excreta. Although the system is primitive, these sound principles of sanitation have been practiced here for centuries.

The visitor to Mexico or Peru today has difficulty in realizing that these two countries had more advanced medical knowledge than any that existed in Europe or among the Moslems at the time these countries were conquered by the Spaniards. Early reports sent back to Spain by Cortez in Mexico and Pizarro in Peru recorded his astonishment at the medical knowledge of these people. "There are houses as it were where they sell medicine made from herbs, both for drinking and for use as ointments and salves."[14] The surgical skill of the Incas is only being duplicated in our time; amputations, trephining, bone transplants, and cauterizations were performed by them.

Archeologists working in Peru have found vast numbers of skulls that had been trephined—some as many as three times. It is not possible to attribute this frequency to blows on the skull to relieve pressure when no fracture is evident. It is possible that trephining may have been done for relief of headache, providing a classic example of where the cure is worse than the disease.

----

[12] Sulfur was well known to the ancient world and is indeed the "brimstone" of the Bible. It is still used for some skin conditions.

[13] Like taxes and bad jokes the enema has always been with us and probably always will be. The Greeks probably learned about enemas from the Egyptians, who seemed to have made a national pastime out of giving themselves enemas. Pliny thought that the Egyptians learned the practice from a constipated Nilotic bird, the ibis, which uses its beak as a rectal syringe.

[14] Emily Walcott Emmart, An Aztec Medical Treatise, the Badianus Manuscript. *Institute of History of Medicine,* Johns Hopkins University, Vol. 3 (Jan. 1935).

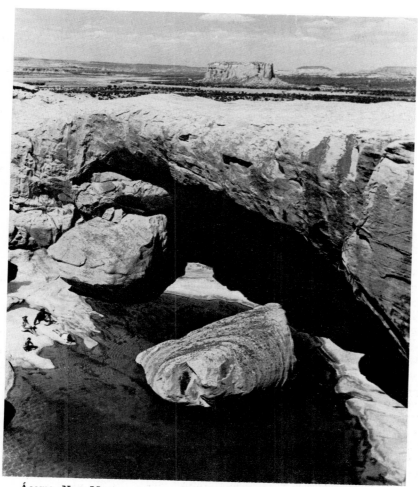

Ácoma, New Mexico. The background shows the great mesa which rises abruptly from the plateau. In the foreground is the natural catch-basin which provides the main water supply for the inhabitants of Ácoma, an ancient Indian village in western New Mexico. Ácoma, the Sky City, was built by Pueblo Indians about a thousand years ago, and it is considered the oldest continually inhabited community in the United States. (Courtesy of the New Mexico State Tourist Bureau.)

Some of the medicines employed by the natives of North and South America, the use of which has been taught to the Europeans, are quinine, cocoa (source of cocaine), cascara, datura, ipecac, and syrup of white pine.[15] The latest

[15] For a detailed list of native drugs, see William Corlett, *The Medicine Man of the American Indian and His Cultural Background.* (Springfield, Ill., Charles C Thomas, 1935), Chap. 16.

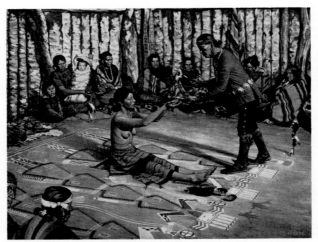

Indian medicine. (Parke, Davis. See list of Acknowledgments.)

drug to be refined and standardized is curare,[16] which has long been employed by South American Indians as an arrow poison.

The conquering Spaniards imposed cruel slavery on the proud Incas and Aztecs. The native religion was suppressed and the Indians were converted to Christianity, which they grafted on to their own beliefs. With suppression and slavery, all initiative in medicine and surgery ceased.

REFERENCES

AUSTIN, ANNE L.: *History of Nursing Source Book.* New York, G. P. Putnam's Sons, 1957.

CLENDENING, LOGAN: *Source Book of Medical History.* New York, Harper & Brothers, 1942.

CORLETT, WILLIAM T.: *The Medicine-Man of the American Indian and His Cultural Background.* Springfield, Ill., Charles C Thomas, 1935.

DURANT, WILL: *Caesar and Christ.* New York, Simon & Schuster, Inc., 1944.

ENCYCLOPAEDIA BRITANNICA. Chicago, Encyclopaedia Britannica, Inc., 1957.

EVANS, JESSIE C.: The Modern Point of View in Teaching History (from the Proceedings of the 20th Annual Convention of the American Nurses' Association). *American Journal of Nursing* 17:952-957, 1917.

FRAZER, JAMES G.: *The Golden Bough: A Study in Religion and Magic.* New York, The Macmillan Co., 1944.

GARRISON, FIELDING H.: *History of Medicine.* Philadelphia, W. B. Saunders Co., 1929.

---

[16] The explorer, Jacques Cartier, made an expedition to Canada in 1534, and the sailors on this voyage developed severe scurvy. The Canadian Indians gave the Frenchmen juices made from the sprouting tips of almeda tree (Hakluyt), which is still an effective remedy for scurvy because of the high vitamin C content.

GOLDBERG, EMANUEL: Men in Nursing. *RN* 22:40, 1959.

GORDON, MAURICE B.: *The Romance of Medicine.* Philadelphia, F. A. Davis Co., 1949.

von HAGEN, VICTOR WOLFGANG: Realm of the Incas. New York, New American Library, 1961 (revised).

HOLY BIBLE (*Leviticus and Deuteronomy*), Revised Standard Version. New York, Thomas Nelson and Sons, 1953.

LETOURNEAU, CHARLES U.: A History of Hospitals. *Hosp. Manag.* 87:58-59, 115, 1957.

LUMMIS, CHARLES F.: *The Land of Poco Tiempo.* Albuquerque, N. M., University of New Mexico Press, 1952.

PAVEY, AGNES E.: *The Story of the Growth of Nursing.* Philadelphia, J. B. Lippincott Co., 1953.

RODGERS, LESTER B., ADAMS, FAY and BROWN, WALKER: *The Story of Nations.* New York, Henry Holt and Co., 1940.

SCRAMUZZA, VINCENT M., AND MacKENDRICK, PAUL L.: *The Ancient World.* New York, Henry Holt and Co., 1958.

CHAPTER 3

The Influence of Christianity

The coming of Christ and His humanizing doctrines exerted a profound influence on many aspects of life; both medicine and nursing were affected. Christianity placed great value on human life. It embodied a fraternal concept of equality and charity which forced the faithful to undergo sometimes severe sacrifices in order to alleviate the suffering of others.

To the Christians, Christ was physician of both soul and body, thereby turning backwards the hands on the clock of pagan Hippocratism. But on nursing's clock the hands moved forward from sunset to sunrise.

With the dawn of Christianity the concept that there was no place or dignity for women outside of marriage was destroyed; Christianity widened the opportunities for single women to pursue useful and active careers. The activities of these early women workers, deaconesses, matrons, and saints laid the foundations for trained nursing. From Christianity's teaching of brotherhood arose a fresh ambition for humanity that spread steadily among the people.

The life and teachings of Christ represent a striking example of how one person can influence all aspects of contemporary civilized life and significantly alter the civilizations of succeeding generations.

During His short, exemplary life Jesus, who was born a Jew, preached a simple rule of true kindness and love, principles which His disciples carried throughout the Near East and eventually to all-powerful Rome. By 395 A.D., Christianity had become the state religion of the whole Roman Empire. It found fertile ground in a Rome tired of wars and plagues and outmoded religions.

Christianity soon developed a body of church laws with such power and influence that the church became a state within the empire. When Rome fell in 476 A.D. and all law and order were abandoned, the Christian or Catholic church assumed control and civilization was saved from complete destruction.

The early Church established bodies and groups within itself to deal with specific tasks. While the work of these groups was interrupted by various social forces, it has had a continuing influence on the care of the sick and the development of nursing. It is in these groups that nurses are particularly interested.

DEACONS AND DEACONESSES

The early Christians had been generous in their charities, and the apostles themselves distributed food to the poor. But this was time-consuming, so the deacons, who understood the business side of church life, were appointed to take over this work so that the apostles could devote their full time to preaching. Later the deacons rather than priests were often chosen bishops.

The earliest orders of women workers in the church were those of deaconesses, women chosen to assist in church work. They were especially concerned with nursing and care of the poor. Christian nursing included men as well as women, each concerned with the care of his or her own sex. It was the special duty of deaconesses to attend the sick in their homes, suggestive of the role played by our visiting nurses today.

St. Paul, writing to the newly established Christian church in Rome, recommended the services of Phoebe (ca. 55 A.D.), saying: "for she has been a helper of many and of myself as well."[1] Phoebe became the first deaconess and the first nurse. It is not likely, however, that deaconesses were an established group at that time, but, at the great ecumenical congress of all the bishops of the church at Nicea in 325 A.D., an organization or order was established.

The deaconess orders flourished throughout the Near East and eastern Europe for five centuries. Beginning about 500 A.D., many sisterhoods were established as philanthropic outlets for women and as security for women made destitute by many wars. These sisterhoods absorbed the deaconess orders, the latter disappearing from recorded history until after the Reformation in 1517. Beginning in the sixteenth century the Christian church limited the activities of the sisterhoods; their members lived under strict discipline within enclosures until the time of St. Vincent de Paul, who established the Sisters of Charity in 1633.

---

[1] Romans 16:1-3.

EARLY HOSPITALS UNDER CHRISTIANITY

The early Christians were encouraged to make pilgrimages to the Holy Land. They provided themselves with neither money nor food, but expected to be given food and shelter by hospitable Christians along the way. This practice led to the establishment of the hospice or inn for travelers. These inns were maintained by the well-to-do as an appreciation for services or as a religious vow for some special blessing.

Hospitals for the care of the sick were established as a result of the First Council of Nicea in 325 A.D. Christianity had been generally accepted by the countries of the Roman Empire, except Palestine. On the initiative of Emperor Constantine the Great, an ecumenical congress was called primarily to decide upon a definite creed or belief and to establish regulations for the propagation of Christianity. This resulted in the formulation of the Nicene Creed. At this council, also, each bishop present was instructed to build a hospital in every city maintaining a cathedral. This was meant to aid in the spread of Christianity and was in keeping with examples set by Jesus in caring for the sick and afflicted.

The first general public hospital, which opened in 380 A.D., is said to have been built by Fabiola, a rich Roman matron. Saint Jerome described this institution as a place where the sick could ''be given nourishment and those medicines of which they might have need.''

The first hospital established by voluntary contributions was Ephrem in Edessa, in what is now western Iraq. This hospital was founded in 375 A.D. for the care of plague victims.

Perhaps one of the best-known early hospitals was the Basilias, established by Saint Basil in 370 A.D. The physical layout of the Basilias appears somewhat similar to our larger hospitals of today. Because of the largeness of the Basilias, it was referred to as a new town. As we can see from James Walsh's description, Saint Basil's health center was not only designed for the prevention and treatment of disease but also for rehabilitation of patients:

The Basilias was not only a hospital in our sense but it also cared for the crippled and the poor of all classes. There was an orphantrophium or orphan's home, a brephotrophium or infant asylum for foundlings, a gerontochium for the old. There was also a nosocomium or house for the ailing; there was a xenodochium, or place of hospitality for strangers, and then there were separate buildings for lepers and those suffering from various contagious diseases. Besides these, Basil had edifices in which those who had been maimed or lamed might learn new trades before they went out to face the world again, in order that they might be able to support themselves properly. Finally, as the climax of Christian thoughtfulness for those in need, there was a building given up to an employment bureau so that employers and employees might be brought together under such circum-

*stances as assured understanding and sympathy. All in all there was
provision for every kind of human need.*[2]

The oldest hospital in continuous use is the Hotel Dieu (house of God's
charity), Lyons, France; this hospital was founded by King Childebert in 542
A.D. to care for pilgrims, the sick, and the infirm. The hospital had large beds,
some capable of accommodating five patients. In 1630, however, the administration ruled that patients must have individual beds. Since the twelfth
century, this hospital has been in charge of the Augustinian nuns.

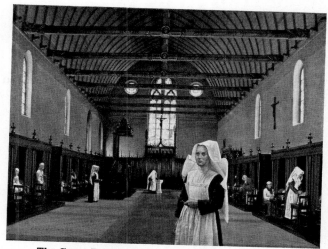

The Great Room of the Poor of Hotel Dieu, Paris.
(Courtesy of Parke, Davis & Company.)

Recalling Victor Robinson's statement that the real foundation of
monasticism was the desire of the human heart to escape the fever of life,[3]
it was paradoxically to the good of the public that Rome did have some
bruised souls among its populace. And nursing took a high place as a
penance for sins and a solace for unhappy lives.

Temporary Military Hospitals. Probably the first temporary hospital at
the scene of battle was that set up by Queen Isabella of Spain. The crusade
of Spain against the Moors began in 1212 and continued intermittently for
nearly two centuries. In 1486 King Ferdinand and Queen Isabella set about
to drive the Moors out of Spain. Only Granada, the southeastern province
of the Spanish peninsula, was still held by the Moors.

Queen Isabella was a student of medicine and understood the need of
trained physicians at home and on the battle field. Peter Martyr (1455-1526),

---

[2] James J. Walsh: *The History of Nursing* (New York, P. J. Kenedy and Sons, 1929),
pp. 14-18. As quoted by Sister Charles Marie Frank, *The Historical Development of Nursing*
(Philadelphia, W. B. Saunders Co., 1953), p. 69.

[3] Victor Robinson, *White Caps* (Philadelphia, J. B. Lippincott Co., 1946), p. 26.

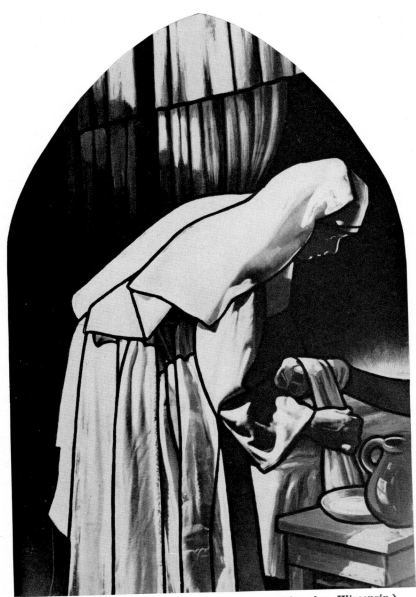

Augustinian nun. (Courtesy of Will Ross, Inc., Milwaukee, Wisconsin.)

her ambassador to Milan, writes that, during the seige of Granada which lasted more than four years, Queen Isabella superintended the construction of four large tent hospitals at Sante Fe near Granada, provided these hospitals with all possible comforts, and appointed physicians, chemists, surgeons, and assistants, some of them women. When the war was over Queen Isabella undertook supervision of the construction of many permanent hospitals all over Spain.

EARLY NURSING LEADERS

Marcella. In the middle of the fourth century there was a group of Roman matrons of noble birth, keen intellect, and great wealth who, because of life's disillusionments, turned their homes into hospitals and centers of almsgiving. The leader of this group of distinguished women was Marcella. Upon the death of her father, Marcella had been left an orphan; she had also lost her husband seven months after their marriage. She then turned to the scriptures to find solace, later introducing the first example of monastic life in Rome. She converted her palace on the Aventine, the most exclusive part of Rome, into a convent. She was a devoted scholar of the scriptures and dedicated her life to the teaching of her followers. For this work, she had been given the title of *Mother of Nuns and Founder of Convents in the West.*

Fabiola. Because of her unhappy experiences in two marriages and perhaps under the influence of Marcella's teachings, Fabiola renounced the worldly life, became a Christian, and in expiation for her former sins she devoted her life to the services of others.

As we have noted, in 380 A.D. she built what is said to have been the first general, public hospital in Rome. This hospital was dedicated to the services of the sick, as distinguished from those who were simply poor.

Saint Jerome recounts vividly of Fabiola's life and work as a nurse among the patients in this hospital:

There she gathered together all the sick from the highways and streets, and herself nursed the unhappy, emaciated victims of hunger and disease. Can I describe here the varied scourges which afflict human beings?—the mutilated, blinded countenances, the partially destroyed limbs, the livid hands, swollen bodies, and wasted extremities? . . . How often have I seen her carrying in her arms these piteous, dirty, and revolting victims of a frightful malady! How often have I seen her wash wounds whose fetid odour prevented everyone else from even looking at them! She fed the sick with her own hands, and revived the dying with small and frequent portions of nourishment. I know that many wealthy persons cannot overcome the repugnance caused by such works of charity; . . . I do not judge them, . . . but if I had a hundred tongues and a clarion voice I could not enumerate the numbers of patients for whom Fabiola provided solace and care. The poor who were well envied those who were sick.[4]

Paula. A friend of Fabiola and reputed to be the most learned woman of her day, Paula also renounced the worldly life. The whole city of Necropolis belonged to her. Following the death of her husband, and at the advice of

---

[4] Nutting and Dock, *op. cit.*, p. 138.

Marcella, Paula became a convert to Christianity; she entered Marcella's monastery, where she had close communication with Fabiola.

After the death of two of her daughters, Paula and her one remaining daughter sailed for Palestine in fulfillment of a long, ardent wish. To make this decision meant breaking one of the tenderest of her family ties—she had to leave her ten year old son with relatives. But making sacrifices was a part of Paula's chosen work.

She and her daughter settled in Bethlehem, where they established a monastery. En route to Bethlehem, Paula built hospices for pilgrims and hospitals for the sick. She and her staff worked diligently in these hospitals, fluffing pillows to comfort patients, rubbing their feet, and boiling water to bathe them.

EARLY NURSING SAINTS

Another group of women and men who worked daily and untiringly as nurses in the hospitals and in the homes of the poor were many who later were canonized saints. It is easy to appreciate what it must have meant to the poor banished leprous victims to have the assurances and practical services of these saints.

As Alban Butler[5] states, "the lives of the saints speak for themselves." We are not concerned so much with the kind of nursing care they gave, but rather with the effect of their work on the future of nursing and women in general.

We know that the care given by the saints was not what we call trained nursing or medical nursing. It was practical nursing, inspired by kindness and charity rather than by science. While the patterns of nursing change, the spirit of these workers that laid the foundations of nursing remains the same.

St. Radegunde (587 A.D.). The daughter of a Thuringian King and a descendant of Theodoric, St. Radegunde was of strong character and brilliant intellect. When she was a little girl, roaming in the forest, she was seized by the ruthless King Clothacar, who took her to his farm and made her the fifth of his seven wives. Radegunde was a queen, she had wealth—all of the material things that contribute to happiness. But she was not happy as queen and failed to carry out her royal and wifely duties. She left the "cruel and licentious prince" and sought refuge in the church. Even while she had been living in her husband's palace, Radegunde had devoted almost all of her time to the sick and needy, particularly the lepers.

She had always been deeply interested in nursing. And after she escaped from King Clothacar's palace, Radegunde established on her estate near Poitiers a settlement where she housed approximiately 200 nuns. She built there gardens, baths, porticoes, galleries, and a church. It is significant that she made provision for baths, because with the fall of the Roman Empire baths disappeared from medieval life. This would suggest that most monastic nursing did not maintain the Roman concept of hygiene.

[5] *The Lives of the Saints* by Alban Butler was published in 1878 as a detailed account of the saints from the beginning of Christianity. This four-volume work has now been abridged and brought up to date. It is available in paper-back form from Benziger Brothers, New York and Chicago.

Radegunde's monastery-hospice was the first institution of its kind to be established by a woman in France. Wearing a nun's dress of undyed wool, she personally bathed the patients in her hospice. In addition to caring for the sick, Radegunde's little community "read the scriptures" and studied literature, transcribed manuscripts, and presented dramatic performances. While Radegunde lived in her convent as any other member, she was regarded by the community as the head and center of activities.

St. Matilda (968 A.D.). Matilda, known as "Mold the Good Queen," was married to the King of England. But like her mother, who was also a saint, she wore a hair shirt and walked barefoot in the vicinity of the church; she renounced worldly things to give care to the lepers. In St. Giles-in-the-Fields she built a hospital for lepers. This hospital, which accommodated forty lepers, a chaplain, a clerk, and a messenger, was England's first institution for the care of the lepers. Historians have failed to give us any details concerning the medical and nursing services rendered at this institution.

Here we have seen the outstanding work in the field of nursing performed by some of the early saints. But they were not alone in developing nursing during the dawn of Christianity, and in the next chapter we shall see the later work of other saints in this area.

REFERENCES

DOLAN, JOSEPHINE A.: *Goodnow's History of Nursing*, 10th ed. Philadelphia, W. B. Saunders Co., 1958.

DURANT, WILL: *Caesar and Christ*. New York, Simon & Schuster, Inc., 1944.

GARRISON, FIELDING H.: *An Introduction to the History of Medicine*, 4th ed. Philadelphia, W. B. Saunders Co., 1929.

GIBBON, EDWARD: *The Decline and Fall of the Roman Empire*. New York, E. P .Dutton & Co., original publication, 1776.

GORDON, BENJAMIN LEE: *The Romance of Medicine*. Philadelphia, F. A. Davis Co., 1949.

GORDON, BENJAMIN LEE: *Medieval and Renaissance Medicine*. New York, Philosophical Library, Inc., 1959.

JAMIESON, ELIZABETH M., SEWELL, MARY F., and GJERTSON, LUCILLE: *Trends in Nursing History*, 5th ed. Philadelphia, W. B. Saunders Co., 1959.

LETOURNEAU, CHARLES U.: A History of Hospitals. *Hospital Management*, 87:58-59, 1959.

MAYNARD, THEODORE: *Too Small a World*. Milwaukee, Bruce Publishing Co., 1945.

PAVEY, AGNES E.: *The Story of the Growth of Nursing*. Philadelphia, J. B. Lippincott Co., 1953.

ROBINSON, VICTOR: *White Caps*. Philadelphia, J. B. Lippincott Co., 1946.

SCRAMUZZA, VINCENT M., and MacKENDRICK, PAUL L.: *Ancient World*. New York, Holt, Rinehart, and Winston, Inc., 1958.

THOMPSON, JAMES W., and JOHNSON, EDGAR N.: *An Introduction to Medieval History of Europe, 300 to 1500*. New York, W. W. Norton & Co., Inc., 1937.

WILSON, FRANK E.: *The Divine Commission*. New York, Morehouse-Gorham, 1940.

CHAPTER 4

The Arabian Empire and
The Crusades

For six centuries the Arabian Empire was a world power in order and extent of government, in refinement of human relations, and in standards of living, literature, science, medicine, and religious tolerance. Its influence on medicine and nursing has purposely been given proportionately greater emphasis in this book than is usual in texts on nursing history, or, as a matter of fact, in the world history texts used in American high schools.

There are three reasons for this: (1) Since the United States is a Christian country, most of its students are familiar with the tenets of Christianity, making it unnecessary to dwell upon the influences of this religion; (2) it is important to become acquainted with the historical heritage of the area encompassed by the ancient Arabian Empire since these lands are at the present time experiencing rejuvenation which will undoubtedly have considerable effect upon modern civilization; (3) we are greatly indebted to the Arabian Empire for the preservation of knowledge of ancient medicine and science. In addition, modern technology, communications, and military interests make it imperative that we appreciate the history and culture of the Near East, Middle East, and Far East.[1]

---

[1] The National Geographic Society has divided the countries of southern Asia into: (a) Near East: Turkey, Cyprus, Syria, Lebanon, Israel, Jordan, Egypt, Iraq, Iran, and Saudi Arabia; (b) Middle East: India, Pakistan, Afghanistan, Nepal, Bhutan, Sikkim, and Ceylon; (c) Far East: China, Mongolia, Korea, Japan, Philippines, Indochina, Thailand, Burma, Malays, and Indonesia.

Accordingly, the United States government has prepared *A Pocket Guide to the Middle East* to promote better relations between personnel assigned to the area and the native inhabitants through understanding of the culture and background. The introductory chapter states: "It (the guide book) will give you glimpses of Saudi Arabia, Iraq, Iran, Egypt, Israel, Jordan, Syria, and Lebanon. You will find it worth while to read more about the history-steeped East where our civilization arose—where West Meets East." [2]

Concerning the preservation of knowledge of ancient medicine, Arturo Castiglioni, in his authoritative book, *A History of Medicine,* states: "Thus the Arabs inherited all the medical patrimony of the past and became the faithful guardians of ancient medicine. When they and their relations disappeared from the theatre of their greatest exploits, and the fall of the Arabian dominations of Spain marked the end of this historic period, the traces that they left were so remarkable that they remain highly significant of the role that the Arabs played in the history of civilization and of medicine." [3]

The walls of the Spanish Room of the Hall of Fame of the International College of Surgeons, dedicated in September, 1960, are decorated with four murals depicting every phase of surgery. The bronze plaque at the entrance to the room bears an inscription, written in both Spanish and English, giving full credit to the Arabs for the glory of Spanish medicine during the Middle Ages.

The Arabian Empire played a hand in Columbus' discovery of America in that Columbus, educated as a sailor in Sicily, which had been under Moslem rule for four centuries, was taught, as the Moslems believed, that the world was round. Thus Columbus became convinced that he could reach the East by sailing west; in his attempt to do so he landed in the West Indies.

Arabia, largest of all peninsulas, covers an area of one million square miles. It is 1400 miles long, and 1200 miles wide at its broadest point along the southern border. The word "arab" means arid. The country is a vast, dry, sandy plateau; the climate of the greatest portion is characterized by burning sun during the day and nights of bitter cold.

In the early days of Christianity, Arabia maintained commerce with India by seagoing vessels along the southern coast, but since some 1200 miles of desert separated Arabia from Egypt, Syria, and Palestine, camel caravans were used to bring goods from Arabia's southern coast to the merchants of Egypt, Syria, and Palestine. Mecca, in western Arabia, was the commercial center for caravans traveling north or south.

The lucrative caravan trade attracted a large number of Jews as merchants; Christians likewise became merchants, and caravan supervisors and drivers along these routes. Another aspect of this trade was bringing worshipers to Mecca, which was the shrine, the Kaaba (the cube), to which pilgrimages have

---

[2] From the introductory chapter of *A Pocket Guide to the Middle East.*

[3] Arturo Castiglioni, *A History of Medicine,* 2nd ed. (New York, Alfred A. Knopf, Inc., 1947), p. 261.

been made from long before the time of Mohammed up to the present.[4] Although Arabia had no definite religion prior to Islamism, each tribe had its own rites, influenced by the religions of the Babylonians, Chaldeans, Assyrians, and Egyptians. Mecca was a city of many faiths but of no established religion.

RELIGION OF THE MOSLEMS

Mohammed, born about 570 A.D., was the son of parents who belonged to one of the poorer clans of the tribe that controlled the city of Mecca. He grew up among caravan merchants and camel drivers, and he himself made several trips to Syria as a camel driver. With an inquisitive mind and an early interest in religion, he absorbed, sorted, rejected, and retained bits of all the religions with which he came in contact. From this background evolved the faith of Islam. According to this religion, there is no God but Allah, and Mohammed is his prophet.

Mohammed compiled a book called the *Koran*, a small holy book about the size of the New Testament. In compiling the *suras*, or scripture lessons, Mohammed assumed that all revelation came from Heaven and that his message would be found in part in the scriptures of the Jews and of the Christians. The reader of the *Koran* will note many resemblances to both the Old and New Testaments.

Mohammed continued to live in Mecca and preach his religion of strict monotheism until 622 A.D., when he fled to Medina to escape death at the hands of his enemies. His flight from Mecca to Medina is known as the *hegira*; it marks the beginning of the Moslem era. The lunar calendar used by Moslems from Spain to Japan is reckoned from the year of the hegira (Anno Hegirae, abbreviated A.H.).

After six years in Medina, Mohammed's attitude changed: "The means of persuasion had been tried, the season of forbearance had elapsed, and he was now commanded to propagate his religion by the sword, to destroy the monuments of idolatry and, without regarding the sanctity of the days or the months, to pursue the unbelieving nations to the ends of the earth."[5]

Mohammed died at the age of sixty-three, but he had lived to see a vast empire held together by the Moslem religion rather than by the Arabian government. The empire extended from Spain on the west to the Indus River on the east.[6] Much of it had been conquered by the sword, but once a country or city had submitted, the people (Jews, Christians, and Moslems)

[4] Carlton S. Coon, *Caravan: the Story of the Middle East* (Holt, Rinehart and Winston, Inc., New York, 1958), pp. 115-118.

[5] Edward Gibbon, *The Decline and Fall of the Roman Empire*, 1781, Chapter 50. (Now published by E. P. Dutton Co., New York.)

[6] "Parts of China, Java, the Celebes, the Philippines and the Malay Peninsula are still strongly Mohammedan, though they have never been part of the political empire of the Arabs or the later Turks." James W. Thompson and Edgar N. Johnson, *An Introduction to Medieval Europe, 300 to 1500* (New York, W. W. Norton & Co., 1937), p. 170.

lived together peacefully. The only requirements made by the conquerors were a special poll tax and the prohibition of arms.

Moslem learning is the religious and cultural tolerance exhibited by the Moslems that makes the glory of the Arabian Empire of special interest to persons in all fields of science, especially medicine. While the Arabs were an illiterate people they were keenly intelligent and displayed a sincere respect for learning. The Moslems put into practice the teaching of the Prophet: "Teach science, which teaches the fear of God. He who desires knowledge adores God, and when he spreads it he is giving alms." They absorbed and cultivated the best in the countries they ruled. From India the Moslem scholars learned arithmetic, algebra, and trigonometry; from the Greeks they learned geometry, astronomy, and medicine. And they translated the works of Hippocrates, which had lain buried for five centuries under Christian asceticism.

When this information was translated into Arabic, schools throughout the empire studied these works and went on to make original contributions in their fields of study. The medical tradition was carried on extensively by Jews and Arabs, who became the best physicians in what is now southern Europe.

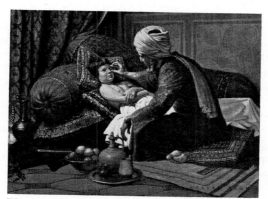

Rhazes. (Courtesy of Parke, Davis & Company.)

Rhazes, a Persian physician, was considered the greatest physician of the Islamic world and his medical books were still being printed as late as 1806. The physician whose medical knowledge produced the greatest effect on European medicine was Avicenna (979-1037). The Jewish physician Moses Maimonides (1135-1204) was born in Cordova, Spain, and later migrated to Egypt where he became court physician to Saladin, the Moslem ruler who completed the union of the Mohammedan east. The prayer of Maimonides[7] could well be the prayer of every doctor and nurse who cares for the sick:

---

[7] The medical writings of Maimonides, written in Arabic, have been in oblivion for 800 years. The Israel Torah Research Institute of the Hebrew University of Jerusalem has selected ten of these medical manuscripts for translation into English and modern Hebrew.

And now I turn unto my calling;
Oh, stand by me, my God, in this truly important task!
Grant me success! For—
Without thy loving counsel and support
Man can avail but naught.
Inspire me with true love for this my art
And for thy cre-a-tures.
Oh, Grant—
That neither greed nor gain, nor thirst for fame, nor vain ambition,
May interfere with my activity.
For these I know, are enemies of Truth and Love of men,
And might beguile one in profession,
From furthering the welfare of Thy creatures.
Oh, strengthen me!
Grant energy into both body and the soul,
That I may e'er unhindered ready be
To mitigate the woes,
Sustain and Help,
The rich and poor, the good and bad, the enemy and friend.
Oh, let me e'er behold in the afflicted and the suffering
Only the human being!

The Moslem religion forbade autopsies, but Moslems excelled in surgery and performed difficult operations. They are credited with the use of catgut, and they induced anesthesia by the use of hemp fumes. They transformed alchemy into chemistry and discovered silver nitrate, potassium, copper sulfate, mercury, and nitric and sulfuric acids.[8]

By 1094 the Arabian Empire was transforming the Mediterranean into a Moslem lake. The Christians in southern France were struggling to keep the Moslems from invading their country, while to the east the Byzantine emperor feared for Constantinople. Such conditions were somewhat similar to the current spread of Communism by the Russians.

The Christian church had been separated in 1054 into the Greek and Roman churches. Now both churches faced a common enemy. Emperor Alexius Comnenus appealed to Pope Urban II for help. The latter had long regretted the schism of the Catholic church and considered a crusade as possibly being the means of uniting the churches again. Pope Urban made a powerful appeal at Clermont, France, to which the people eagerly responded, "It is the will of God." They took the Crusader's oath and sewed the emblem of the cross on their garments. The propaganda used by Pope Urban resembles that used by the United States in our great crusade of World War I, "To make the world safe for democracy." There have been crusades in every age; it seems to be necessary to the human mind as part of the spirit of adventure.

---

[8] These scholars produced another kind of medical book—the "cram book"—in the form of questions and answers which have survived in hundreds of medical manuscripts. Such books are still used by doctors and nurses in the form of state board review books.

Western Europe was greatly concerned with the fate of Syria and Palestine because the origin of the Christian faith was in Palestine and it was the ambition of every Christian to make at least one visit to the Holy Land during his lifetime. The Moslems in Palestine were tolerant and the pilgrimages continued as they had since early Christianity. These tourists were profitable visitors to Palestine and the Moslems were good businessmen. If Constantinople fell, however, Italy and France might well be next and Christianity would be lost.

THE CRUSADES

There were seven major crusades and several minor ones. The first crusade began in April, 1095. It consisted of a great horde of untrained and undisciplined people under no unified command; they were bands of vassals pledged to their respective lords who hoped somehow to get to Jerusalem and rescue the Holy Land. Some 12,000 to 15,000 armed men finally reached Syria, accompanied by such noncombatants as women and children, monks, clerks, and priests. Three years later Jerusalem was captured, "when the slaughter was so great that men waded in blood up to their ankles." Jerusalem remained in Christian control until 1187, when it again returned to Moslem rule and remained so until World War I.

The second crusade began in the spring of 1147, but nothing was accomplished and the five successive campaigns resulted only in loss of life. By 1250 the Mongols from the far northeast, led by the nephew of Jenghiz Khan, were in control of the Near East. It was then only a question of time until the Christian states in Syria and Palestine would be destroyed. This was carried out by the Turks in 1291 by destroying both Tripolis and Acre; they slaughtered every inhabitant and filled the port with the debris of the fortifications.

HOSPITALS OF THE CRUSADES

Long before the crusades the Christian church had urged pilgrimages to Palestine. The faithful making these journeys often became ill and needed medical care and nursing. A hospital for sick pilgrims had been built in 1048. This hospital was organized as a monastic order in 1120 with the objective of protecting Christians in Palestine; Knights of the Hospital of St. John was the name given this order. These men served both as warriors in battle and nurses in the hospital, and were therefore called Knights Hospitallers. During the crusades this order built hospitals both at Malta and at Rhodes. These were again used during World War I as military hospitals.

Another military nursing order, the Knights Templars, was organized in 1119. Their residence was near Solomon's temple, hence the name Knights Templar. They, too, cared for the sick and injured and went into battle with other crusaders.

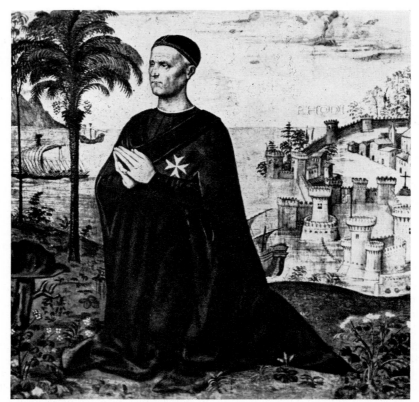

Knights Hospitallers, famed initiators of nursing hospitals during the Crusades. Painting by Pinturicchio (1454-1513). (Bettmann Archive.)

A third important order was the Teutonic Knights. In 1187, Saladin laid siege to the Christian city of Acre, an important seaport in what is now northwest Israel. A night attack by the Hospitallers and Templars scattered the Moslems. A group of German knights, camped nearby, converted their tents into emergency hospitals and cared for the wounded. These men formed the order of the Teutonic Knights; they vowed to build hospitals, care for the sick, and defend the faith.

All were monastic orders, but for the first time their members left the cloister and fought in open battle. When the fighting was over, they acted as stretcher bearers, took the wounded to the hospital, and cared for them. These orders detested each other religiously, yet they presented a united front before the Moslem enemy. They all wore the traditional armor or coat of mail in battle, but, because of the rivalry, none wanted to be mistaken for a member of another order. This led to a distinctive outer cloak: the Templars wore a white robe decorated with a red cross; the Hospitallers wore a black robe with a white cross; the Teutonics wore a white robe with a black cross.

The military nursing during the two centuries of the crusades strongly influenced nursing, even to the present day, both in uniform and discipline.

It established definite rank, unquestioned obedience, promotion for superiors, and penalties for broken rules that now seem absurd.

Lazarettos. The crusades, extending over 200 years, brought leprosy to all of Europe. The disease appears to have been leprosy (Hansen's disease) as we know it today. It was early recognized as communicable, and hospitals were built to isolate those afflicted. These hospitals, forerunners of our pest-houses and now known as communicable disease hospitals, were called lazarettos. There is a pathetic story about the derivation of the word lazaretto: "There was a rich man, who was clothed in purple and fine linen and who feasted sumptuously every day. And at his gate lay a poor man named Lazarus, full of sores, who desired to be fed with that which fell from the rich man's table; moreover, the dogs came and licked his sores."[9]

Approximately 19,000 lazarettos were established throughout Europe, and were occupied by leprous victims until the appearance of the Black Death in 1349. Lepers, as well as healthy persons, died during this plague, and the lazarettos were emptied of their patients. By 1400, leprosy was rarely seen and the lazarettos were used for other communicable diseases.

EFFECTS OF THE CRUSADES

Thousands of Europeans had been stationed in the Near East over a period of 200 years. They lived in rich and prosperous countries with luxuries and refinements of which the European had never dreamed. The cities were clean;

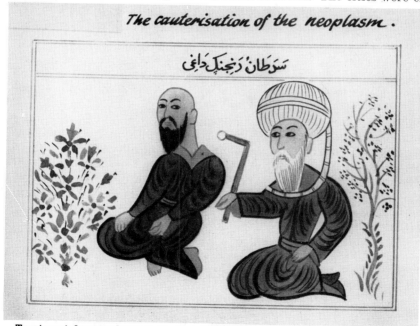

Treatment for neoplasm in Turkey during the fifteenth century. (Courtesy of the Hall of Fame, Museum of Surgical Science, International College of Surgeons, Chicago. From the collection on Turkey.)

[9] Luke 16:19-22.

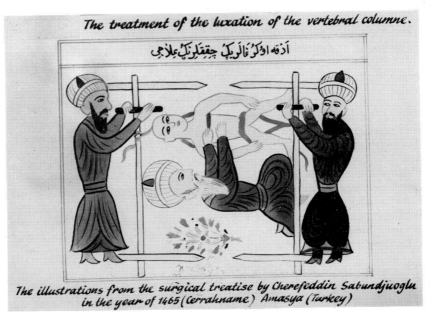

The treatment of the luxation of the vertebral columne.

أدقه اوكُرُ غاكُريكَ چققكُرنِكَ علاجِى

The illustrations from the surgical treatise by Cherefeddin Sabundjuoglu in the year of 1465 (Cerrahname) Amasya (Turkey)

Orthopedic practice in Turkey. (Courtesy of the Hall of Fame, Museum of Surgical Science, International College of Surgeons, Chicago. From the collection on Turkey.)

instead of using coarse woolens and leather for clothes the inhabitants wore cool cottons and rich silks. The crusaders learned to like peaches, apricots, bananas, rice, and sugar; intermarriage was common; there was no religious persecution. Because of the superiority of the Moslem physician, he was called to treat the European's family when ill.

Although the crusades did not accomplish their main objectives they did have several important effects on European history. They influenced the development of monarchy by weakening feudal nobility, hastened the liberation of the common people of town and country, and sped up the urbanization of Western Europe.

As a result of the crusades, new ideas of siege tactics were adopted into Western military science, and there was a general increase of scientific knowledge.

As new scientific facts filtered into Europe from Spain and Sicily, a wave of interest and enthusiasm stimulated the European scholars and paved the way for the great period of exploration that marked the end of the Medieval period of history.

Hospitals, erected to care for the sick poor, transferred from ecclesiastic to secular control. Medicine, which declined considerably in the early Medieval period, had now established two conflicting trends: diagnosis and treatment were determined largely by speculation, with no search for new facts or truths; yet the foundation for scientific medicine was being established through the use of dissection of human anatomy. Previously the study of anatomy had been based largely on Galen's study of animal dissections.

But the era was not altogether dark. The people were blessed in that a number of saints came to their rescue.

NURSING SAINTS

St. Hildegarde (1098-1179 A.D.). Hildegarde, called the Prophetess and Sibyl of the Rhine, was one of the greatest figures of the twelfth century. She was the first of the great Roman mystics, a poet, prophet, physician, and political moralist. Hildegarde wrote extensively, including two books on medicine and natural history. In her medical books she focused on the causes, symptoms, and treatment of ailments. She also discussed normal and morbid psychology, referred to frenzy, insanity, dreads, obsessions, and idiocy. She mentions that "when headache, vapours, and giddiness attack a patient simultaneously they make him foolish and upset his reason. This makes people think he is possessed by an evil spirit, but this is not true."[10]

Although Hildegarde combined the arts of medicine and nursing, her work was more outstanding as a physician.

Sts. Francis and Clara (1181-1226 A.D.). "And as ye go, preach, saying, 'The kingdom of heaven is at hand.' Heal the sick, cleanse the lepers, raise the dead, cast out devils: Freely ye have received, freely give. Provide neither gold nor silver, nor brass in your purses, nor script for your journey, neither two coats, neither shoes, nor yet staves: for the workman is worthy of his meat."[11] This was the message heard by Francesco Bernadone in the little chapel of Santa Maria degli Angeli, the message that changed the course of his life.

As scion of a cloth-merchant, Francis gave no thought to education; instead, he spent his evenings in caroling serenades with other young men through the streets of Assisi. He was known as king of the revelers. But he renounced the life of ease and wealth. Upon making his decision, he dressed in rags and made a farewell visit to the home of his parents. At this meeting he disowned his father and renounced his mother.

He immediately went to a leper settlement and lived there until his plans materialized. For this act, the people of the town labeled him a madman. But through perseverance and courageous leadership Francis obtained official sanction of his crusade to help lepers. When the Cathedral of Assisi opened its doors to the barefooted friar, he was no longer considered to be a madman. The people clamored to hear his sermon, and among those in the audience was sixteen-year-old Clara who became his disciple. She, too, made her decision as suddenly as Francis had done.

Clara prevailed upon Francis to let her live as he lived. After she had received her vows of poverty, chastity, and obedience, he instructed her to

---

[10] Alban Butler, *The Lives of the Saints*, ed. and rev. by Thurston and Attwater (London, Burns, Oates, and Washburne, Ltd., 1934), p. 580.

[11] St. Matthew 10:7-10.

dress in sackcloth and go through the streets begging gifts for the poor. She followed his instructions and upheld the Franciscan ideal wherever she went. Francis installed her in the San Damiano convent, whose abbess she remained for forty years. Clara established the Franciscan nuns, later known as Poor Clares. Their duties consisted of taking care of the sick and afflicted.

Francis slept and ate in the lazar-houses; he also dressed the sores of the lepers. He referred the diseased and deformed to Clara and her nuns, who attended them in little houses made of mud and branches. Later, Clara's most important patient was Francis himself. Sick and exhausted from the hardships he had endured, Francis failed to respond to drug therapy. He was subjected to the cruelty of cauterization before his death. A rod of white-hot iron was drawn across his forehead. The physicians even made incisions in the cauterized wound and then applied plasters and salves. The agonizing treatment he received in his last days is one of the most pathetic stories ever recorded in history.

Francis died in 1226, but his work lived on. One of the most important of his creations was the Third Order or Tertiaries. Clara survived Francis for some years. After her death, the Order underwent modifications and nursing was no longer carried out by her nuns.

St. Elisabeth of Hungary (1207-1231 A.D.). Elisabeth, the patroness of nurses, was the daughter of a Hungarian King. In her cradle she was betrothed to Ludwig, son of the Landgrave of Thuringia. At the age of four Elisabeth was transferred from her home to the Wartburg, where she was to be brought up in the castle and educated under the supervision of Ludwig's parents. However, they soon felt that she was a poor choice for their son and suggested that she be sent home or placed in a convent. She was beautiful, though frail of physique, and had rare mental and spiritual qualities. Ludwig, who succeeded his father as Landgrave of Thuringia, refused to let her leave.

Ludwig and Elisabeth were married when he was twenty years of age and she fourteen. Their marriage was happy and they had a family of three children. Elisabeth used all of her wealth to make the lives of the poor more happy and useful. Ludwig was one of the few people who understood Elisabeth; together they built a hospital for the sick and needy. She often fed the sick with her own hands, made their beds, and otherwise attended them in the hot summers. Orphan children were provided for at her expense, and she established another hospital in which twenty-eight patients received constant care. Elisabeth fed from 300 to 900 persons daily at her gate.

To discourage idleness, Elisabeth employed those who were able to work. Although she was wealthy, she lived frugally; she worked continually in her hospice and in the homes of the poor; and went fishing in the streams to help provide for the many sufferers. Even when ill herself she would try to spin or card wool. Finally her health gave way after Ludwig's death, and she died on November 17, 1231, before her twenty-fourth birthday.

St. Agnes of Bohemia (1317 A.D.). Although she had been betrothed by her royal father to the Hohenstaufen, Friedrich II, German monarch, Roman Emperor, and King of Sicily and Jerusalem, Agnes was not interested in titles nor the man bearing these titles. Instead of wearing the crown of a queen, she preferred to patch and wash clothes of leprous beggars. She was able to pursue this work, because her father died before her wedding day, and she cancelled the wedding arrangements. She left the castle on Hradcany Hill and built a hospital in Prague, where she gave nursing care to the sick and distressed and performed such servile duties as making fires, cleaning dirty rooms, making beds, and preparing and cooking foods that would be tasty for the patients.

St. Catherine of Siena (1347-1380 A.D.).

Born of humble Italian parents, Catherine was the twenty-fifth child of dyer Giacomo Benincasa. Her twin sister died during delivery. Catherine was a child prodigy; at the age of seven she pledged her life to the service of Christ and was referred to as a little saint.

In the short thirty-four years of her life, Catherine was a hospital nurse, prophetess, preacher, and reformer of society and of the church. She was also a skilled politician in matters of state. The Florentines, who had quarreled with the Pope and had been excommunicated by him, turned to Catherine because of her renowned position. She visited the Pope in behalf of her fellow citizens, accompanied him to Rome, and was received reverentially by the entire papal court. The Pope not only appointed her as his arbitress with the Florentines, but he accepted her advice and restored the papacy (from Avignon) to Rome.

St. Bridget of Sweden (1373 A.D.).

The Order of St. Bridget of Sweden established the House of Syon near Ilseworth on the Thames, England, which became one of the wealthiest of convents. Her instructions to the nurses in caring for the sick seem remarkably modern. The practice of psychosomatic medicine—and perhaps even the development of its concept—was still four centuries away, but St. Bridget wanted her nurses to understand that "there be some sickness vexing them so greatly and provoking them to ire that the matter drawn up to the brain alienates the mind." The House of Syon had become a popular institution by the time of the Reformation in 1517. Nevertheless it, too, was a victim of the wrath of the Reformation when only four English hospitals were permitted to remain open. Saint Bridget moved her nurses as a group to Holland and from there many Brigittine communities were established.

St. Frances of Rome (1440 A.D.).

This gentle saint, a widow known as St. Frances the Roman, devoted all of her time to visiting the sick, ministering to their needs, and relieving their distress. Her work, however, was interrupted for one year by a serious illness. After she recovered, St. Frances went daily to the hospital Santo Spirito to nurse the patients, particularly those suffering from the most repellent diseases.

When the plague and starvation were destroying Rome, St. Frances, in the face of insults and rebuffs, went from door to door begging for food for the poor; she even sold her jewels to get money to buy food. Weakened from overwork, St. Frances herself became a victim of the plague, but she finally regained her health and was able to carry out a project she had had in mind for a long time—that of forming a society of women who would devote themselves to the sick and the poor. She followed this work until her death.

In the Medieval era, despite wars and plagues, the world—particularly the world of nursing—made considerable progress under the influence of Christianity. I think it may be said that nursing owes its foundation to the work of benevolent men and women, the crusades, and the guilds. But this progress in nursing is brought to a halt in the period which follows—the Dark Period in Nursing.

REFERENCES

ARNOLD, THOMAS, and GUILLANE, ALFRED: *The Leprosy of Israel.* London, Oxford University Press, 1952.

AUSTIN, ANNE L.: *History of Nursing Source Book.* New York, G. P. Putnam's Sons, 1950.

CASTIGLIONI, ARTURO: *History of Medicine.* New York, Alfred A. Knopf, Inc., 1941.

CHESTERTON, G. K.: *St. Francis of Assisi.* New York, George H. Doran Co., 1924.

CLENDENING, LOGAN: *Source Book of Medical History.* New York, Paul B. Hoeber, 1942, Chap. 11.

DOLAN, JOSEPHINE A.: *Goodnow's History of Nursing,* 10th ed. Philadelphia, W. B. Saunders Company, 1958.

DURANT, WILL: *The Age of Faith.* New York, Simon & Schuster, Inc., 1950.

GIBBON, EDWARD: *The Decline and Fall of the Roman Empire.* New York, E. P. Dutton & Co., Inc., original publication, 1776.

GORDON, BENJAMIN LEE: *The Romance of Medicine.* Philadelphia, F. A. Davis Co., 1949.

NUTTING, M. ADELAIDE, and DOCK, LAVINIA L.: *A History of Nursing,* Vol. 1. New York, G. P. Putnam's Sons, 1935.

SLATTERY, MARGARET: *New Paths Through Old Palestine.* Boston, Pilgrim Press, 1921.

THOMPSON, JAMES W., and JOHNSON, EDGAR N.: *Introduction to Medieval Europe, 300 to 1500.* New York, W. W. Norton & Co., Inc., 1937.

CHAPTER 5

The Renaissance and the Reformation

The Renaissance marks the period of transition from medieval to modern civilization. But, what, exactly, was this great movement that affected the lives of so many people, and when did it start? Since it is impossible to set a specific time as to when things happen in history, the word "Renaissance" as used here is given wide meaning. It includes the cultural developments of European society between 1300 and 1600 A.D. It not only encompasses achievements in art, music, literature, and science, but also the drastic changes in the economic and social structure of society, as well as organization of the states. Lucas outlines these accomplishments as follows:

Basic Economic Changes. Life in the earlier Middle Ages was organized around the simple agricultural ways of the manor, which attempted to be self-supporting. What little trade existed was exchanged on the basis of barter. But the Renaissance changed all of this; the use of coined money, commerce, and industry became prominent features in the more progressive centers of Europe. An economic revolution was in process: a capitalist society was emerging.

Basic Social Changes. As the use of coined money increased and commerce and industry progressed, there was a shift in the social life; the manor, the nobleman's castle, and the bishop's palace were superseded by busy towns and crowded streets. The people abandoned agricultural life and migrated to the towns.

Basic Political Changes. These economic and social transformations brought significant political changes. Previously, the princes and vassals had things under control and managed the affairs of their states as they wished. But with the availability of coined money and with the growth of trade and industry, the states themselves could tax their subjects and fill their treasuries with cash.

Great Cultural Changes. The religious dramas of the Middle Ages were replaced with secular works; a new kind of art flourished and sculpture attained a respectable place among the classics. Other significant social changes included expansion of scientific thought, the appearance of mercantilism, and the use of the system of vocational education and the invention of printing as the means of popularizing educational advancements. And lastly, all of these changes called for a new attitude toward the world.[1] In the Middle Ages men adhered largely to ascetic ideals, but with the Renaissance men took on a more secular outlook, revolting against the idea that life beyond was more important than life in this world.

The viewpoint of some historians indicates that this knowledge was born during the Renaissance, not reborn, as some claim. They feel that this birth, together with the many social and economic transformations, had disadvantages. Two classes of society developed: the wealthy intelligentsia who lived in luxury, and the poor uneducated class whose members found themselves wearing the shackles. There was a lowering of moral values and witchcraft and superstition were revived.

In medicine, the Renaissance brought about significant progress in the fields of anatomy and physiology, particularly in the study of the circulation of the blood, and also in the concepts of communicable diseases, surgery, obstetrics, ophthalmology, and pharmacology. But this new knowledge seems to have had no influence on improving patient care. Apparently, since nursing was a religious vocation, it was not considered in the reform movement. At least there is no mention of nurses.

THE REFORMATION

What was the Reformation? The term "Reformation" applies to the religious upheaval of the sixteenth century which destroyed the unity of the Christian faith in western Europe. It is impossible to present all of the contributory causes of the Reformation. The major causes however, according to Lucas, fall into six broad headings: (1) the rise of political absolutism produced a secular state of mind; (2) the medieval church organization clashed with the absolute states of Europe; (3) many popular religious practices and ecclesiastical habits urgently needed reform; (4) the Renaissance

---

[1] Henry H. Lucas, *The Renaissance and the Reformation* (New York, Harper & Brothers, 1934), pp. 3-6.

contributed its share to the Reformation; (5) it was impossible for the church to adjust itself at once to the needs of the new age; (6) a tense and explosive state of mind was developed.[2]

Europe had lived under the feudal system since the collapse of the Roman Empire in 476 A.D. Under this system a strong warlord established himself in a well-fortified castle. The poor people, as security for themselves, swore allegiance to this lord who, in turn, promised them protection. In return for this protection the peasants tilled the surrounding land. This master-servant relationship, known as the feudal system, persisted in Europe for seven centuries. The Europeans carried the feudal system to Mexico, where it continued in its original form until 1920.

By the fourteenth century life had become safer and the peasant no longer needed to live near the castle walls in order to survive. The crusades provided an opportunity for the serf to leave the castle with his master, but he never returned in the same capacity. Women obtained more freedom than they had known since the Roman Empire; the crusades had taken the men, both serf and master, and the women necessarily had to assume managerial responsibilities.

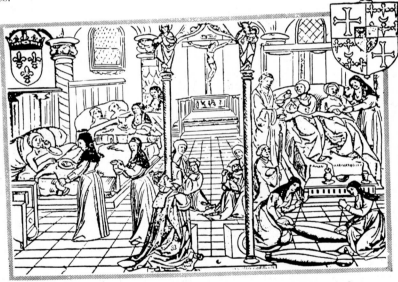

A Ward in Hotel Dieu of Paris. From a wood engraving of the 16th Century

In Europe there were no cities as we know cities today. A city at that time was a fort or seat of the bishop's church, situated around a natural harbor or at the head of a navigable river. In fact, during the seventeenth and eighteenth centuries, towns in the United States developed in a similar manner.

When the crusaders came back from the East they could not return to the old life; they demanded eastern foods and a higher standard of living.

[2] Ibid., pp. 419-22.

With the fall of the Roman Empire in 476 A.D., Rome became a wide-open anarchy. The Christian church, with a strong, well-disciplined organization from parish priest to the bishop of Rome, took the place of the Roman Imperial government as the authority of law and order. The church was a potent medium of higher culture; it sponsored the development of music and art and beautiful churches, which even today are attractions for tourists. And this development of churches contributed a great deal to the formation of literary and intellectual culture. The growth of education was a significant factor of the age.

The convents cared for the sick and destitute, provided refuge for widows and unmarried women, and directed their energies into worthwhile social service. For centuries these convents provided the only means of formal education for girls. But life in general was organized on a family basis and the home was considered to be the seat of culture. The family as a whole was responsible for the conduct of its members. Because of this close relationship much informal education was acquired in the home.

As the thirteenth and fourteenth centuries saw the weakening of the feudal system, they also saw the weakening of the Roman Catholic church. (The Christian church had been separated into the Roman and Eastern churches in 1054.) The Roman Catholic church was the most powerful institution in all of Europe. Everyone belonged to it, as now all belong to some nation, and contributions to the church were collected as a regular tax is collected today. The medieval church performed many services that are now carried on by other institutions: it dispensed charity to the poor; cared for the sick as hospitals do today, and was responsible for all teaching, since there were no public schools.

By the time of the Reformation the church had gained enormous wealth and had great intellectual and social influence. But discontent had long been brewing against the church and alleged abuses within it. Such men as John Wycliffe in England, John Huss in Bohemia, and Meno Simons in Germany, began laying the groundwork for the activation of this long accumulated resentment against feudalism and the church; this flamed into open rebellion in 1517.

The rebellion against the church was led by Martin Luther, an Augustinian monk who had been educated at Eufurt, Germany. He had differed with some of the doctrines of the established church for some time and, in 1517, posted on the church door in Wittenberg a list of ninety-five theses or arguments of an ecclesiastical nature, as an invitation to debate. These were supposed to be not so much denunciations as the basis for discussion with other scholars. Debates were popular and Luther enjoyed this matching of wits.

But the air was charged with dissatisfaction, both social and religious. Everyone wanted copies of the arguments, and the presses worked overtime to supply the demand. The Reformation had begun and the resulting religious wars continued until the middle of the sixteenth century when the ruler of each German state could decide whether his subjects would follow Roman Catholicism or Protestantism.

The revolt was not limited to Germany. The Protestant church that developed in Scotland was called Presbyterian, while in England, King

Henry VIII set himself up as head of the English church and called that form of Christianity, Anglicanism. The many religious denominations which we have today had their origin in the Reformation, the most significant event of the sixteenth century.

THE DARK PERIOD OF NURSING

The Reformation had a devastating effect upon nursing. Since the Council of Nicaea in 325 A.D., the Christian church and hospitals had been companion projects; the nuns cared for the sick as a matter of course. But the wrath of Protestantism swept away everything connected with Roman Catholicism in schools, orphanages, and hospitals. The property of hospitals and schools was confiscated and used to compensate political friends or given to schools benefiting men.

Nurses fled for their lives. The entire personnel of a hospital often fled as a group to avoid persecution, some traveled to Mexico to open missions and hospitals after the Spanish conquest. In England the dissolution of the monasteries was drastic, more than a hundred hospitals were completely put out of existence. Only four were permitted to remain open.

Imagine our situation in the United States if a decree went out that one month hence *all* hospitals would be closed. There would be no nurses available to care for the ill. Such were the conditions in England and in many other European countries. No provision was made for the sick poor, there was no lay organization to replace those who had fled, and no one to develop or teach others to carry on.

Beginning in the sixth century women had been restricted to life behind monastery walls. This became even more limited when Pope Innocent IV (1243-54) opposed self-government for any body of religious women. Martin Luther had grown up in a culture that limited women's activities to the home and family. He was trained as a monk in the doctrines of the Roman Catholic church, whose view was that women belonged either at home or in the convent. This outlook prevented new women's organizations from filling the gap left by closing monasteries. Luther's philosophy of faith rather than good works as the means of salvation gave little inducement to men or women to help the sick and needy.

The records of the English hospitals, more complete than those of hospitals on the Continent, present a clear picture of English monasticism: "There was the reasoned and intelligent discipline—perfect like the military discipline, but infused by a more thoughtful and ethical purpose, gaining therefrom a different tradition, one wholly humane. There was the practical efficiency, the cheerful balanced poise, the ability to control the situation, the entire devotion called today keenness in professional work. The loss of this system left English nursing in a depth from which secular authorities for a long time did little or nothing to extricate it."[3]

---

[3] Lavinia L. Dock and Isabel M. Stewart, *A Short History of Nursing*, 4th ed. (New York, G. P. Putnam's Sons, 1938), p. 95.

Education for girls, which had been the province of the nuns, was lost. There was no one to pass on the information about the care of the sick; the religious motive of devotion to the sick, which always had given us the best hospital service, was entirely lacking. The municipal authorities managed all of the surviving hospitals. Women entering nursing service came more frequently from the illiterate classes, until eventually women serving jail sentences were ordered to care for the sick in hospitals instead of serving their sentences in the city prison.

The nineteenth century novelist Charles Dickens was popular toward the end of the dark period of nursing, and was no doubt instrumental in hastening the end of this period. Although Dickens was a writer, his influence on social reform was great—his novels were entertaining and popular, and therefore widely read. They presented social conditions as they were lived in the very time of the reader, in the age when "children were seen but not heard." Dickens, in *Oliver Twist,* was the first author to make a child the chief character of a book.

Dickens vividly portrayed the deplorable status of nursing at that time, and his interpretation in his book titled *Martin Chuzzlewit,* published in 1844, has immortalized the public's image of the nurse. Dickens describes the selfish and cruel conduct of two private duty nurses, Sairey Gamp and Betsy Prig, who cared for one of the characters in this book. Chapters XXV and XXIX in *Martin Chuzzlewit* should be read in full to appreciate the selfish, uncouth women who cared for the sick:

"Anthin' to tell afore you goes, my dear?"
"The pickled salmon is quire delicious. I can partick'ler recommend it. Don't have nothink to say to the cold meat, for it tastes of the stable. The drinks is all good."
Mrs. Gamp expressed herself much gratified.
"The physic and them things is on the drawers and mankle-shelf. He took his last slime draught at seven. The easy chair ain't soft enough. You'll need his piller."

This picture of nurses was not a part of Mr. Dickens' imagination. Mrs. Gamp was in reality a person hired by a friend of Dickens to care for an invalid very dear to her. "A regular Sairey Gamp" became a byword for the undesirable nurse and it is still used as a term of contempt for the uncouth, ill-bred nurse.

Today it seems unbelievable that these conditions could have existed for 200 years. As the United States and Canada became settled, the same conditions were common in both countries. The social and political attitudes during those centuries expressed indifference to suffering. New hospitals were built by municipalities, but they were cheerless, dreary places without any regard for sanitation or fresh air. The hospitals built by the Christians and Moslems were beautiful buildings set in spacious gardens with fountains in the courtyards that gave an air of graciousness completely lacking in the hospitals that followed the Reformation.

At that time the medical profession was beginning to show a scientific interest in medicine. Research was being carried out, yet there was no intelligent staff to assist in this. Bathing was not permitted, but bleeding and purging were considered necessary for most medical conditions.

This low status of nursing, which in history is known as the Dark Period, continued roughly from the Reformation until our Civil War. Some attempts were made to improve conditions, but there was no visible improvement.

REFERENCES

ARNOLD, THOMAS, and GUILLAUME, ALFRED: *The Legacy of Islam.* London, Oxford University Press, 1931.

AUSTIN, ANNE L.: *History of Nursing Source Book.* New York, G. P. Putnam's Sons, 1957.

BAINTON, ROLAND H.: *Here I Stand—A Life of Martin Luther.* New York, Abingdon-Cokesbury Press, 1950.

DOCK, LAVINIA L., and STEWART, ISABEL M.: *A Short History of Nursing,* 4th ed. New York, G. P. Putnam's Sons, 1938.

DURANT, WILL: *The Reformation.* New York, Simon & Schuster, Inc., 1957.

HAYES, CARLTON: *The Political and Cultural History of Modern Europe.* New York, The Macmillan Co., 1938.

NUTTING, M. ADELAIDE, and DOCK, LAVINIA L.: *A History of Nursing.* New York G. P. Putnam's Sons, 1935.

PAVEY, AGNES E.: *The Story of the Growth of Nursing.* Philadelphia, J. B. Lippincott Co., 1953.

PELIKAN, JARASLAV: *The Riddle of Roman Catholicism.* Nashville, Tenn., Abingdon Press, 1959.

THOMPSON, JAMES W., and JOHNSON, EDGAR N.: *An Introduction to Medieval Europe, 300 to 1500.* New York, W. W. Norton & Co., 1937.

WILSON, FRANK E.: *The Divine Commission.* New York, Morehouse-Gorham Co., 1940.

CHAPTER 6

Leaders for Reform

The Intellectual Revolution affected the lives of rich and poor, king and peasant, the learned and the less informed, and greatly improved the social status of women. Its influence was felt in all of Europe—and eventually the whole world. It was, indeed, a revolution and affected every phase of human life: it gave the modern vogue to natural science and produced such intellectual giants as Robert Boyle, René Descartes, Isaac Newton, and Joseph Priestly; it profoundly influenced religion; it originated modern social science and a respect for history.

This revolution emphasized humanitarianism, and medicine rose from its lethargy and superstition. During this period Morgagni summed up his studies on morbid anatomy and became regarded as the father of pathology. Thomas Willis made a complete and accurate account of the cranial nerves, and the hexagonal network of arteries at the base of the brain is still called the circle of Willis. Francis Glisson was known for his classic account of rickets, the capsule of the liver, and his use of suspension in spinal deformities. Anton van Leeuwenhoek devoted his life to the study of microorganisms, using his improved microscope. Also transfusions and intravenous injections were begun during this period of widespread interest in medicine.

Along with the development of natural science, medicine, and the arts, the Intellectual Revolution developed an interest in human beings and their welfare, but this interest was not primarily motivated by Christian principles. Jean Jacques Rousseau of France probably had more influence in developing this attitude than any other person; he wrote and lectured on equality and democracy, and advocated outlawing the aristocrats and plutocrats. These ideals were eagerly assimilated by others interested in social improvement and were eventually the seeds from which sprang the French Revolution.

But what did all of these social improvements do for nursing? Actually, nursing benefited greatly from the Intellectual Revolution. In France, Germany, and England individuals became interested in the improvement of nursing conditions and some hospitals developed in both the United States and Canada. Some of these institutions were short-lived, but many flourished and still remain today.

St. John of God (1495-1550). In Spain there was significant improvement in the care of the sick because the religious orders intensified their efforts to serve the ill. Outstanding among those who responded to the needs of the sick poor was St. John of God, founder of the Brothers Hospitallers or Hospitaller of St. John of God, an order which has since spread over Christendom. At the age of forty, remorseful for his past conduct, John resolved to amend his life, and decided to devote his life and work toward helping the sick and the poor. He sold wood in the marketplace to earn money for feeding the destitute, and even rented a house in which to care for the sick.

During the day John tended to his patients, at night he sought new sources of charity. But soon this became unnecessary because people recognized the value of his great work and brought everything he needed for his little hospital. He did not, however, confine his charity to his own hospital, giving freely to all distressed persons whom he met.

Worn out by years of hard work, John became ill; he died on March 8, 1550, at the age of fifty-five. He was canonized in 1690, and in 1886 Pope Leo XIII ''declared him the heavenly patron of all hospitals and sick folk.'' Pope Pius XI in 1930 added nurses of both sexes to this order.[1]

St. Vincent de Paul (1580-1660). A parish priest and a social reformer, Vincent was well aware of the hordes of desperately poor people living throughout central and southern Europe. Nothing had been done about it because poverty was considered a divine chastisement or spiritual discipline. Vincent, however, developed a revolutionary idea: he believed that poverty could be abolished. He advocated education in manual training and skilled trades, and had farm camps organized for beggars, who were as numerous as flies. Vincent realized that there always would be a small number of persons unable to provide for themselves, but these would be given constructive aid by organized charity. These ideas to reduce poverty were not armchair theorizing—many were put into use, and the men and women who worked under his council formed the first societies organized specifically for charity.

Among these organizations was an excellent social service group called the Dames of Charity who worked in the Hotel Dieu of Paris. One of these women, Mme. de Gaussault, saw the need for actual nursing aid to supplement

---

[1] Alban Butler, *The Lives of the Saints*, Vol. 2, pp. 517-20.

the overworked Augustinian nuns, so she persuaded Vincent to organize a nursing service. In 1633 he recruited a vigorous group of young women whom he called *Filles de Charité,* and whom he placed under the supervision of Mlle. de Gras (nee Louise de Marillac). From this group developed what has become the famous nursing order of the Sisters of Charity (Daughters of Charity of St. Vincent de Paul). These nuns did not take vows until 1642, and then for only one year at a time; the vow is still renewed annually on March 26. The foundation of this order marked the beginning of freedom for nuns, who had a cloistered life since the sixth century. Vincent admonished his daughters: "Nuns must need have a cloister, but the Sisters of Charity needs go everywhere." And indeed, they have gone everywhere—they were the only order not suppressed during the French Revolution, and the Sisters of Charity cared for both Union and Confederate soldiers during the Civil War.

Under the auspices of Mother Elizabeth Seton, a branch of the Sisters of Charity was founded in the United States in 1812; thirteen years later these nuns accepted the responsibility for the nursing service in what is now the University of Maryland Hospital in Baltimore.

George Fox (1624-1691). This man, the founder of the sect known as the Society of Friends (Quakers), traveled in England, Scotland, and America preaching his doctrine that Christianity was a strictly personal experience, an "inner light," independent of church, state, and clergy. He advocated plain living and plain speaking. The Friends refused to take oath or bear arms.

One factor in the Friends' doctrine—equality of men and women—was indeed revolutionary, for women's activities had been restricted since the fall of the Roman Empire. They were held to be of inferior intelligence, incapable of carrying responsibility, and unable to conduct affairs of business, nor had women been permitted to own property. Fox, by advocating equality, made it easier for women to become active in nursing.

John Howard (1726-1790). Among the foremost pioneers of the public health movement was John Howard, who possessed ample means to enjoy the good things of life. Yet he spent his life in England and on the Continent making journeys into "hells on earth": prisons, communicable disease hospitals, orphanages, cells of galley slaves, hospitals, and infirmaries. Although uneducated, Howard collected data and statistics; he had his statistical studies published at his own expense which he gave to rulers and others in authority. Howard incurred the wrath of the medical profession by insisting on fresh air and plenty of water in the institutions that he visited. Because the physicians of Messina did not consider the plague contagious and did not request isolation, John Howard blamed them for the deaths of 43,000 persons in three months.

His interest in public health led him to investigate the lazarettoes, and he at one time had himself confined to the lazaretto in Venice in order to get first-hand information on conditions there.[2]

---

[2] Anne L. Austin, *History of Nursing Source Book* (New York, G. P. Putnam's Sons, 1957), pp. 81-83.

As a result of the work of John Howard, prison reforms were carried out in Europe and America, fresh air was permitted in hospitals—"enough to slightly bend the flame of the candle—," and the public was made aware of the low standards of nurses and nursing.

Philippe Pinel (1745-1826). Philippe Pinel was the son of a doctor in the village of Tarn, France. At the age of forty-eight Pinel was appointed medical director of the Bicêtre and the Salpêtrière—the two great hospitals of Paris.

The belief that mental illness was caused by demons had held sway for many centuries; even in biblical times "there met him a man from the city who had demons; for a long time he had worn no clothes and he lived not in a house but among the tombs."[3]

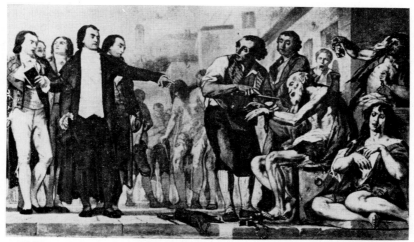

Philippe Pinel (1745-1826), French physician, demanding the removal of chains from the insane of the Bicêtre Hospital in Paris. (Painting by Charles Muller. Bettmann Archive.)

Philippe Pinel earned everlasting fame through his modern open-door treatment of the mentally ill. But only in fiction does a person rise to fame entirely on his own merits. Beside Pinel's name in psychiatry's hall of fame should be that of Jean-Baptiste Pussin, an obscure tanner's apprentice. Pussin had been employed at the Bicêtre to care for the mentally ill before the appointment of Dr. Pinel. He was uneducated and untrained, but his intelligence, innate kindness, tact, and sincerity made him unloosen the chains of some of the patients before Pinel became the director of the Bicêtre.

When Pinel saw what could be done through kindly understanding, he said, "I abandoned the dogmatic tone of the physician." Pinel brought Pussin and his equally sympathetic wife to the Salpêtrière as his assistants. There, with Pinel's authority, the experiment was tried on more patients. In 1793 Pinel obtained permission from the National Assembly to loosen the chains of forty-

[3] St. Luke 8:27.

nine patients and thereby proved that the insane were sick: they were not queer, immoral, or possessed of devils. These persons suffered from sick minds in the same manner that other parts of the body became diseased.

Elizabeth Gurney Fry (1780-1845). A member of one of the best known families of the Society of Friends, Elizabeth Gurney Fry stands next in importance to John Howard as a prison reformer. Although she was concerned with the duties of her home and eleven children, Mrs. Fry still had time to be interested in the women prisoners of Newgate prison, not far from her home. In 1817 she established schools and sewing classes among women prisoners and greatly improved prison conditions by developing work for the prisoners and the segregation of the sexes.

After visiting Theodor Fliedner, pastor at Kaiserswerth, where the first school for deaconesses was established in 1840, Mrs. Fry returned to England to establish the Institute of Nursing Sisters. This was the first organization of women to be trained as district or private duty nurses. They were carefully selected as to character and were required to be able to read and write. They had little of what we call training; they went daily for several months to Guy's Hospital to observe and learn what they could from the untrained ward nurses. They were, however, devoted and respectable women which in itself was an important improvement.

These women visited and cared for the poor in their homes, but they also gave nursing care to people who paid regular fees to the Institute for their services.

The Institute of Nursing Sisters continued under the royal patronage until the house was bombed during World War II and the nurses were absorbed by the staffs of other institutions.

Mother Mary Catherine McAuley (1787-1841). Mary Catherine McAuley was born near Dublin, Ireland, into a home of considerable wealth. Her father died when she was quite small and her mother and the three children lived with relatives and friends. Following the death of her mother when Catherine was twenty, she lived with a druggist, William Calligan, and his wife. The Calligans amply supplied her with all she cared to use of this world's goods and took pleasure in witnessing her almsgiving and the sweetness which enhanced the value of whatever she did to relieve the distressed.[4]

Mrs. Calligan was an invalid during the last two years of her life. Catherine cared for her and for the husband who survived his wife by three years. The family had no children and William Calligan felt that his all-but-adopted daughter would use his great wealth wisely. His bequest to Catherine in current values was $700,000.

With this great wealth Catherine designed and, in 1827, built a large house on Baggot Street in Dublin as a school for the education of hundreds of poor girls and instruction for the women who lived in the home. This group took no vows until December, 1831, when the order of the Sisters of Mercy was founded.

---

[4] Sr. Mary Beata Bauman, *A Way of Mercy* (New York, Vantage Press, 1958), p. 23.

Mother McAuley listed "visitation and care of the sick" as one of the good works of the group living on Baggot Street. There were no nursing schools in that day and professional nursing was unknown. Medical science had not even caught up with Hippocrates (400 B.C.) or King Asoka (250 B.C.); asepsis, anesthesia, surgery (except amputations) were unknown. Nursing consisted of comfort and nutrition for the patient. Mother McAuley had had twenty years of experience in caring for the sick. She had lived most of her life among physicians and pharmacists: her brother, brother-in-law, and uncle were doctors; her benefactor was a pharmacist.

In 1829 the plague of Asiatic cholera, spreading westward, reached Dublin. Mother McAuley and her sisters were placed in charge of a cholera hospital set up in the Townsend Street Depot. Bleeding was the usual treatment for the first stage of cholera, followed by calomel and large doses of opium, but the treatment used at the Townsend Street Depot was brandy, laudanum, and applications of heat.

Although Mother McAuley had passed away, the Sisters of Mercy answered the call to the Crimean War in the spring of 1854. By fall, shocking stories reached England concerning lack of supplies and inadequate medical and nursing personnel to care for the sick and wounded. Sir Sidney Herbert, then Secretary of War, appealed to Florence Nightingale to take a group of nurses to Scutari. Among those who went with Miss Nightingale were five Sisters of Mercy, who were already in Paris when Miss Nightingale issued her appeal for nurses. The War Office requested the sisters to wait in Paris for Miss Nightingale's party. By the time the nurses reached Turkey, another group of fifteen sisters from Mercy convents in Ireland were responding to an appeal from the Motherhouse in Dublin and they, too, cared for the sick and wounded at Balaklava. The sisters remained until peace was declared in April, 1856. When they returned to London, they received a triumphant ovation for their heroic services in the Crimean War.

Mother Mary McAuley had died in November, 1841, but the Sisters of Mercy continued to carry out her plans. Mercy Hospital in Pittsburgh was opened in 1847 and Mercy Hospital in Chicago in 1851. Today this order is second largest of the Roman Catholic orders and has built a chain of hospitals that encircles the globe.

Theodor Fliedner (1800-1864). A silk factory in Kaiserswerth (near Dusseldorf), Germany, failed shortly after Reverend Theodor Fliedner arrived to assume his duties as pastor of the small Lutheran parish. More than a century later this failure seemed providential. In order to maintain the church Reverend Fliedner set out to solicit funds for his work. In Holland he saw the work being done by the Mennonite Deaconesses, and in England he met Elizabeth Fry and saw the humanitarian work that she was carrying on in prison reform. The young pastor, then twenty-three, returned to his parish in Germany full of zeal to carry out these good works. In 1826 he founded the Rhenish-Westphalian Prison Association, the first of its kind in Germany.

With this accomplished, he began to investigate the possibilities of deaconess work that he had seen in Holland. Deaconess work had been well organized in the apostolic church until about 500 A.D. ''When he (Fliedner) visited the Amsterdam church to raise funds he became acquainted with a deaconess system that had nearly died out, and was thereby inspired to establish his own deaconess system, which developed into a flourishing institution.''[5]

But he was a man, and to train deaconesses a woman would be necessary, a special kind of woman: one experienced with sickness, with a spirit of Christian service, executive ability, and with grace and dignity to meet all types of people.

Friederika Munster (1800-1842). This woman was ''destined to become the mother of the revived apostolic order of deaconesses, and the immediate ancestor of modern nursing was born in the year 1800.''[6] Friederika's father was a schoolmaster and later comptroller on the estate of Prince Solms Braunfels. The death of her mother left Friederika in charge of the home and the care of smaller brothers and sisters. When she was twenty-five her father married again; by this time the children were grown and she was no longer needed at home, so she volunteered her services to a newly founded orphanage near Dusseldorf. After working for two years, she became ill. During her convalescence in the home of a friend she met Theodor Fliedner. Friederika and Fliedner had much in common since both were interested in the poor and underprivileged. When Fliedner asked Friederika to go to Kaiserswerth and take charge of his prison work, Friederika was willing, but her father refused to give her permission. Theodor Fliedner, however, was resourceful. He asked Friederika to marry him. Her father consented to this and she went to the parsonage to use her talents for convicts, orphans, schools, and the training of nurses.

We are particularly interested in Friederika Fliedner's work in the education of nurses, which began in 1836. In that year, the Fliedners opened a hospital. Their staff consisted of one patient, one nurse, and one cook. Although Mrs. Fliedner had had two years of experience in an orphanage, she had no training in nursing and especially in the development and administration of a school for nurses; further, there was no one to instruct her. Her talents for organization, personnel direction, teaching, and humanitarian interest could only have been found in a person of extraordinary mental endowment.

In one year's time, twelve young girls made their applications to enter a three-year training course as deaconesses. They were assigned to cooking and housekeeping, laundry and linen, women's ward, men's ward, and children's ward. Periodically these assignments were rotated so that all had the same experience. They were given formal classes by a doctor and, strangely enough, they were also given classes in pharmacology and required to pass a state examination in this subject. Mrs. Fliedner gave nearly all the nursing instruction; she compiled her notes in a journal which became the standard of teaching at Kaiserswerth, and which may be regarded as the first textbook

---

[5] The Mennonite Encyclopedia. Vol. II (Scottdale, Pa., Mennonite Publishing Co., 1956), p. 23.

[6] M. Adelaide Nutting and Lavinia L. Dock, *A History of Nursing*, Vol. II (New York, G. P. Putnam's Sons, 1935), p. 7.

of nursing. When students finished their studies, they could do hospital work, private duty, or district nursing.

Mrs. Fliedner continued to be the head of the school during her lifetime. Both she and her husband hoped that some of the deaconesses could be trained to take over that responsibility, but as soon as one proved capable she was sent to open a branch hospital and school.

Mrs. Fliedner had not only the management of the hospital and school, but also of the orphanage, children's school, and the convict refuge. Pastor Fliedner made many journeys to establish hospitals in other countries and assumed little of the administrative duties at Kaiserswerth.

In addition to her duties at Kaiserswerth, Mrs. Fliedner was the mother of nine children, four of whom died in infancy or at birth. Life was a constant conflict between her duty to her children and her work at the mother house. Although she was a woman of remarkable physical stamina, she was unable to carry the double burden. She died at the age of forty-two after giving premature birth to a dead infant.

A year later Pastor Fliedner went to Hamburg seeking a superintendent for his work at Kaiserswerth and again found a wife as capable and devoted as his first wife had been: Caroline Bertheau, director of nursing at the general hospital at Hamburg. After their marriage the second Mrs. Fliedner took charge of the household and children, together with the rapidly growing institution, and brought up eight children of her own. Pastor Fliedner died in 1864, but Caroline continued as the heart and soul of the work for twenty years after his death.

The Model for Nursing. The Kaiserswerth has been the model for nursing to the present day. Elizabeth Fry visited this hospital and founded the Nursing Sisters Institute along the same lines. Florence Nightingale spent three months at Kaiserswerth in 1850 and used the same pattern for St. Thomas's Hospital School of Nursing in 1860. Susan Dimcock and Marie Zakrzewska were doctors educated in Germany and were familiar with Kaiserswerth and its methods. They put these into effect in founding the nursing school of the New England Hospital for Women and Children in Boston in 1872.

The deaconess schools gave a small allowance or stipend to students. This practice was common in the United States and Canada until the depression began in 1929.

The preliminary school period of three to six months has been called by various names; perhaps the term ''probation'' was longest in use. This was a period in which the student could become acquainted with nursing and decide if she wished to continue; at the same time the student proved to the school that she either had or did not have the qualifications for developing into a satisfactory nurse. This period is now called the ''first semester'' and the students are known as ''freshmen,'' but the purpose of this period has not changed from the original one as instigated by Mrs. Fliedner in 1836.

Rev. William Alfred Passavant (1821-1894). Reverend William Passavant was requested by his parish in Baltimore, Maryland, to serve as a representative at a church convention in London in 1846. While there he learned of the work being done at Kaiserswerth through the deaconesses working at the German Hospital in London. He visited Kaiserwerth, talked to Pastor Fliedner, and left a sum of money to pay the passage of four deaconesses to be sent to the United States as soon as Mr. Passavant could obtain a suitable building.

The Passavant Hospital and School of Nursing in Pittsburgh, opened in 1849, was the first school of nursing under Protestant auspices in the western hemisphere.

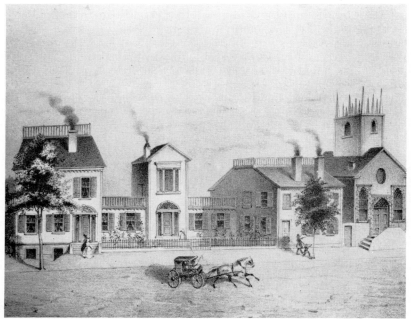

Original Passavant Hospital, Pittsburgh, 1849. First Protestant hospital in the western hemisphere. (Courtesy of Community Relations Department, Passavant Hospital.)

In 1863 a second hospital and school was opened in Milwaukee, admitting persons of all nationalities and religions. This hospital was long known as Passavant Hospital, but the name has now been changed to Milwaukee General Hospital.

With these two hospitals established, Rev. William Passavant and his family spent a summer vacation in Chicago. While there, Rev. Passavant learned of the pitiful condition of the Lutheran immigrants exposed to poor living conditions and without hospital facilities when ill. He therefore began plans for a third deaconess hospital and school. William Ogden, a wealthy Chicagoan, shared Rev. Passavant's interest and donated a site for the project between Clark Street and Lake Michigan. The hospital was burned in the great Chicago fire of 1871 and the new hospital was not opened until 1885.

The fourth deaconess institution founded by Rev. Passavant was opened in Jacksonville, Illinois, in 1869. This was an orphanage, but two weeks after opening, the State School for the Blind was burned and the eighty children from the school were housed in the orphanage. Later the orphanage, unable to find any needy children, was converted into a hospital. Sister Louisa, a graduate of the Passavant Hospital in Pittsburgh and America's first trained deaconess, and Sister Caroline were sent from Pittsburgh to take charge of the hospital.

Florence Nightingale (1820-1910).   The name, Florence Nightingale, symbolizes modern nursing. Perhaps no name of the exciting nineteenth century is as well known as Miss Nightingale's. No one has formulated a satisfactory definition of a genius, yet all agree that one of the requirements for this high classification is the extent of influence on the lives of others. That factor alone puts her in the category of the genius. Her influence affects the lives of every human being almost daily.

Miss Nightingale was born of a wealthy family at a time when nursing was performed by the least desirable of women. She was educated in Greek, Latin, and higher mathematics when education for women was only elementary because women were thought to be incapable of higher learning. She worked for the welfare of enlisted soldiers at a time when they literally were considered to be "cannon fodder." During her long life (ninety years), Florence Nightingale saw women of refinement enter nursing schools, higher education for women become generally accepted, and military conditions improve greatly.

Florence Nightingale was born May 12, 1820, in Florence, Italy, for which city she was named. Her parents were English—her father was an English country gentleman and her mother was a gay, pleasure-loving woman who never was able to understand her serious daughter.

Miss Nightingale, reared in wealth, enjoyed all the gaiety of the English aristocracy and no doubt accepted it as thoroughly as any young woman would. Then, in 1842, occurred the "hungry forties." In towns and villages there was general starvation; workhouses, hospitals, and prisons overflowed; immigration to the United States was high. Although Miss Nightingale did not keep a diary, she wrote hundreds of private notes, many of which have been preserved. One written in the spring of 1842 showed that she was keenly aware of the misery and suffering of the people: "My mind is absorbed with the sufferings of man, it besets me behind and before . . . All that the poets sing of the glories of this world seems to me untrue. All the people that I see are eaten up with care or poverty or disease."[7] She was aware that her destiny lay among the miserable of the world. Life was a conflict between the gaiety which she enjoyed and the misery which she was unable to alleviate.

At the age of twenty-four Florence Nightingale became convinced that her mission in life was among the sick. During the next seven years she made repeated efforts to study nursing, but her parents sternly refused. (This may

---

[7] Cecil Woodham-Smith, *Florence Nightingale* (New York, Mc-Graw-Hill Book Co., Inc., 1951), p. 31.

be humiliating to the modern student who enters a nursing school with her parents' blessing.)

Hospitals at that time were places of degradation and squalor. The "hospital smell" resulted from dirt and poor sanitation, not from antiseptics. Hospitals were constructed in long wards of fifty or sixty beds two feet apart, and the windows were nailed shut, for this was the age of the fear of fresh air. The well-to-do cared for the sick in their own homes, but those who came to the hospitals were from the poor tenements and cellars. The beds were dirty; a new patient was put between the same sheets used by the last patient. The ward was the nurse's only home. She lived, slept, and often cooked her meals there. Her bed was a cage on the stair-landing where it was impossible for the night nurse to sleep during the day. Discipline and supervision were unknown.

The seven years of disappointment and frustration during which Miss Nightingale sought to win over her parents were not wasted. She had a good background in mathematics and statistics; she spent five years collecting facts on public health and hospitals, and had an enormous mass of detailed information readily available. She became known as an expert on hospitals and in 1859 wrote a book, *Notes on Hospitals,* about the construction of civilian hospitals.

By 1850 the public became aroused to the dreadful conditions of hospitals and nurses. The Sisters of Charity, Kaiserswerth, Sisters of Mercy, Charles Dickens' novels, the humanitarianism that had spawned the French Revolution—all were having their effect on the general public who was becoming aware that something must be done.

In June, 1851, Miss Nightingale took her life in her own hands and announced to her parents that she was going to Kaiserswerth to study nursing. Her mother had hysterics (at that time it was quite proper for women to have hysterics) and scene followed scene. Her father "retreated into the shadows," and her sister felt that the family name was forever disgraced.

Mrs. Nightingale forbade Florence to tell anyone where she was going or to write any letters from Kaiserswerth. Everything was to be done in secret. Florence spent three months with the deaconesses in Kaiserswerth, then in September of 1853 she became administrator and director of nurses of an "Establishment for Gentlewomen during illness."[8] Her seven years of visiting hospitals gave her some revolutionary ideas which she put into practice, much to the consternation of the hospital board.

Miss Nightingale remained at this institution for about a year, until the Crimean War broke out. There had been a series of hostilities between Great Britain and Russia for several months, and France had allied herself with England to protect Turkey. The base for the war was established at Scutari, a town on the Asian shore of the Bosphorus. It was well known that the allies planned to attack Sebastopol, but the commissary department had received no official notification. Consequently, 30,000 men were sent into action, but cooking equipment, medicine chests, bedding, stretchers, and hospital wagons

[8] Sir Edward Cook, *The Life of Florence Nightingale* (New York, Macmillan Company, 1942), p. 133.

had all been left behind. The British won the battle of Alma at great sacrifice. When the wounded reached the great Barracks Hospital there were no beds, no food, no cups and buckets to bring water, no bandages. There were no nurses and only a few army surgeons.

Covering this campaign was the first war correspondent to follow an army— William Howard Russell of the *London Times*. When Russell sent in his reports describing the sufferings of the sick and wounded and the lack of provisions for care or food, the public seethed with rage. Sir Sidney Herbert, Secretary of War, knew that he was in danger of losing his office and he appealed to Miss Nightingale, whom he knew personally, to recruit nurses and to go at once to the Crimea to care for the wounded and the thousands who were dying of cholera.

This was the opportunity for which Miss Nightingale had waited to make full use of her many talents. Forty nurses were secured: twenty-six Roman Catholic and Anglican nursing sisters and fourteen nurses recruited from various English hospitals. The journey to the Crimea took a month. They arrived at Istanbul and were taken to Scutari the same day. By this time the hospital equipment had arrived but nothing had been done. The nurses set about to install five kitchens; they set up laundries, and cleaned the barracks of filth and lice. The soldiers were given such luxuries as clean bedding, hot soup, and hospital shirts. The death rate fell amazingly.

Miss Nightingale had never accepted the germ theory; she could not be convinced that microscopic organisms could cause the death of a strong man. But she demanded clean dressings, clean bedding, well-cooked, edible food, proper sanitation, and fresh air. It was to these improvements that she attributed the low death rate.[9]

The Crimean War ended in March, 1856, but Miss Nightingale stayed until July to care for the wounded. After a short rest she plunged into a program of military reform for the British Army. She had seen such unnecessary loss of life that she wrote: "While I live I fight for their cause." Using the public's rage and indignation as a wedge, she was successful in having appointed a Royal Commission for the Health of the Army, and she spent the next three years working with this commission which greatly improved the care and sanitation of military personnel.

The public's appreciation of Miss Nightingale's work was one of deep and lasting gratitude. A fund was started and, by the time Miss Nightingale returned to England, the fund had reached 44,000 pounds. Miss Nightingale was too concerned with military reforms to give attention to the ultimate use of this money, but in 1859 she made plans for the establishment of a school of nursing, using the Kaiserswerth school as a model. Florence Nightingale's school was opened at St. Thomas's Hospital because the medical director there

---

[9] Miss Nightingale's biographers do not agree upon the death rate or upon its reduction. It is not likely that an accurate account was kept. Great loss of life to the god of war was expected, and little effort was made to alleviate the suffering of the wounded. Even during the Civil War, 1861-65, an accurate figure of the death rate was seldom kept. For the Crimean War it was variously estimated at 42 to 73 per cent. Miss Nightingale is credited with reducing this rate to 2 per cent. This low rate may have been estimated for battle casualties only. Asiatic cholera was prevalent during the entire war, with a high death rate.

was interested in her project, and the matron of St. Thomas's, Mrs. Ward-roper, was a woman Miss Nightingale greatly admired. The school opened in June, 1860, with fifteen students who enrolled for one year. The students' uniform consisted of a brown dress with white cap and apron. Miss Nightingale had published a small book, *Notes on Nursing,* which was used as a textbook and, even to this day, may be found in all nursing school libraries.

Miss Nightingale never expected her graduates to be staff nurses. She knew the need for these graduates as missionary nurses who could go into other hospitals and other countries to establish schools and improve nursing. The graduates fulfilled their appointed missions and this legacy has come as a gift to every civilized country through the influence of one person.[10]

REFERENCES

AUSTIN, ANNE L.: *History of Nursing Source Book.* New York, G. P. Putnam's Sons, 1957.

BAUMAN, SISTER MARY BEATA: *A Way of Mercy.* New York, Vantage Press, 1958.

COOK, SIR EDWARD: *Life of Florence Nightingale.* New York, The Macmillan Co., 1913.

"DEACONESS." *The Mennonite Encyclopedia,* Vol. II. Scottdale, Pa., Mennonite Publishing House, 1956.

DOYLE, ANN: Nursing by religious orders in the United States. *Amer. J. Nurs.* 29:1197 (Oct.) 1929.

GERBERING, G. A.: Life and Letters of William A. Passavant, 4th ed. Greenville, Pa., The Young Lutheran Co., 1906.

NUTTING, M. ADELAIDE, and DOCK, LAVINIA L.: *A History of Nursing,* Vol. II. New York, G. P. Putnam's Sons, 1935.

PAVEY, AGNES E.: *The Story of the Growth of Nursing.* Philadelphia, J. B. Lippincott Co., 1953.

PENNOCK, META RUTTER: *Makers of Nursing History.* New York, Lakeside Publishing Co., 1940.

ROBINSON, VICTOR: *White Caps.* Philadelphia, J. B. Lippincott Co., 1946.

SEYMER, LUCY RIDGELY: Mary Crossland of the Nightingale Training School. *Amer. J. Nurs.* 61:85 (May) 1961.

"THE NIGHTINGALE COMMUNION SERVICE." *Amer. J. Nurs.* 48:288 (May) 1948.

WHITNEY, JANET: Elizabeth Fry goes to Newgate. *Atlantic Monthly* 158:614 (Nov.) 1936.

WILLIAMS, CECELIA BARKER: Stories from Scutari. *Amer. J. Nurs.* 61:88 (May) 1961.

WOODHAM-SMITH, CECIL: *Florence Nightingale.* New York, McGraw-Hill Book Co., Inc., 1951.

[10] The Bulletin given by St. Thomas's Hospital School of Nursing in 1859 to prospective students was described in considerable detail by Sarah Tooley in her book, *Life of Florence Nightingale,* 1905.

CHAPTER 7

Scientific Strides

A new era evolved with the dawn of scientific liberty. In the early part of the nineteenth century, medicine was greatly influenced by the intellectual, political, social developments. There was a freer atmosphere. Together with the marked increase in material and cultural growth, a deeper sense of human dignity prevailed among all classes.

The medical discoveries of the nineteenth century were influenced by the Intellectual Revolution of the seventeenth century and the Age of Enlightenment of the eighteenth century. The alchemy[1] of the Moslems developed into the science of chemistry during the nineteenth century: Priestly discovered oxygen, Scheele discovered chlorine, and Lavoisier established quantitative analysis. Newton's discoveries in physics had shaken the scientific world by proving the universality of a natural law of gravitation. Chemistry and physics proved to medicine that laboratories and clinical teaching were necessary for the education of physicians. Leyden University in Leyden, Holland, was the first medical school to equip laboratories and provide clinical instruction for medical students.

The amazing advances in all branches of medicine during the nineteenth century were made possible by the preceding two centuries of intense investi-

---

[1] "Alchemy," from a Greek word meaning juices, was originally the art of extracting medicinal juices from plants.

gation, experimentation, clinical observation, and a truly humanitarian interest in the alleviation of suffering.

It is not possible to list all of the great persons; also, it is difficult to decide which were most important, and whose contribution was most beneficial. But there are several persons whose work stands out.

EARLY HEALTH PIONEERS

Leyden was the great medical center of the eighteenth century. Many Scotch graduates of this school returned to Scotland and developed a famous medical center in Edinburgh during the latter part of the eighteenth century. Many bold operations were performed, plastic surgery was revived, large blood vessels were successfully ligated, amputations were performed with greater skill. Anesthetics, however, were still unknown, and operations within the cranium, abdomen, and the female pelvis were not generally attempted until the second half of the nineteenth century.

Ephraim McDowell (1771-1830). This young Virginia doctor went to Edinburgh for a year (1793-94) of study under the renowned surgeon, John Bell. Dr. Bell was concerned with the fate of women afflicted with ovarian disease, and imparted his interest and despair to his students.

When Dr. McDowell returned to America, he established his medical practice at Danville, Kentucky, then a raw, pioneer town on the outskirts of civilization. He soon became known as a skillful surgeon, especially in lithotomies.

Ephraim McDowell's fame as Father of Ovariotomy was the result of one of the most dramatic events in American medical history. In December, 1809, Dr. McDowell was called in consultation to see Mrs. Jane Todd Crawford who thought she was in labor. The patient's abdomen was greatly distended and her "pregnancy" was considered to be beyond term. Her own physician, realizing that this was no ordinary labor, called upon Dr. McDowell, then thirty-eight years of age, to assist in the delivery. Dr. McDowell performed a vaginal examination and found the uterus empty. He recognized the disease as being one of the ovary, a condition which Dr. Bell considered to be somewhat unresponsive to treatment. The patient was forty-seven years of age and the mother of several children. If nothing could be done for her she would die. Dr. McDowell made a decision. Although he had neither seen nor heard of such an operation, he felt that removal of the tumor, though extremely hazardous, might save the patient's life. He frankly discussed with Mrs. Crawford the seriousness of her condition, and of the alternatives. He told her that although he had never performed such an operation if she would come to his office in Danville he would do his best to cure her by surgery. He must have inspired Mrs. Crawford's confidence for she made the sixty-mile trip from her home in Motley's Glen to Danville on horseback, resting the tumor on the horn of the saddle.

Dr. McDowell had no anesthesia to give his patient, because it was not discovered until 1842-46. He had no cap, gown, or mask. He simply covered his suit coat with a butcher's apron, picked up his scalpel and made a long incision. Because of the pressure of the tumor the intestines rushed out upon the table and remained there during the twenty-five-minute operation. The germ theory was unknown at the time; there was no warm saline solution to cover the intestines as there would be today under such circumstances. Dr. McDowell opened the tumor and removed fifteen pounds of gelatinous material. Then he removed the sack and its contents (which weighed twenty-two pounds), closed the incision, applied a binder and put the patient to bed. There was no nurse, only kindly neighbors to give instinctive nursing care.

To the modern nurse, Mrs. Crawford's operation appears crude, even horrifying, but Mrs. Crawford survived and lived to be seventy-eight years of age.

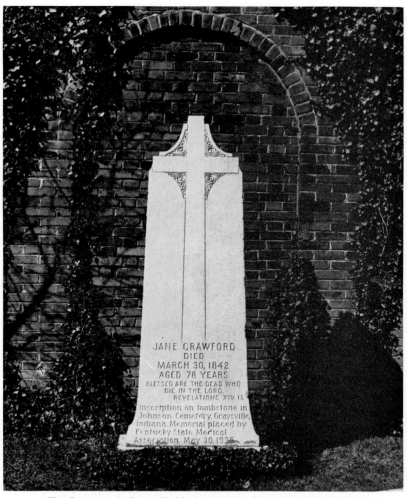

Headstone of Jane Todd Crawford, Danville, Kentucky.

Although this was the first known successful ovariotomy, Dr. McDowell did not report it until eight years later (1817), when he described his procedure and findings in the *Eclectic Repertory and Analytic Review,* published in Philadelphia. In this report he skipped the immediate postoperative period. Instead, he stated: ''In five days I visited her, and much to my astonishment found her making up her bed.''

William Beaumont (1785-1853). William Beaumont, a surgeon in the United States Army, was stationed at the fort on Mackinac Island, a small island in Mackinac Strait which separates Lake Huron from Lake Michigan. There, in June of 1822, when thousands of fur traders brought their winter trappings to be sold to the fur-trading companies, a young half-breed Indian, named Alexis St. Martin, was accidentally shot in the stomach, leaving a hole as large as the palm of a hand. But because Alexis St. Martin refused to permit Dr. Beaumont to close the wound, it healed with a permanent fistula.

One year later Dr. Beaumont conceived the idea of making digestive experiments through the fistula directly into the stomach, since at the time the stomach was an unexplored region. Over a period of eleven years he conducted 236 experiments, using such primitive tools as a spool of thread, a gum elastic tube, and cheese cloth compresses.

Dr. Beaumont carefully noted the time needed for the digestion of hash, steaks, fats, and raw and cooked foods. He recorded the reactions to emotions when food was eaten, proving that gastric digestion was delayed under emotional stress. As a result of his studies, Dr. Beaumont gave an accurate description of the normal action of the gastric mucosa, described the movements of the stomach to the completion of gastric digestion, and showed that gastric juices are secreted only when food is present. His chemical analysis of the gastric juice led him to the conclusion that it contained free hydrochloric acid, plus some other active chemical substance which later investigators found to be pepsin.

Dr. Beaumont's experiments on different foods laid the foundation for gastric physiology dietetics.[2] The results of these experiments were published in 1833, under the title *Experiments and Observations on the Gastric Juice and the Physiology of Digestion.* This has been called ''the most notable and original classic in American medicine.''[3]

CONQUEST OF PAIN

Today, anesthetics are taken for granted, without realizing that the conquest of pain is little more than a century old. Opium and whisky to dull the pain and four strong men to hold the patient were the only efforts made to

---

[2] Most of these experiments were done at Fort Crawford, Prairie du Chien, Wisconsin. The old military hospital has been restored as a museum and widely scattered relics of Dr. Beaumont have been collected and are on display.

[3] A service occasionally rendered to lovers of rare books by modern publishers is the publication of a facsimile edition of famous works. Dr. Beaumont's research on the physiology of digestion is now available in a facsimile edition.

relieve pain during earlier operations. When ether and chloroform were discovered there was a dreadful outcry against their use. Many believed that man was supposed to suffer. Chloroform was denounced from the pulpit when it was used at childbirth: "In sorrow shalt thou bring forth children." When Sir James Simpson (1811-1870), the discoverer of chloroform, learned that his discovery was called "the decoy of Satan," he quoted the first operation to be carried out under deep anesthesia: "So the Lord God caused a deep sleep to fall upon the man, and while he slept took one of his ribs and closed up its place with flesh."[4] Queen Victoria ended the controversy by having chloroform administered during the delivery of her seventh child.

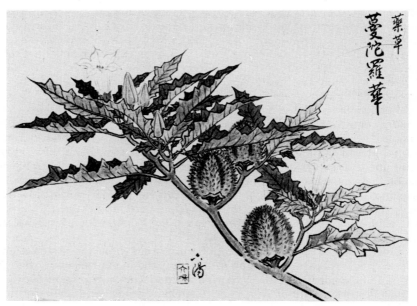

Datura alba or datura stramonium used in 1805 as an anesthetic by the Japanese. (Courtesy of the Hall of Fame, International College of Surgeons.)

Sir Humphrey Davey (1778-1829), in England, had become aware of the pain-relieving properties of nitrous oxide while trying to ease the pain of an infected tooth. Nitrous oxide, or laughing gas, became popular but was abandoned because the effect was too short.

Ether, however, was an American discovery. In 1842, Dr. Crawford Long (1815-1878) of Danielsville, Georgia, used ether for several operations, but Danielsville was a frontier town and no publicity was given the event.

---

[4] Genesis 2:21, Revised Standard Version.

Three years later, Horace Wells (1815-1848), a dentist from Hartford, Connecticut, went to New Haven to hear a lecture on nitrous oxide. The next day Wells described this lecture to a fellow student, William T. G. Morton (1819-1868). Both dentists were interested in finding an agent that would relieve the pain of tooth extraction. Wells tried nitrous oxide but was unsuccessful. Morton, as a student at the Harvard Medical School, became acquainted with Dr. Charles Jackson (b. 1844), professor of chemistry. Morton explained to Dr. Jackson that he was searching for something to relieve pain for extractions, and Dr. Jackson suggested that sulfuric ether, when inhaled, had properties similar to nitrous oxide. Morton tried it on his dog, on himself, and in his dental practice. Later he called on Dr. John Collins Warren of Massachusetts General Hospital to give Dr. Warren permission to use ether for a surgical operation. Ether was used as a surgical anesthetic on October 16, 1846. After Dr. Warren had completed the operation he turned to his incredulous audience and said: "Gentlemen, this is no humbug."

Insensibility to pain was something new—there was no word for it. The word "anesthesia" was coined from the Greek *an* meaning not, and *aisthesis,* feeling.

Oliver Wendell Holmes and Ignaz Philipp Semmelweis.

Oliver Wendell Holmes (1809-1894), well known as an American poet,[5] is less known for his great contribution to American medicine. It was he who coined the word "anesthesia." In his early career as professor of anatomy at Harvard Medical School he recommended that women in maternity hospitals should never be attended by a physician who had been conducting post-mortem examinations or visiting patients with puerperal fever without carefully washing his hands; he believed that disease may be conveyed in this manner from doctor to patient.

At this time, 1842, the cause of infections was still unknown. Holmes based his assertions upon observations. He noticed that there was less puerperal fever among women attended by midwives than among those attended by physicians. In searching for the reason he concluded that the midwives washed their hands more frequently and that they did not perform autopsies. His paper on the *Contagiousness of Puerperal Fever,* read to the Boston Society for Medical Improvement, created such violent opposition that Dr. Holmes was considered fanatical and his professorship was endangered.

At the same time a Hungarian physician in the first obstetric ward at the Allgemeines Krankenhaus, Vienna, made the same observation. This physician, Ignaz Philipp Semmelweis, was in charge of the ward used for obstetrical experience for student physicians. Students came into this ward directly from the autopsy room, often making vaginal examinations with unwashed hands. In the ward devoted to the instruction of midwives greater attention was given to personal cleanliness. Semmelweis became aware of a much higher mortality rate among the mothers in the medical students' ward than in the ward for midwife instruction.

[5] "Old Ironsides," "The Chambered Nautilus," "Contentment," and "The Autocrat of the Breakfast Table" are familiar to every grade school student.

Through this observation he developed a theory of the transfer of puerperal fever from unclean hands to the obstetrical patient. While studying this idea a member of the hospital staff died of a wound accidentally incurred while performing an autopsy examination. Semmelweis, at the post-mortem examination of the staff member, observed that the diseased tissue had the same appearance as that of the unfortunate mothers in the medical students' ward. He immediately instituted handwashing for all medical students.

Such practice met with fierce opposition, even persecution, from the orthodox obstetricians of that day. Semmelweis was not equal to the strain of violent controversy, and brooding over the wrongs that had been done to him by his colleagues brought on insanity and subsequent death. He is one of medicine's martyrs and always will be one of its far-shining names, for every child-bearing woman owes him a debt of gratitude.[6]

THE CONTROL OF INFECTION

The microscope has been a revolutionary tool in the development of medicine and has aided in the introduction of much of the scientific aspect of modern nursing. Everyone is aware of the invisible world of microorganisms, yet proof that these highly important organisms existed for both good and evil is less than a hundred years old. Since these organisms could not be seen with the unaided eye, it remained for the ingenuity of man to invent something that would make them visible. During the great plague of Rome in 1655, a Jesuit priest, Athanasius Kircher, who was also an optician, examined the blood of patients and "found that the blood of plague patients was filled with a countless brood of 'worms,' not perceptible to the naked eye, but to be seen in all putrefying matter through the microscope."[7]

Antoni van Leeuwenhoek (1632-1723). Born in Delft, Holland, van Leeuwenhoek had time, money, industry, and a great intellectual curiosity about natural history; he saw and described a variety of microbes, blood cells, capillaries, plain and striated muscles, bacterial chains, and clumps. He conducted these investigations for half a century and in 1863 gave this information to the Royal Society, of which he was a Fellow. He left 247 microscopes with lenses that he had ground himself. He made available a wealth of material for reading and for examination.

Yet nothing happened; nearly 200 years went by. This was the age of "laudable pus," during which suppuration was expected, even encouraged as being essential to the healing process. Because the stench in the hospital wards was so nauseating, a physician visited his patients as little as possible and when he did he held a perfumed handkerchief to his nose. Nurses were criticized for drinking alcoholic beverages, but only a person half stupefied by drink could endure the odor.

---

[6] Every nurse student should be required to read *The Cry and the Covenant* by Morton Thompson.

[7] Fielding H. Garrison, *An Introduction to the History of Medicine*, 4th ed. (Philadelphia, W. B. Saunders Co., 1929), p. 252.

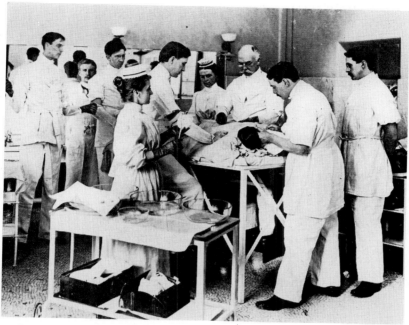

Professor Charles McBurney (1845-1913), famous for his discovery of "McBurney's Point," operated in Roosevelt Hospital, New York. (After a rare photograph made in 1901. Bettmann Archive.)

Although the nineteenth century was the age when pus-producing organisms were praised, it was also the century that saw the error of such therapeutics recognized and corrected. This medical revolution was due to the work of many men, each adding his bit which made possible the final result.

The proof of the germ theory and its application in the care of the sick in all branches of medicine was attributed to the initiative and observations of four men: Louis Pasteur, Joseph Lister, Robert Koch, and Edwin Klebs.

Louis Pasteur (1822-1895). A French chemist, Pasteur first became interested in pathogenic organisms through his studies of the diseases of wines. Pasteur's discovery that heating the wine to a temperature of 55° to 60° C. (pasteurization) killed microorganisms which caused the wines to spoil was of great economic value to the wine industry, and this led Pasteur to investigate many fields. The inscription on the arches over the tomb of Pasteur enumerates, among his notable achievements, activities in the areas of molecular dyssymmetry, fermentation, spontaneous generation, diseases of the wines, diseases of silkworms, microorganisms in beer, virulent diseases—anthrax and chicken cholera, and preventive vaccines—particularly for hydrophobia.[8]

Joseph Lister (1827-1912). The son of a wine merchant and the first physician to be raised to the peerage, Joseph Lister made some outstanding improvements on the compound microscope. As a young student in the hospitals of London, Lister was disturbed by the high surgical mortality rate caused by septicemia, pyemia, erysipelas, tetanus, and hospital gangrene. He compiled his own statistics on amputations and found that 45 per cent were fatal, although he had changed the dressing frequently and was scrupulously clean. "... Yet Lister had already begun to think of the old Hippocratic healing by first intention as the surgeon's ideal. Noticing that, when attainable, this was always disassociated from putrefaction, his attention was accidentally drawn to Pasteur's work, and, grasping its tendency, he set out to prevent the development of microorganisms in wounds. Perceiving that Pasteur's heat sterilizations would avail nothing here, he turned to chemical antiseptics. After trying out zinc chloride and the sulphites, he hit, by lucky chance, upon carbolic acid, which had been employed, previously, in the disinfection of sewage at Carlisle."[9]

Lister, regarded as the father of modern surgery, practiced antiseptic surgery with excellent results. In operating room experience, today's nurse must constantly carry out aseptic technics; the Listerian principles of avoiding sepsis are the same.

Robert Koch (1843-1910). In his first position, as district physician at Wollstein, Koch made long monotonous journeys over the country roads and observed cattle lying dead in the pastures. His curiosity was aroused; he was told that the cattle were dying of anthrax. Later his wife, Emma, bought him a microscope for his birthday. This opened the way for a lifetime of investigation but the gift of the microscope also brought sadness into Koch's home. Mrs. Koch divorced the doctor because he carried his experiments too far when he brought tissues of dead cattle into the house, fed and kept small animals in the home, and ignored well-cooked meals.

Koch is known as the father of microbiology because of the technic he devised for examining and attaining cultures, and his well-known postulates. In addition, he and his numerous assistants—later famous in their own right— discovered *Vibrio cholerae* and demonstrated its transmission by water, food, and clothing; they also discovered the cause of infectious conjunctivitis.

Edwin Klebs (1834-1913). The fourth member of this famous quartet— Pasteur, Lister, Koch, and Klebs—proved and firmly established that germs are the cause of infectious diseases. Klebs became professor of pathology at Bern, Switzerland, in 1866 and later held the same position at Wurzburg, Prague, and Zurich. He also served as professor of pathology at Rush Medical College, Chicago, in 1896.

---

[8] Garrison, *op. cit.*, pp. 589-90.

[9] Rene-Valey Radet, *The Life of Pasteur*, trans. from French (New York, Doubleday and Co., 1924), p. 429.

Louis Pasteur was a chemist, not a physician, yet he worked with physicians during his professional life. Nevertheless, because of professional jealousy he was not accepted by the medical profession. Dr. Klebs, as a contemporary of Pasteur and having wide acclaim as a pathologist, took up the cause in behalf of Pasteur and did much to win pathologists over to the idea that bacteria caused infectious diseases.

The discovery of the bacterial origin of diseases may be considered the greatest achievement of the nineteenth century. Although the microscope had been known for two centuries it remained for Lister, Pasteur, and Koch to provide the "missing link."

TREATMENT OF MENTAL ILLNESS

Philippe Pinel, during the French Revolution, demonstrated the open-door treatment of the mentally ill. Four years later, William Tuke (1732-1822), of the Society of Friends in England, inaugurated the same system without any knowledge of the Pinel experiment. With his own private fortune Tuke built The Retreat in New York and personally controlled the hospital. Despite opposition and ridicule he proved that the mentally ill should be treated as human beings.

In 1800 there were only four mental hospitals in all of the United States: Philadelphia (1752), Williamsburg, Virginia (1773), New York (1791), and Baltimore (1797). The Society of Friends, Philadelphia, learned of the work of the Quaker, William Tuke, in England, and in 1817 opened a mental hospital in Philadelphia, where the mentally ill were "regarded as men and brethren." In 1818 the McLean Asylum was opened at Somerville, Massachusetts; the hospital at Worcester, Massachusetts, was opened in 1833; and The Retreat at Hartford in 1836.

The nineteenth century that saw the control of pain and infection also witnessed a revolution in the care of the mentally ill, which continues to this day.

Dorothea Linde Dix (1802-1887). Miss Dix, a Boston schoolteacher, was asked to teach a Sunday school class in the House of Correction at Cambridge by one of the seminary students. It was here that Miss Dix saw the overcrowding, filth, and herding together of the criminals and the mentally ill. She could not feel pity without doing something constructive about it. Did the condition exist only in East Cambridge jail or was it common practice throughout the state? Notebook in hand she visited every jail and almshouse from Cape Cod to Berkshire during the next two years. With her accumulated mass of statistics and eyewitness reports, she addressed the venerable, majestic legislature of Massachusetts: "I proceed gentlemen, briefly, to call your attention to the *present* state of insane persons confined within this Commonwealth, in *cages, closets, cellars, stalls, pens; chained, naked, beaten with rods, and lashed* into obedience!"[10]

---

[10] Francis Tiffany, *The Life of Dorothea Linde Dix* (Boston, Houghton, Mifflin Co., 1890), p. 76.

Her report was devastating. Boston was scandalized; what had been regarded as the most enlightened state in the Union was now ridiculed. It was charged that the story was incredible, a pack of sensational lies. But Miss Dix had expected this and she had fortified her position by presenting letters from sheriffs all over the state who declared that they were unable to provide anything better under the existing system of caring for the mentally ill. The city fathers of the Massachusetts towns were shocked and humiliated; the legislature voted to allocate money to build state hospitals.

Miss Dix was fired with the spirit of the crusader. To her the treatment of the insane represented nothing less than crucified humanity. She spent the next thirty years in personal investigations of prisons and almshouses. From these surveys she prepared memorials, addressed to the state legislatures, on conditions of the treatment of the mentally ill in their states.

Dorothea Dix had an uncanny gift in dealing with legislators. With the memorial prepared, she went to the state capitol and acquainted herself with the legislators. She did not make the address to the assembly, but she was unerring in her selection of the right legislator to introduce the bill for funds for a state hospital and to "father" successfully the bill through both houses.

Thirty-four state hospitals stand as her monument. Furthermore, she carried her crusade to Scotland, the Channel Islands, Europe, and Japan. With our present rate of one in ten persons needing psychiatric treatment and care at some period in life,[11] we can be thankful for the constructive work of the spinster schoolteacher of Boston.

THE CONQUEST OF OPHTHALMIA NEONATORUM

Loss of sight, complete or partial, through ophthalmia neonatorum, has long been a scourge of mankind and, as the population increased, the number of blind babies increased. "Doctors explained to mothers of babies who had lost their eyesight at birth that this condition was due to such causes as peculiar constitution of the atmosphere or sudden changes of temperature. Colds were assumed to be the cause of inflamed eyes. This belief was so widespread that Cortez, the Spaniard, in 1537, decreed that all babies should be baptized with warm water instead of cold water."[12]

From time to time through the centuries some unusually observant person would suggest that possibly leukorrhea in the mother had some association with ophthalmia in the newborn baby, but no investigations were made. The blind children learned to beg; the state provided an asylum or refuge (no schools) for those who could not be cared for by parents or relatives. Gonorrheal ophthalmia was the chief cause of the blindness.

Carl Siegmund Franz Credé (1819-1892). Dr. Credé became professor of obstetrics and gynecology at the University of Leipzig in 1856, at the age of thirty-seven. He was deeply concerned over the condition then known as "babies'

---

[11] Statistics furnished by the Mental Health Society of Greater Chicago, 1959.

[12] C. A. Smith and L. Halse, "Ophthalmia Neonatorum," *Public Health Reports* (May, 1955), p. 463.

sore eyes.'' With hundreds of babies born in the maternity department each year, Dr. Credé tried numerous experiments. But in 1856, germs, as the cause of disease, were unknown. Then his contemporaries—Pasteur, Koch, and Lister—demonstrated a relationship between microorganisms and infection. Bacteriology developed into an exact science; numerous investigators began research. A. Neisser (1855-1914 A.D.) discovered the gonococcus in 1879, and two years later other researchers demonstrated gonococcus in parents with ophthalmia neonatorum.

With this information Dr. Credé began searching for a chemical disinfectant that would destroy the organisms in the eye without harming the delicate conjunctiva. He found that gonococcus had a low resistance to silver nitrate, even in a weak solution. After animal experimentation, Dr. Credé began trials with newborn babies.

In his report entitled *The Prevention of Ophthalmia Neonatorum,* published in 1884, Dr. Credé stated that ''within a period of almost three years, there occurred in 1160 children only one or at the most two cases of blennorhea gonorrhea.'' The general procedure described by Dr. Credé in 1884 has remained unchanged to this day: ''All the sebaceous matter clinging to the eyelids was removed. Then on the table where the child is swathed before clothes are put on the child, each eye is opened by means of two fingers, a single drop of a 2 per cent solution of silver nitrate hanging on a little glass rod is brought close to the cornea until it touches it, and is dropped on the middle of it. There is no further care given to the eyes.''[13] It has since been found that a 1 per cent silver nitrate solution is equally effective; this is in common use today.

Credé's report and demonstration met with widespread opposition. The cause of babies' sore eyes had been proved; a simple and effective measure had been demonstrated yet babies continued to become blind because of the general apathy of the public and the medical profession. The reason for this indifference, no doubt, was the public's attitude toward venereal disease. It was considered to be highly improper to mention sex or social hygiene in any form. The cause of ophthalmia neonatorum is gonorrhea in the mother, yet this could not be mentioned by the campaigners for preventive legislation. Newspapers and pamphlets could not print the word gonorrhea; they could only cite the great number of children that were ''needlessly blind because of lack of proper medical care.''

Forty years after Credé's announcement, only twenty states in this country had definite enactments requiring the prophylactic treatment of the eyes of every newborn. Various state groups prepared and introduced bills for the enforcement of such treatment but these bills were fought bitterly by antimedical groups whose opposition to medical treatment was based on religious grounds and whose members flooded the legislature with protests. Slowly the states learned that the passage of such a bill required the education of every physician and legislator as well as every citizen. This meant an active and dedicated committee working in each legislative district.

[13] Logan Clendening, *Source Book of Medical History* (New York, Paul B. Hoeber, Inc., 1942), p. 185.

Prophylactic law against ophthalmia neonatorum is now in effect in every state. In 1908, gonorrhea was the cause of 28 per cent of blindness in the United States; preventive medicine has reduced this to 1 per cent.

THE FIGHT AGAINST TUBERCULOSIS

Tuberculosis was known to the ancients, but it was apparently unknown in the western hemisphere until the arrival of the Europeans, following the discovery of the West Indies in 1492. It was not until the latter part of the nineteenth century that the disease was known to be communicable. Plagues had ravaged the Eastern and European countries for centuries, and lazarettos and pesthouses had been built to segregate infected persons. The "great white plague," however, was generally considered to be a familial disease, somehow being transferred from one generation to another by an inheritance factor. The communicability of this disease is so well known to us that it seems self-evident, yet August Flint and William H. Welch, authors of *The Principles and Practice of Medicine,* revised and published in 1881, stated that "The doctrine of the contagiousness of the disease (tuberculosis) has . . . its advocates but general belief is in its non-communicability." The following year, 1882, the tubercle bacillus was discovered by Koch and proved to medical science that tuberculosis was caused by a specific organism.

Nothing had been found to be effective in the treatment of tuberculosis, and the death rate continued to rise. Most physicians agreed that rest was beneficial, but this was only an empirical assumption. Because the patient complained of fatigue, rest was taken for granted, but that fresh air could have been helpful was never suggested. To the modern student the fear of fresh air that prevailed for hundreds of years, even through the nineteenth century, seems unbelievable.

During the nineteenth century new ideas of sanitation were developing as a sort of sanitary awakening—it was recognized that fresh air, pure water, and good food were essential to healthful living—but the medical profession continued to consider fresh air and plenty of food as harmful to the tuberculous patient.

Then in 1853 Herman Brehmer (1826-1889), upon graduation from medical school, devoted his doctoral thesis to the theme that pulmonary tuberculosis was curable, and a year later he established a sanitarium in Silesia, Prussia, where he advised his patients to rest in open-air balconies. This was the turning point in the treatment of tuberculosis.

Edward Livingston Trudeau (1848-1915). Edward Trudeau descended from a line of physicians as far back as the family can be traced. His father, James Trudeau, was a New Orleans physician who probably practiced medicine very little, because he is remembered mostly for his work with John James Audubon in anatomy of birds; his expedition to the Rocky Mountains with General Fremont; and, after two years spent with the Osage Indians, his study of their customs and language. This same love of nature and wild life was carried to his son, Edward, and is credited by him as saving his life.

Edward Trudeau's brother developed tuberculosis. He was ill from four to five months, and since there were no nurses in those days, Edward cared for his brother both day and night. "Not only did the doctor never advise any precautions to protect me against infection, but he told me repeatedly never to open the windows as it would aggravate the cough, and I never did, until toward the end my brother was so short of breath that he asked for fresh air."[14]

After the death of his brother, Edward studied medicine, married, and developed an extensive medical practice in New York City. He, too, contracted tuberculosis, first manifested by a "cold" abscess and later by scrofula. Although he was a graduate physician at the time, neither he nor his colleagues associated these conditions with tuberculosis. Seven years after the death of his brother, Dr. Trudeau learned that the upper two-thirds of his own left lung was involved in an active tuberculous process.

At that time the mortality rate of tuberculosis was extremely high and, as he recalled the illness and death of his brother, he felt that he was doomed to an early death. Since he thought his life was to be short, Dr. Trudeau decided to spend the remainder in the environment that would be most pleasant for him. He loved the wild primitive outdoors, as had his father. Two years earlier he had spent a hunting vacation in the Adirondack Mountains in upper New York State where he had stayed at a hunting lodge owned by Paul Smith.

After two years at Paul Smith's lodge, the doctor had gained weight and strength and began to practice a little medicine by treating guides and resort guests. He had become bored with waiting to die. He subscribed to four medical journals and began to take an active interest in his practice—and especially in tuberculosis. In 1882 he read of Dr. H. Brehmer's Goerbersdorf Sanitarium in Silesia, and became interested in founding such an institution in the United States.

Tuberculosis sanitariums were unknown in the United States. There were no existing plans to use as a guide. Tuberculosis was not considered a transmissible disease, and in the wards of the hospitals these patients were admitted to beds in rooms with patients having noncontagious diseases.

Dr. Trudeau, in his autobiography, explains why he adopted the cottage plan: "I felt that segregation, such as could be secured by the cottage plan, would be preferable for many reasons. By adopting this plan an abundance of fresh air could be secured for the patient, the irritation of constant close contact with many strangers would be avoided, and I knew that it would be easier to get some of my patients to give a little cottage which would be their own individual gift, rather than a corresponding sum of money toward the erection of larger buildings." The first cottage, called "Little Red," was opened in 1884. A picture of this cottage was used on the Christmas seals of 1934. The cottage plan for sanatariums continued into the twentieth century.

Dr. Trudeau, who is known as the father of tuberculosis sanatariums in America, lived to the age of sixty-seven years in spite of tuberculosis from which he never recovered and which ultimately caused his death. He probably

---

[14] Edward Livingston Trudeau, *An Autobiography* (New York, Doubleday and Co., 1930), p. 30.

made a greater contribution toward the treatment and reduction of the number of deaths from tuberculosis than did any other person.

A REVOLUTIONARY DISCOVERY

The glorious nineteenth century that had seen pain conquered and infections controlled also saw human tissue made visible. A poster in the Medical Section of the Smithsonian Institute, Washington, D.C., states, ''If only the human body had been transparent what a world of unset and wrongly set bones and mistaken diagnoses of other troubles would have been saved in the early days.''

Wilhelm Conrad Roentgen (1845-1923). Wilhelm Roentgen, a German physicist, educated at the University of Utrecht, Germany, became director of the Physical Institute of the University of Wurzburg and professor of experimental physics.

The physics laboratory at Wurzburg was well equipped, and as Roentgen experimented with the Crookes tube with reference to cathode and other rays, he became aware of a luminescence on a barium platinocyanide screen some nine feet away. Subsequent experiments proved this to be a new kind of ray which passed through various dense substances, such as human tissue.

Roentgen called these X rays—X for the unknown; however, they also are called Roentgen rays. For this discovery Roentgen was awarded the Nobel Prize in 1901.

The discovery of X rays had a revolutionary effect on medicine, especially in diagnosis. The reactions of doctors ranged from extreme skepticism to surprising optimism. Laymen were impressed and excited; the press gave the discovery wide publicity—a machine had been invented by which the doctor could see the bones, even through the skin and flesh. Medical men saw a new horizon: they would be able to see structures which hitherto could only be seen in surgery or on the autopsy table. Within one month after the announcement, patients were being examined by this method. ''The roentgen-ray examination as a helpful diagnostic measure is thoroughly established. It has probably done more than any other one thing for the remarkable advancement in diagnosis and treatment which has occurred during the last twenty-five years and its value in certain diseases cannot be too highly emphasized.''[15]

The discovery was announced on December 28, 1895. Seven weeks later, *The Journal of the American Medical Association* took notice in the editorial, ''The Roentgen Rays.'' A quotation from this editorial asks that enthusiasm be guided by moderation:

The general interest in the recent discovery of PROF. ROENTGEN, the details of which now fill the daily press and which were at first received with incredulity by the public as a scientific hoax, seems to call for some notice....

---

[15] Leo G. Rigler, ''Nature and Value of Roentgen Examination,'' *Outline of Roentgen Examination* (Philadelphia, J. B. Lippincott Co., 1938), p. 1.

The fact that we have, however, a force, for that is what it may be called, that will act on sensitive chemicals of the photographic plate through flesh, cartilage, skin, and other tissues of the animal body, is enough to be fertile of practical suggestions to any thinking physician or surgeon . . . but enthusiasm as to its future should be tempered by a scientific spirit of moderation that proves all things before building its faith upon them.[16]

In the early experiments only the bones were visible; then a seamstress broke off a needle in her wrist and by X-ray examination the fragment became visible among the carpal bones. A child swallowed a coin; a metal bead lodged in a bronchial tube; a bullet was located accurately, and the use of the X ray to locate dense foreign bodies became established.

Roentgen himself and some of his early medical colleagues were aware that the nature of any tissue would determine the degree of its opacity, and experiments in contrast media began within a year after the original discovery. Lead solutions were used in cadavers. Then iodide solutions were used on experimental animals. Reduced iron and small rubber bags containing lead were used unsuccessfully in an attempt to visualize the esophagus. The "bismuth metal" was used for some time. Later came barium sulfate which is still in use because it is inert and cheap. The iodide solutions and oils are used to visualize kidneys, gallbladder, gastrointestinal tract, spinal cord lesions, bronchial tree, and paranasal sinuses—in fact, it is now almost possible to duplicate autopsy findings in a living person by this method.

Many of the early workers who experimented with the use of X rays paid dearly for the privilege of playing a role in medical progress, for it became apparent that, if improperly used, X ray could cause cancer and leukemia. But, paradoxically, it became evident that X rays could be used effectively in the treatment of many forms of cancer. In fact, twenty-three days after the newspaper announcement of the discovery of X ray, treatment was started on a patient with breast cancer. Since then great progress has been made in controlling the production, delivery, and quality of X rays to cure thousands of patients with cancer and to give relief to many more. Cancer of the skin, breast, cervix, and testes has proved most sensitive to X-ray therapy; cancer in other organs has been treated with varying degrees of success. X-ray therapy, however, is not reserved for cancer only; it is also effective in various inflammatory and metabolic disorders.

The X ray has become a universal tool in diagnosis and treatment; it is used in every specialty. Eighty per cent of patients in hospitals submit to some form of Roentgen study during the course of their illness.

THE EFFECT ON NURSING

It is only natural that the century which had produced so many great scientists and physicians should also see the rebirth of nursing which had laid dormant for three centuries. Nursing was essential to further medical and

---

[16] Editorial, "The Roentgen Rays," *The Journal of the American Medical Association*, Vol. 26 (Feb. 15, 1896), p. 336.

surgical development; therefore, the older nursing orders were revived; Mother Seton brought the Sisters of Charity to Baltimore in 1809; the Fliedners of Kaiserswerth opened their school of nursing in 1836; Florence Nightingale opened a school of nursing at St. Thomas in London in 1860. And in the latter part of the nineteenth century the nurse became recognized as a *trained* nurse, and nursing was in the process of achieving professional status.

REFERENCES

BEAUMONT, WILLIAM: *Experiments and Observations on the Gastric Juice on the Physiology of Digestion*, facsimile ed. New York, W. W. Norton & Co., 1960.

CASTIGLIONI, ARTURO: *A History of Medicine*. New York, Alfred A. Knopf, Inc., 1941.

CLENDENING, LOGAN: *Source Book of Medical History*. New York, Paul B. Hoeber, Inc., 1942.

DE KRUIF, PAUL: *Microbe Hunters*. New York, Harcourt, Brace & Co., 1926.

DEUTSCH, ALBERT: Dorothea Linde Dix: Apostle to the insane. *Amer. J. Nurs.* 36:987 (Oct.) 1936.

DUBOS, RENE and JEAN: *The White Plague*. Boston, Little, Brown & Co., 1952.

FLEXNER, SIMON F. and JAMES T.: *William Henry Welch and the Heroic Age of Medicine*. New York, The Viking Press, 1941.

GARRISON, FIELDING H.: *An Introduction to the History of Medicine*, 4th ed. Philadelphia, W. B. Saunders Co., 1929.

GHENT, PERCY: *Roentgen: A Brief Biography*. New York, Hunter-Rose Co., 1929.

GLASSER, OTTO: *On Conrad Roentgen*. Springfield, Ill., Charles C Thomas, 1934.

HAGGARD, HOWARD W.: *The Lame, the Halt, and the Blind*. New York, Harper & Bros., 1929.

HOLBROOK, STEWART W.: Angel of the madhouse. (Condensed from *The Lost Men of History*.) Pleasantville, N. Y., *Reader's Digest*, 1955.

PELTIER, LEONARD F.: The impact of Roentgen's discovery upon the treatment of fractures. *Surgery* 33:579 (Apr.) 1953.

ROBINSON, VICTOR: *The Story of Medicine*. New York, Tudor Publishing Co., 1932.

ROBINSON, VICTOR: *White Caps*. Philadelphia, J. B. Lippincott Co., 1946.

TIFFANY, FRANCIS: *Life of Dorothea Dix*. Boston, Houghton Mifflin Co., 1918.

TRUDEAU, EDWARD LIVINGSTON: *An Autobiography*. New York, Doubleday and Co., 1930.

VALEY-RADOT, RENE: *The Life of Pasteur*. (Trans. from the French ed.) New York, Doubleday and Co., 1924.

CHAPTER 8

Early American Hospitals

A hospital has been defined as an institution for the treatment and care of the sick and injured. If we keep this definition in mind, Charity Hospital of New Orleans can be considered to be the first hospital in the United States.

Charity Hospital (1737). The early colonists of New Orleans, founded in 1718, were for the most part adventurous young men seeking their fortunes in the New World. Not many had homes or wives to care for them during the frequent epidemics caused by poor sanitation and insects. Consequently the hospital was recognized early as a necessary institution. In 1736, Jean Louis, a sailor, left a bequest of 10,000 livres (about $2000) "to serve in perpetuity for the founding of a hospital for the sick of the city of New Orleans . . . and to secure the things necessary to succor the sick." This hospital was opened in 1737 and named L'Hospital des pauvres de La Charité (popularly referred to as St. John's Hospital). Forty-two years later it was destroyed by a hurricane. A larger hospital, called St. Charles Hospital, was built; it burned down in 1809. This left the sick without any place to go when hospitalization was required. The local government took action and in 1813 a new hospital, called Charity Hospital, was incorporated as a state institution. Today it is one of the largest hospitals in the country. Both Tulane University and

Louisiana University Medical School utilize the valuable clinical material in the wards of Charity Hospital.

Pennsylvania Hospital (1751). Still defining a hospital as an institution for the care and treatment of the sick and injured, Pennsylvania Hospital in Philadelphia is the oldest hospital in continuous use in the continental United States.

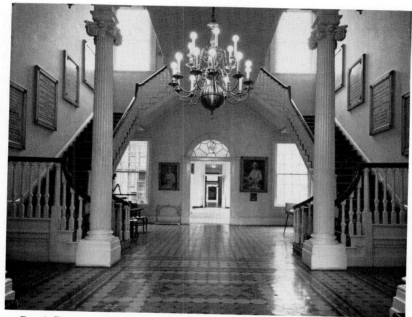

Great Court of Pennsylvania Hospital, Philadelphia. (Courtesy, Public Relations Department, Pennsylvania Hospital.)

Philadelphia was settled by the Quakers, led by William Penn in 1682. The Society of Friends, founded by George Fox, had been aware of human suffering and considered alleviation of misery and poverty to be a religious duty. It is not surprising, therefore, to find that a committee of Philadelphia citizens presented to the Colonial Assembly in 1751 a petition to build a hospital. The governor granted a charter for a hospital and allotted 2000 pounds toward its erection, provided the citizens would raise a like amount. A prominent physician, Dr. Thomas Bond, and Benjamin Franklin were on this committee. Franklin, with his usual ingenuity, soon raised 2000 pounds from the townspeople. He made a copy of the floor plans and visited well-to-do persons in Philadelphia, explaining that by making a generous contribution to the new hospital, the contributor's name would be inscribed on a plaque placed on the door. Franklin's idea is still used today.

Patients were admitted to the hospital in 1756. The board of managers consisted of twelve members (men) and a treasurer. Benjamin Franklin was the first president of the board. These members, called attending members, were divided into pairs and each pair served two months. They did all the purchasing, saw that repairs were made, employed the nurses, and did the many things that are now done by the hospital administrator.

Philadelphia Dispensary (1786). In 1786 the Revolutionary War was over and the colonists had won their independence. But many of the soldiers who returned were without jobs and in poor health. These soldiers, as well as the poor that we always have with us, needed care.

To provide this care, the Philadelphia Dispensary was opened. Like the Pennsylvania Hospital, it owed its origin to the enlightened philosophy of the Quakers. The Dispensary was an independent organization and in no way connected with the hospitals of Philadelphia. The sponsors advanced the idea that many persons need not go to the hospital: they could be cared for in the home—without separating them from their families—and could go to the Dispensary for medicines and medical advice. Funds were solicited by appealing to public sympathy. Each person who gave one guinea (about $5) was called a contributor. Those who paid ten guineas became life members. The board of managers annually appointed six attending men, all of whom gave their services free and were on duty at the Dispensary two months each year.

The Dispensary was an immediate success. One of the first projects was vaccination against smallpox, then one of the most frequent causes of epidemics. The Dispensary, which merged with the Pennsylvania Hospital in 1923, was the forerunner of the outpatient departments and clinics of our modern hospitals. It laid the foundation for health laws to control sanitation and epidemics in both cities and states.

New York Hospital (1771). In 1769 Dr. Samuel Bard, professor of the practice of medicine at King's College, New York, delivered the commencement address to the first graduating class of the college's medical department. The exercises were held in Trinity Church before a distinguished audience. In this address Dr. Bard made a strong plea for a hospital as "the best and only means of properly instructing pupils in the practice of medicine. . . . Nor would the good Effects of the Hospital be wholly confined to the poor; they would extend to every Rank, and greatly contribute to the Safety and Welfare of the whole Community."[1]

The Society of the Hospital in the City of New York was granted a charter by King George III in 1771. When the building was constructed, the first patients, five American soldiers who had been wounded in one of the early battles of the Revolutionary War, were admitted on July 12, 1776.

From the beginning, nurses were of a better quality than those who cared for the almshouse patients. Twenty-two years later a radical change in nurses and nursing was made by Dr. Valentine Seaman, attending surgeon at the hospital. He instituted a series of lectures for nurses and attendants,

---

[1] Helene Jamieson Jordan, *Cornell University-New York Hospital.* (New York, The Society of New York Hospital, 1952), pp. 3-4.

and for the midwives in the city almshouses. This was the first organized teaching for nurses on record.

Because of the enlightened board of directors and well-informed medical staff, the New York Hospital has several "firsts" to its credit. It established the first hospital pension plan, the first pharmacopeia, the first hospital in New York State for mental disorders, and the first hospital to use iron bedsteads, as "they do not retain dirt, are not apt to retain infection, nor do they harbour vermine like wood." A school of nursing was opened by the hospital in 1877.

ALMSHOUSES WITH INFIRMARIES

Blockley (Now Philadelphia General Hospital).   Quakers, with their characteristic concern for social welfare, had established an almshouse in Philadelphia in 1713 for Quakers only. The Philadelphia City Council saw the need for such an institution for all the people and in 1731 established a city almshouse, with a ward to be used as an infirmary. As the city grew the need for more space for the indigent became necessary. In 1834 new buildings were constructed in Blockley township and the institution was called Blockley.

All of the work of the institution including nursing was supposed to be done by the inmates. In the annual reports to the city council over a period of sixty years no mention was made of nurses. In 1793 an epidemic of yellow fever raged in Philadelphia. It was impossible to procure suitable nurses, hence only the most depraved creatures could be employed.

Through the years Blockley became less an almshouse and more a hospital. It contained wards for the mentally ill, smallpox wards, a refuge for abandoned children, and an almshouse for the blind, lame, and incurables. The wards were overcrowded and had no laundry, no toilets, and only small hand lamps for use at night. It is unbelievable that such conditions could have existed for 150 years.

In 1884 Alice Fisher, one of Miss Nightingale's nurses, opened a school of nursing at Blockley and achieved reforms that astonished the city. An incident related by Miss Fisher in the early days of the school furnishes food for thought for modern students: "When young women of refinement came as students to care for a pauper class of patients, some were uneasy and hesitant. Then the patients were wont to say, 'Remember if it warn't for we 'uns, you 'uns wouldn't be here.' "

Bellevue (1794).   The Dutch West Indies Company had set up headquarters in New Amsterdam, New York. When sick sailors and slaves came into port the sailors were billeted by the citizens but the slaves were left to shift for themselves. When the town had grown to a thriving population of 1000 by 1658 the citizens petitioned the town council to provide a shelter to care for the sailors and slaves and to free the townspeople from this responsibility. Mrs. Hillege Wilbruch, the first midwife of the colony, cared for them for a salary of fifty dollars a year.

After the British took over in 1674 and renamed the city New York the old shelter was abandoned and the indigent sick were farmed out at city expense.

In 1735 an epidemic of smallpox struck the city, and the overseers of the poor petitioned the city council to build an almshouse. A new building was constructed to serve as a public workhouse and house of correction. The building had an infirmary of six beds, and was the immediate ancestor of the present Bellevue Hospital.

The first Bellevue Hospital was purchased by the city in 1794 to be used as a communicable disease hospital for a threatened epidemic of yellow fever. For many years it was used only as a communicable disease hospital—at that time it was called a pest house. In 1816 the second Bellevue Hospital was built with quarters for the indigent, a penitentiary, and an infirmary, all in the same building, with apartments for the resident physician and the warden.

Epidemics resulting from unsanitary conditions and overcrowding were frequent, and typhus fever, carried by rats, was common. The so-called nurses—"ten-day women" who were detailed from the jail—cared for the patients.

Twenty years later, after a condemning investigation of conditions, the prisoners were moved to Blackwell Island. The almshouse and hospital continued together until 1848 when Bellevue began its career as a hospital with the creation of a hospital board.

WESTWARD MOVEMENT OF HOSPITALS

The early settlement of the United States was along the Atlantic coast. The Indians resisted, and rightly so, attempts by the white men to take lands farther west. But after wars and treaties the frontier moved west beyond the Allegheny Mountains and into the Ohio Valley, through the Cumberland Gap into Kentucky and Tennessee. The acquisition of the Louisiana Territory in 1803 opened homestead opportunities for people from the Atlantic coast and for immigrants from overcrowded Europe.

The migration required transportation and the Ohio and Mississippi Rivers and their tributaries offered the only means of getting to the widely opened lands. On these long journeys many people became ill; cholera was especially prevalent, malaria was endemic, and smallpox and diphtheria were uncontrolled. But disease was not the only foe—the way was dangerous and accidents were common.

Cincinnati General Hospital (1823). River trade and migration from Pittsburgh down the Ohio River made Cincinnati a natural geographical location for a permanent city. Its early activity was the river trade and the boatmen and settlers going farther west. In 1815 the township trustee rented a house on Vine Street above Sixth Street for "the care of sick and injured persons."

Dr. Daniel Drake, who was granted the first medical diploma west of the Allegheny Mountains, was the most influential citizen in the Ohio Valley. He founded the Medical College of Ohio in 1817, which later became the Medical College of the University of Cincinnati. Dr. Drake at once began the promotion of a hospital to provide clinical experience for the medical students.

By 1821 there were three incentives for building a hospital: to provide for the sick poor of the city, to care for the boatmen on the Ohio River, and to provide clinical experience for medical students. As a result of this appeal the Commercial Hospital and Lunatic Asylum of Ohio was opened in 1823.

The first structure of the Commercial Hospital and Lunatic Asylum was three stories high, eighteen wards or compartments, and a tenantable basement. On the top floor was a lecture room with a seating capacity for one hundred students. The basement, eight feet in height, was used for the accommodation of the aged, infirm, indigent, and orphan inmates.

For ten years the building served as general hospital, mental hospital, almshouse, and orphanage. In 1833 the Cincinnati Orphans Asylum was opened and the children were moved from the basement of the Commercial Hospital. Twenty years later a mental hospital was established and the mental patients were moved from the basement.

A completely new hospital was opened in 1869 and was named Cincinnati Hospital, but the next thirty years saw that an additional hospital was needed as keenly as the original hospital had been. A new site was selected and plans were made for a hospital that would be large enough to meet the increasing demands. The contagious disease unit was opened first, then the main hospital was opened in 1915. At that time the name was changed from Cincinnati Hospital to Cincinnati General Hospital.

The College of Nursing and Health of the University of Cincinnati and Cincinnati General Hospital was established in 1893, although Cincinnati Hospital had had affiliate students from the Hospital for Sick Children as early as 1883.

Louisville General Hospital (1823). When Louisville, Kentucky, was founded in 1780 it had a population of thirty. Twenty-three years later the Louisiana Territory was added to the United States and the Mississippi River and its tributaries were opened for trade. Steamboat navigation was introduced in 1811. Louisville, on the falls of the Ohio River, played an important role in the commerce and navigation of the river. When the river was low all boats and barges were unloaded at the head of the falls and the materials transported on land to the foot of the falls, where they were again put on boats and barges.

The mariners on the Ohio River, because of the long voyages, exposure in open boats, and prevalence of malaria, often fell sick and were taken care of by the citizens of Louisville. In 1817, with a population of 4000, the pioneer community saw the urgent need of a hospital. Seven acres of land on what is now Preston and Chestnut Streets were donated as a site for the hospital. The hospital, however, was not opened for patients until 1823.

The Federal government made a yearly grant-in-aid to the hospital of $500, which was mainly supported by a 2 per cent tax levied on all auction sales, except on articles grown or manufactured in the state. This unique way of raising funds brought an annual revenue of about $3000.

In 1822 Louisville was hit by a severe epidemic of yellow fever, and the town was called "the graveyard of the west." A board of health was set up to cope with this situation. Successive outbreaks of smallpox, yellow fever, and cholera continued to plague the city. A permanent board of health was established with power to appoint a health officer and establish regulations for the health of the city. This board considered the protection of the public health as one of the first duties of the government. Sickness had long been associated with swampy, marshy land. After the swamps were drained, sanitation improved.

Louisville General Hospital was a city-county institution under city-county public health administration. From 1823 until 1836 it was organized to meet a specific need—to care for mariners—and was called the Louisville Hospital Company. By 1836 the city council was aware that municipal institutions must be set up and maintained. The Louisville Marine Hospital was given over to the mayor and city council; there persons other than mariners, and including the sick poor of the city, could be admitted. The mariners were removed to the United States Marine Hospital when it was opened in 1873. The Louisville Marine Hospital, however, has continued to function as the city hospital, primarily for the indigent sick of the community.

The hospital's report of 1880 gave the mortality rate as 16 per cent (as compared with present mortality rate in general hospitals of 2 or 3 per cent). The reasons given for this high death rate were common to hospitals in general and make us aware of the improvements made in medicine, nursing, and public welfare: many accident victims, often resulting in speedy death, were brought to the hospital; many patients in the ward died from old age; patients brought there after several weeks of illness died in the hospital, not so much from the original disease as from previous bad nursing and neglect; the hospital was, and of necessity had been for many years, the home of the homeless consumptive for whom there was no cure.

An important event in the long history of the United States Marine Hospital was the Ohio River flood in 1937. During the flood the hospital was surrounded by water, but it continued to function. Bulkheads were placed in the doors to keep water from seeping into the engine room where the hospital generated its own electricity. This hospital was the only building in the city that had electricity and elevator service during the entire flood. Within three days 1756 patients were admitted and furnished with beds. Again, as in all national disasters, the Red Cross responded to the emergency call and by boats delivered supplies to the hospital.

In 1942 the city hospital came under new management and the name was changed to Louisville General Hospital. This hospital is affiliated with the University of Louisville School of Medicine. By an act of the state legislature the Jefferson County Health Department, the City of Louisville Health Department, and the Waverly Hills Sanatorium were removed from politics and placed under a nonpartisan board. The school of nursing was founded in 1886.

De Paul Hospital (1828). This was the first hospital to be established west of the Mississippi and the oldest extant Catholic hospital in the United States; it was opened in 1828 in St. Louis, Missouri.

Immigrants from the eastern states and especially from Europe were streaming into the midwest. California also attracted new settlers who followed the Santa Fe Trail westward from Independence, Missouri. St. Louis was a natural stopover as a place to replenish provisions before pushing on by boat on the Mississippi or the Missouri rivers or by wagon train along the Santa Fe Trail.

The Most Rev. Joseph Rosati, Bishop of St. Louis, was concerned about the great number of ill travelers arriving in St. Louis. With financial aid from Bishop Rosati and a donation of land by John Mullanphy, a three-room log cabin was built at Third and Spruce Streets.

These men appealed to Mother Seton of the Sisters of Charity to assign four nurses to staff the tiny hospital. Nurses arrived in October, 1828, after having traveled 1500 miles by stage coach and steamboat to reach St. Louis, then a thriving town with a population of 6000.

The new hospital was simply called The Sisters Hospital. Hospitals, as such, were unknown to St. Louis and the travelers, but as they learned to trust the Sisters and appreciate their care, more and more availed themselves of the hospital's services. Soon the hospital became too small, and in 1832 a new three-story brick hospital was erected on Spruce Street and called St. Louis Hospital. This was the year of the epidemic of Asiatic cholera and the hospital was immediately crowded with the sick and dying. Hundreds of patients were brought to the hospital by frightened relatives. But the Sisters went about their duties calmly and efficiently. The City of St. Louis then realized its debt to the Sisters and gave the hospital the position of the City Hospital of St. Louis; in the hospital the Sisters cared for all government and city patients.

In 1849 cholera struck again—with a blow more deadly than before. Entire families fell victims of the plague and four nurses from the Sisters of Charity died. In the midst of the epidemic a steamboat fire swept and destroyed half of the city, but the hospital, directly in the path of the fire, was miraculously saved.

In 1874 a still larger hospital was built on Montgomery Street, and was named St. Louis Mullanphy Hospital. It served for fifty years and it was there that the school of nursing was founded in 1894, begining with a class of six students.

Although it had survived the steamboat fire, De Paul Hospital did not survive a later tornado. In the mid-afternoon of Sept. 29, 1927, the quiet that follows the activity of the noon meal was disturbed by a dazzling flash of lightning and a deafening clap of thunder announced a devastating tornado which ripped through the building, destroying it beyond repair. Some looked at the damage as a blessing from the skies. It was time for a new and more modern hospital farther west in the city. A new hospital of 400 beds was opened in 1930 and given the name of De Paul Hospital.

Lutheran Hospital (1858). The first Protestant hospital west of Pittsburgh, Lutheran Hospital, was founded by German immigrants in St. Louis, Missouri, in 1858. The great Saxon immigration had begun nineteen years earlier. Saxony, a province of eastern Germany with Dresden as the capital, was predominantly Lutheran and the state-supported church was Lutheran, but it had become strongly influenced by the philosophy of rationalism that followed the French Revolution. During the Napoleonic Wars, rationalism became so involved with Lutheran doctrine that parents were concerned for the religious beliefs of their children.

In 1837 plans were made by many Saxons to emigrate to the central United States where they could be assured of freedom of conscience and religious liberty. These immigrants were professional men, craftsmen, farmers, and businessmen. The sacrifices they made and the hardships they endured make the hardships of the Pilgrims of Plymouth seem mild by comparison.

The initial group of 650 persons landed in New Orleans in January, 1839, and were taken by river boats to St. Louis where poor housing, malaria, small-pox, cholera, dysentery, and hard pioneer labor took a heavy toll of lives. These immigrants had come from Europe where both medicine and nursing were crude. They cared for the sick in their homes as they had in Saxony; they did not feel the need of hospitals.

Emigration from Germany to the United States was heavy from 1840 until 1876, when the Federal government assumed control of immigration. The Industrial Revolution, comparable to our present automation revolution, found home industries in Germany no longer in demand. This, coupled with a decade of agrarian crises, made people restless and willing to seek homes in less well-developed countries of which the United States seemed to offer the greatest hope.

Many of those who came were young men who had no homes or families to care for them when they became ill. Finally, in 1858, the Lutheran Hospital of St. Louis was opened. It consisted of three rooms: one for the attendant, one for men and one for women. Two years later two additional rooms were added.

MENTAL HOSPITALS

The early American hospitals for the mentally ill were not built as hospitals for the care and treatment of mentally ill persons, but for the protection of the public against violently disturbed persons. These buildings were called asylums and resembled prisons—in fact, the patients were even regarded as criminals. The first hospital of this type was the State Hospital, Williamsburg, Virginia, built in 1773.

The effectiveness of humane treatment of the mentally ill was demonstrated by Philippe Pinel in Paris on that memorable May 24, 1798, when he removed the chains of fifty-nine patients, one of whom on that very day saved the life of Dr. Pinel. Pinel's new approach was studied by English physicians emigrating to the American colonies. The McLean Hospital, founded in 1811 in Waverly, Massachusetts, was the first of these progressive mental hospitals. This was followed by the Friends Asylum in Philadelphia, opened in 1871. Here, too, the mentally ill received humane treatment.

The Eastern State Hospital, formerly known as the State Lunatic Asylum in Lexington, Kentucky, was the first mental hospital west of the Allegheny Mountains; the cornerstone was laid in 1817. This hospital was designed not only for custodial care, but also for treatment and occupational therapy.

Many other states sent patients to Lexington, and by 1850 this mental hospital was used for clinical experience for the medical students of Transylvania University (now Transylvania College).

Nurses and hospitals are inevitably linked together. The increase in population and the new emphasis on the concept of preventive medicine have necessitated a spectacular increase in the number of hospitals in the United States.

According to the American Medical Association, the number of hospitals in the United States increased from 178 in 1873 to 4000 in 1909; by 1950 these figures had jumped to 6430. But in all of these hospitals it is the nurse who co-ordinates the activities related to patient care. The doctor makes his requests for specific things to be done for the patient, the nurse sees that his instructions are carried out accurately and efficiently. She is the interpreter and the co-ordinator for both hospital and physician.

In the beginning, with nothing more than domestic training, the nurse gave care to patients in almshouses, twenty-two years later she received her first formal instruction in nursing. In 1884 she studied and worked in a hospital school of nursing and became a trained nurse. Since that date her formal instruction in hospital schools of nursing has become more inclusive. Finally, she became a registered nurse entitled to work in both general and specialized hospitals. In the twentieth century the hospital may or may not be her center of learning; it may be a university, a college of nursing, or a junior college. Regardless of where she studies, the hospital is her laboratory. Whatever the level at which she performs, the nurse, today, is in the process of achieving professional status—a boon to herself, to her profession, and to her hospital.

REFERENCES

COOPER, PAGE: *The Bellevue Story*. New York, Thomas Y. Crowell Co., 1948.

DOYLE, ANN: Nursing by religious orders in the United States. *Amer. J. Nurs.* 29:775 (July) 1929.

FORESTER, WALTER O.: *Zion on the Mississippi*. St. Louis, Mo., Concordia Publishing House, 1953.

HENRIETTA, SISTER: A famous New Orleans hospital. *Amer. J. Nurs.* 39:249 (Mar.) 1939.

JORDAN, HELENE JAMIESON: *Cornell University-New York Hospital*. New York, The Society of New York Hospital, 1952.

MORTON, THOMAS J.: *History of Pennsylvania Hospital, 1751-1895*. Philadelphia, Philadelphia Times Printing House, 1895.

NUTTING, M. ADELAIDE, and DOCK, LAVINIA L.: *A History of Nursing*, Vol. II. New York, G. P. Putnam's Sons, 1935.

PACKARD, FRANCIS R.: *History of Medicine in the United States*, Vol. I. New York, Paul B. Hoeber, Inc., 1932, Chap. 4.

POLACK, W. G.: *Fathers and Founders*. St. Louis, Mo., Concordia Publishing House, 1938.

SILVERTHORNE, NELLES: My Most Unforgettable Character. (Toronto Hospital for Sick Children.) *Reader's Digest*, April, 1962, p. 126.

CHAPTER 9

Life and Thought in Early Schools of Nursing

If we stop today and look back to see the progress that has been made in nursing since America's first trained nurse received her diploma, we will be proud to be members of the profession and we will be encouraged to continue our work.

In 1873 there were no graduate nurses in the United States until Linda Richards graduated from the New England Hospital for Women and Children. By 1880 there were 15 schools and 157 graduates; in 1890 there were 35 schools and 471 graduates, and by 1900 there were 432 schools and 3456 graduate nurses.[1]

What were the conditions in these early nursing schools? How do they compare with the nursing schools of today? What are the threads to follow? What was life like for Linda Richards and her peers?

FIRST SCHOOLS OF NURSING

It is difficult for the student of today, born and raised in a society granting wide rights to women, to appreciate fully the courageous leadership of the

---

[1]Ella M. Rafuse, ''Nursing Education—What is the Challenge? 1888-1938,'' *The Trained Nurse and Hospital Review*, Vol. 50 (Apr., 1938), p. 426.

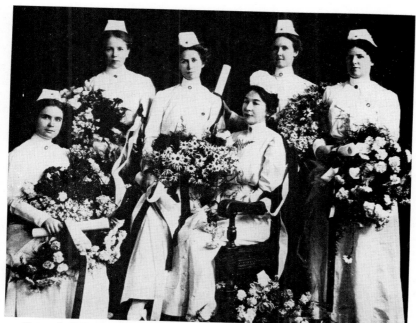

Class of 1910, St. Luke's Hospital, Jacksonville, Florida. First school of nursing in Florida, 1885. Also the first hospital in Florida, 1873.

"founding mothers" who established the first schools of nursing.

The first nursing schools were established along the eastern seacoast. Afterwards such schools were opened in the midwest and San Francisco.

Woman's Hospital of Philadelphia (1861). Since women physicians were not permitted to practice in the established hospitals, Dr. Ann Preston interested ten Quaker women in forming a board of managers to provide a hospital with a three-fold purpose: to provide a hospital and dispensary for women and children, to advance the careers of women physicians, and to establish a school of nursing.

Because of war conditions the school did not flourish. In 1872 it was reorganized on principles which most schools did not recognize for half a century. It was to be maintained for the benefit of the student and was endowed to make this possible—the first endowed school in the United States. A nursing school committee was appointed by the board of managers, and the first diet kitchen for instruction of nurses was equipped.

New England Hospital for Women and Children (1872). This hospital, with ten beds, was founded in 1863 by Dr. Marie Zakrzewski; her primary purpose for establishing the hospital was to provide facilities for women physicians in Boston. Dr. Marie Zakrzewski (affectionately known as Dr. Zak) had studied medicine in Berlin and had spent some time at Kaiswerswerth, Germany, with the Fliedners. She was greatly impressed with the Fliedners' school of nursing. Although the school of nursing was not opened at the New England Hospital for Women and Children until 1872, plans for the school were included in the original hospital charter of 1862.

At first a six-month nursing course was given at New England Hospital for Women and Children; later the length of the course was extended to one year. Within ten years Dr. Zakrzewski had trained thirty-two nurses. The training, for the most part, consisted of clinical work. It was from this school that Linda Richards (Melinda Ann Judson Richards), America's first trained nurse, was graduated.

If we could turn the clock back to 1872 and visit with student Linda Richards at the New England Hospital for Women and Children, we would find her pursuing a strenuous program. As stated in the managers report of 1871, these were the admission requirements she had to meet:

Young women of suitable acquirements and character will be admitted to the hospital as school nurses for one year. This year will be divided into four periods: three months will be given respectively to the practical study of nursing in the medical, surgical, and maternity wards, and night nursing. Here the pupil will aid the head nurse in all the care and work of the ward under the direction of the attending and resident physicians and medical students. In order to enable women entirely dependent upon their work for support to obtain a thorough training, the nurses will be paid for their work from one to four dollars per week after the first fortnight, according to the actual value of their services to the hospital. A course of lectures will be given to nurses at the hospital by physicians connected with the institution, beginning January 21st. Other nurses desirous of attending these lectures may obtain permits from our physicians. Certificates will be given to such nurses as have satisfactorily passed a year in practical training in the hospital.[2]

And if we asked Miss Richards how she liked her training program and how it actually was carried out, her answer would be:

Of the five nurses in our class I first entered the school on the day it was opened, the other four coming within six weeks. Even though the course was far too short, and the advantages few, we five nurses of the first class were very happy, very united, and pretty well instructed. We had no superintendent of nurses —in our ignorance we did not know that such an officer was necessary. As I look back, I wonder that we were as well taught as was really the case, and I sometimes feel that we nurses, eager as we were to learn, instructed the physicians nearly as much as they instructed us.[3]

If we really want to know how well off we are today and how much we have progressed, let's go on a tour of duty with Linda Richards. As she says, we will start early and return late:

Our days were not eight hours; they were nearer twice eight. We arose at 5:30 A.M. and left the wards at 9:00 P.M. to go to our beds, which were in

² M. Adelaide Nutting and Lavinia L. Dock, *A History of Nursing*, Vol. II (New York, G. P. Putnam's Sons, 1935), p. 350.

³ *Ibid.*, pp. 351-52.

little rooms between the wards. Each nurse took care of her ward of six patients both day and night. Many a time I got up nine times in the night; often I did not get to sleep before the next call came. . . . Every second week we were off duty one afternoon from two to five o'clock. We had no evenings out, no hours for study or recreation, and no regular leave on Sunday. Only twice during the year was I given the opportunity to go to church. We were supposed to understand and act. Great care was taken that we should not know the names of the medicines given. All bottles were numbered, but not labeled. We had no text-books, nor did we have entrance or final examinations.[4]

The Three Schools of 1873.   The year that Miss Richards graduated from the New England Hospital for Women and Children School of Nursing, three other schools were founded: Bellevue Hospital School of Nursing, New York City; the Connecticut Training School, New Haven, Connecticut; and the Boston Training School of Massachusetts General Hospital.

This was the era when the population in general considered women incapable of political investigations and organization of institutions. But it had not reckoned with Louisa Lee Schuyler, great grand-daughter of Alexander Hamilton. Miss Schuyler provided the kind of leadership required to mold together the many loose ends which helped to create the U. S. Sanitary Commission during the Civil War and, seven years later, she organized the Charities Aid Association of New York. This association was formed in May, 1872, and the Committee to visit the sick began its activities at once. This Committee of fifty-three members visited the poorhouses and hospitals to learn the conditions under which New York cared for its poor and destitute sick.

It was a notable day in the history of Bellevue Hospital when Mrs. Joseph Hobson, chairman of the committee, visited the hospital and made the acquaintance of the young southern surgeon, Dr. Gill Wylie. Mrs. Hobson introduced herself and explained the reason for her presence. Dr. Wylie said, "Don't appear to be with me; just follow around after me."

Bellevue Hospital School of Nursing began under the direction of Sister Helen, a member of the Protestant All Saints Sisterhood, who had been trained at University College Library, London. A year later Linda Richards became night supervisor. Miss Richards made notes concerning seriously ill patients in order to make a report to Sister Helen in the morning. The doctors, learning of these notes, requested to see them. From these brief notes began our system of medical records.

The Connecticut Training School originated with a committee of men— three doctors and a layman. Dr. Wylie's work in organizing a school at Bellevue Hospital had attracted the attention of the doctors in New Haven. This committee recommended a separate school, with the hospital as a laboratory or practice field.

The school, however, had difficulty in obtaining students. It advertised for probationers in the country newspapers and the missionary society papers; posters were displayed in railroad stations and post offices. But it was hard

---

[4] Linda Richards, *Reminiscences of Linda Richards: America's First Trained Nurse*, 2nd ed. (Boston, Whitcomb & Barrows, 1915), pp. 10-12.

to convince young women that it required a full year to learn to care for the sick.

The school opened with only three students. Later enrollment increased to eight. The school was popular with the doctors and the public, and in 1878 the school and the doctors collaborated in publishing a *Handbook of Nursing.* The Connecticut Training School was incorporated into the Yale School of Nursing in 1924.

The third school to be founded in 1873 was the *Boston Training School* (now the *Massachusetts General Training School*). The Women's Education Association of Boston was concerned with finding some respectable type of work that would give young women a chance to be self-supporting. They learned of the school that had been established at the New England Hospital for Women and Children by women physicians, and the association became anxious to explore the possibility of establishing something similar for Massachusetts General Hospital, which had opened in 1807.

A group of socially prominent women were appointed to present the matter to the hospital trustees. These trustees and the medical staff did not approve of a school of nursing, but the social standing of the committee members made it difficult to refuse permission to try the experiment.

But the committee could find no qualified nurse for the position of superintendent. The medical staff, which had been opposed to the school from the beginning, told the school committee that if a graduate nurse could not be obtained to be put in charge within one year the school must be abandoned.

It was at this critical period that Linda Richards became director of nurses. She organized the work, employed maids for kitchen and laundry service, and organized classes which she taught herself. She was aware that the whole idea of nursing schools depended upon the success or failure of this school in a hospital that was considered one of the best for its time. She gave her personal attention to all seriously ill patients, especially at night. By the end of three months the hospital administrator told her: ''The school is safe. Before another year comes round you will have the nursing of the entire hospital in charge.'' When Miss Richards left two and a half years later the school was on a firm basis. Since 1898 it has been known as the Massachusetts General Training School.

On the occasion of the second annual meeting, in 1895, of the National League of Nursing Education, Miss Richards delivered the address of welcome. In this address Miss Richards described the work plan at the Boston Training School and the bitter tears that were shed when she reorganized it:

The plan of the work in the wards was so unique that I will give a little sketch of the duties of one nurse for five days. This will describe the duties of each, as it was a rotary system. Nurse A, on Monday, had charge of the ward, attending to the duties of a head male nurse; on Tuesday she had entire charge of the ward, with the usual rounds, also of pantry, washing all dishes, etc.; Wednesday she attended to the general cleanliness of the ward and linen closet; Thursday she stood at the sink in the bathroom till noon and washed poultice cloths and bandages; in the afternoon she slept, and went on night duty Thursday night. Her hours, when on night duty, were

*supposed to be from 8 P.M. to 7 A.M., but she reported on duty when she felt
like doing so, at any time before 10 P.M.; on Friday she rested, to be ready to
start the round again on Saturday.*[5]

The Battle Creek Training School for Nurses. The Battle Creek Training
School for Nurses of the Battle Creek Health Center, Battle Creek, Mich.,
was opened in 1883. Records of the school give the present day nurse an idea
of how the student lived in the early days of modern nursing. The following
quotation is from the notebook of Mary Staines Foy, director of nurses from
1899 to 1933. The conditions described are representative of those existent
in many early schools:

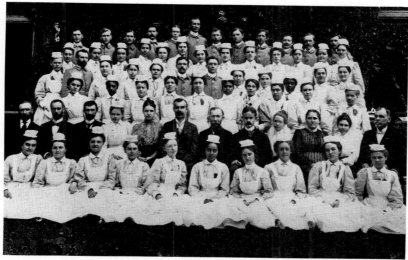

School of Nursing of Battle Creek Hospital, Battle Creek, Michigan. In
this integrated school, men as well as women were accepted. (Courtesy of
Battle Creek Hospital.)

*The first nurses did their studying by a kerosene lamp and each room was
heated by a small wood stove. All winter they had to bring in their own wood
and build their own fire. . . . They ironed their own uniforms at the laundry,
certain evenings a week being set aside for this. Classes were held in the
evenings from seven to nine o'clock. Studying for the next day's recitation
came after that.*

School of Nursing of the Lutheran Hospital of St. Louis. The Lutheran
Hospital of St. Louis opened its school of nursing in 1898, with a hospital of
thirty beds. Eight students were admitted for a two-year course. Four rooms
were furnished as a dormitory. The school grew rapidly and another building
was purchased but even then,

[5] Linda Richards, "Progress in Twenty Years," *The Trained Nurse and Hospital
Review,* Vol. 50 (Apr., 1938), p. 360.

Five in a room we often were, one locker for us all; and sometimes when a probie came she slept out in the hall.

Johns Hopkins School of Nursing (1893). Medical advances came rapidly during the second half of the nineteenth century. Both Europe and the United States found it necessary to increase their educational facilities in medicine and to find ways by which incompetent students could be eliminated. Beginning in 1870, state boards of medical examiners were established, but this was not enough; medical schools needed a model by which to set their standards. A large endowment from the estate of Johns Hopkins, an American financier, made it possible to establish the Johns Hopkins Medical School in Baltimore in 1893.

The leaders in medical education were aware that a model medical school should have a superior nursing school in the same hospital in which the medical students would receive their clinical experience. As a result, in 1889 the board of trustees invited Isabel Hampton to come to the school as director.

Miss Hampton, at the age of twenty-nine, had distinguished herself as director of nurses at the Illinois Training School in Chicago, where she became known as a young woman of high educational ideals. She eagerly accepted the new position as a challenge to demonstrate her belief that nursing education could be a balanced development between education and manual skills. This had been Miss Nightingale's ideal for nursing, but already the pressure for nursing service—the patient comes first—was undermining the student's opportunity for a nursing education.

The Johns Hopkins School of Nursing, with Mrs. Isabel Hampton Robb as principal, attracted women of higher education as head nurses and as students. To be a Hopkins graduate carried considerable prestige.

Women's and Children's Hospital of Chicago School of Nursing (1874). This school, later known as the Mary Thompson Hospital, was the first school of nursing in the midwest. It opened in 1874 and closed in 1949.

Dr. Mary Thompson had graduated from the New England Female Medical College in Boston in 1863. She went to Chicago and found the city crowded with widows and children of veterans of the Civil War. In spite of the disapproval and disbelief of the men doctors, she established within two years the first hospital in the midwest, staffed by women physicians and designed to care for women and children, to provide a free dispensary, and to educate nurses.

The Illinois Training School for Nurses founded in Chicago, 1880, was the first school in the midwest to be organized under the Nightingale plan. ''The purpose was two-fold: first, to train young women to care scientifically for the sick, establishing a new and dignified profession for women and at the same time making available to the public a valuable service; second, to give the patients in Cook County Hospital care far better than that rendered by the untrained and politically chosen attendants then employed.''[6]

The board of directors wanted the school to be independent of the county hospital and politics, and they consulted Miss Nightingale as to how this could best be done. At her suggestion the school was to be autonomous and the hospital wards were to be laboratories for clinical experience. The Illinois Training School signed a contract with the county commissioners for this experience. This plan continued until the school closed in 1929.

Cook County Hospital School of Nursing (1929). A new committee was formed and a board of directors was chosen. This board recommended to the board of county commissioners of Cook County that a new school be formed to carry on the work of the Illinois Training School with equally high standards of service to the sick and with the same careful planning for nurse education.

In this manner the Cook County Hospital School of Nursing came into existence in June, 1929, with the same contractual agreement as the original school. Both the Illinois Training School and the Cook County School have had strong and independent boards of directors who have never permitted politics to enter into the administration of the school.

St. Luke's Hospital School of Nursing, Chicago (1885). A small group of women of Grace Episcopal Church, Chicago, had worked as volunteers for the military hospital at Camp Douglas during the Civil War. In 1864 Rector Clinton J. Locke of Grace Church made a plea to his parish for a ''clean, free Christian place where the sick poor might be cared for.''

This parish group, with the rector and Dr. Walter Huey, met in February, 1864, and drew up a charter; its objectives were to provide for the sick and needy poor of Chicago.

The first hospital was a small home of seven beds on State Street near Eldridge Court. The following year the hospital was moved into a building large enough for fifteen beds. Twenty years later, 1885, a new hospital was built on Michigan Avenue. This building was the result of careful planning and it was considered to be the best designed hospital of the midwest.

The school of nursing was opened the same year in April (1885) with the objective: ''the training and education of young women as nurses.'' The first class graduated in 1887.

Catherine L. Lett, a graduate of Bellevue Hospital School of Nursing, became director of the school in 1888. This was the same Miss Lett who was hostess to the superintendents of training schools for the formation of our present National League for Nursing.

Other Chicago Schools. Three well-known schools of nursing on the south side of Chicago were founded within an eighteen-month period: Mercy Hospital School of Nursing (now St. Xavier College of Nursing) was opened in August, 1889; Michael Reese Hospital School of Nursing, September,

---

[6] Grace Faye Schryver, *A History of the Illinois Training School*, (published by the Board of Directors, 1930) p. 1.

1890; and Provident Hospital School of Nursing, January, 1891. These schools have continued to the present day. The Provident School was the first school in the world to be founded solely for the education of Negro nurses.

Children's Hospital Training School for Nurses (1880). In 1875, three women physicians, Dr. Charlotte Brown, Dr. Martha Bucknell, and Dr. Sara E. Brown, were instrumental in establishing the Pacific Dispensary for Women and Children in San Francisco. In 1880 the Training School for Nurses, the first west of the Rockies, was established. The course was one year and the one pupil, Miss Jessie Astrede, was always on duty. In 1881, a uniform of gray with white cap and apron was adopted and the course was extended to two years.

In 1884, there were eight pupils. The following year the name of the hospital was changed to Children's Hospital for the Care of Women and Children and a Training School for Nurses. In 1888, the first mention of a superintendent of nurses is found in the minutes and an appeal was made to build a nurses' residence. The Children's Hospital School of Nursing, from which 1198 nurses had graduated, closed in 1957.

In bringing to a close the disheartening as well as the heartening aspects of nineteenth century nursing, the voice of Linda Richards in 1898 revealed the progress made by these early schools:

How vastly different are the hospitals of today from those same hospitals a score of years ago. . . Today a visit to these same hospitals is an inspiration. Visit Bellevue, Blackwell's Island, Tewksbury, and many others. They all tell the same story. The perfect cleanliness and order of the wards; the home-like appearance; the contented faces of the patients, make even hospital workers wonder how much can be done; surely, a truly wonderful work is this which we are permitted to have a part in.[7]

REFERENCES

BUCKLER, HELEN: *Doctor Dan.* Boston, Little, Brown, & Co., 1954.

COOPER, PAGE: *The Bellevue Story.* New York, Thomas W. Crowell Co., 1948.

DIETZ, LENA DIXON: *Professional Adjustments I.* Philadelphia, F. A. Davis Co., 1957.

DOLAN, JOSEPHINE A.: *Goodnow's History of Nursing*, 10th ed. Philadelphia, W. B. Saunders Co., 1958.

DREVES, KATHERINE DENSFORD: University of Minnesota School of Nursing. *Nurs. Outlook* 9:14 (Jan.) 1961.

GILES, DOROTHY: *A Candle in Her Hand.* New York, G. P. Putnam's Sons, 1949.

HOLBROOK, STEWART H.: *Dreamers of the American Dream.* Garden City, N. Y., Doubleday and Co., 1957.

---

[7] Linda Richards, ''Progress in Twenty Years,'' *The Trained Nurse and Hospital Review*, Vol. 7 (Mar., 1895), pp. 162-64.

JORDAN, HELENE JAMIESON: *Cornell University-New York Hospital School of Nursing, 1877-1952*. New York, The Society of the New York Hospital, 1952.

"LADY WITH A COMPOUND." *Amer. J. Nurs.*, 59:854 (June) 1959.

NUTTING, M. ADELAIDE, and DOCK, LAVINIA L.: *A History of Nursing*, Vol. II. New York, G. P. Putnam's Sons, 1935.

RICHARDS, LINDA: *Reminiscences of America's First Trained Nurse*. Boston, M. Barrows and Co., 1935.

ROBERTS, MARY M.: *American Nursing: History and Interpretation*. New York, The Macmillan Co., 1594.

SCHRYVER, GRACE FAY: *A History of the Illinois Training School for Nurses, 1880-1929*. Chicago, Board of Directors, 1930.

SLEEPER, RUTH: Nursing's contribution to a famous hospital. (Massachusetts General Hospital) *Nurs. Outlook* 9:276 (May) 1960.

STACK, MARGARET K.: Résumé of the history of the Connecticut Training School for Nurses. *Amer. J. Nurs.* 23:825 (Aug.) 1923.

"TWO EARLY SCHOOLS OF NURSING (MASSACHUSETTS GENERAL AND BELLEVUE)." *Amer. J. Nurs.* 48:612 (Oct.) 1948.

YOUNG, AGATHA: *Women and the Crisis*. New York, McDowell and Oblensky, Inc., 1960.

CHAPTER 10

Development of American Nursing

Although nursing is as old as the human race, productive efforts to achieve professional status dates back little more than a century. The organized system of nursing in the United States dates from 1871.

There are several probable reasons for this lag in the development of nursing in America. A prime reason is that nursing then and now is an adjunct to the medical profession, which did little to promote the development of nursing. By comparison, nursing did not progress as did the allied health professions. The discrepancy is brought out in the fact that some areas of nursing advanced more rapidly than others. For example, much greater progress was made in psychiatric nursing, tuberculosis nursing, and public health nursing than nursing in general. This suggests that the associations concerned with these specialties, such as the American Psychiatric Association, the National Tuberculosis Association, and the American Public Health Association, were influential in promoting the interests of these areas of nursing.

As mentioned in Chapter 1, nursing is interwoven with general history. And as society moves, so must nursing move; the social forces that affect society also affect nursing. War, for instance, with all of its horrors, destruction, and depravity has never failed to influence not only the course of nursing history but of all human endeavors.

The establishment of trained nursing in the United States came as a result of the pioneering work done by women during the Civil War. These women had no training, as nurses, but they developed a high degree of practical skill in giving care to the sick and wounded soldiers. This was the beginning also of organized concentration of women in public duties in the United States.

The first three schools established for the training of American nurses are monuments to the creativity of organized women who earned recognition and a measure of power during the Civil War. After the war, in 1885, schools of nursing began to develop rapidly. A new hospital meant a new school of nursing. The heads of the schools had educational ideals, but they had no permanent independent budget on which to operate, and so they had to follow the dictates of hospital authorities. Hospital authorities had to face the problem of whether to spend funds allocated for the care of the sick or to use the money to educate nurses. The heads of the schools had a lonely struggle; they worked out their own problems and made the best adjustment they could for their students. The exigencies of the ward prevented the student from attending day classes; she attended evening classes and worked a twenty-four hour day. It was considered that students formed a more stable nursing service, because they were easier to control and because their services cost less than the services of graduate nurses.

During the 1890's hospitals were opened as profitable business enterprises; a many-roomed mansion which was bought and equipped as a hospital was not the expensive investment that it is today. A graduate nurse was placed in charge and students were recruited. By the second year the students were assigned to patients as special nurses in the hospital and also in the home; the salary for their services was collected by the hospital.

Nursing leaders, however, quickly realized that the development of short-course nursing schools would have detrimental effects on both students and patients, and they decided to do something about this unhealthy situation.

In 1893, at the World's Fair in Chicago, a group of spirited nursing leaders met to consider the development of national standards and administrative practices of schools. Before the historic meeting adjourned, the group explored the possibilities of organizing a national nursing society. As a result of these talks, a national society, the American Society of Superintendents of Training Schools of the United States, was established to promote fellowship among its members and to establish a universal standard of training.

Action was also taken at this meeting to develop a second organization which would be concerned with membership. The action taken by the Society of Superintendents of Training Schools resulted in the organization called Nurses' Associated Alumnae of the United States and Canada. In 1911 this organization was renamed the American Nurses' Association.

This epochal meeting was the genesis of organized nursing in America; it set the over-all pattern which nurses and nursing have followed to the present time.

This was the age of the "gospel of hard work." In America, an agricultural nation, the day was long. As industry increased the same pattern was taken for granted. Nurses carried a double burden. Nursing had been considered a dedicated, selfless type of work since the beginning of Christianity, and the American tradition of hard work meant twenty-four-hour nursing in the beginning. Later, night nurses were introduced, but both day duty and night duty continued as twelve-hour periods until the turn of the century.

Both hospital boards and physicians argued that frequent changes of nurses would be disturbing to the patient. The eight-hour day was generally not accepted until after 1925, and much later for private duty nurses.

As for age, the Nightingale Training School for Nurses required students to be twenty-five. This was the general pattern in the United States and continued well into the twentieth century, but many of the schools failed to grasp the meaning of Miss Nightingale's education principles and they did not have competent graduates to direct them. And, as Louise Darche pointed out at the Chicago meeting, the American system was not in accord with several points in the criteria developed by Miss Nightingale. The disagreement between the two systems concerned the opportunity for advancement. Advancement, according to the Nightingale plan, was reserved for the hospital's head nurse. The head nurse was the person selected to teach in the school—this was a foregone conclusion. The American plan held that advancement should be based on demonstrable ability and that advanced selection of head nurse as teacher was undemocratic.

The courses in the early schools were only for one year. Nursing was solely "the care and comfort of the sick without remedial measures." Hypodermics were not in use; blood-pressure readings were not done; surgery was limited; orthopedics and pediatrics were unknown specialties; and few maternity patients went to the hospital. The life span was less than thirty-five years, hence there were few degenerative diseases. But there was a great deal of typhoid fever and malaria in the summer and pneumonia in the winter, with a high rate of tuberculosis at all times.

In view of the meager nursing care required, one year was sufficient to learn poultice-making, cupping and bandaging, how to help the doctor with blood-letting, and to prepare gruels, beef tea, and milk toast. Later, another year was added to provide experience and to benefit the hospital financially. Since the turn of the century the nursing course in diploma schools has been a three-year one.

NATIONAL CURRICULUM

Since the beginning of early nursing schools in the 1870's the content of formal classes and bedside teaching had been decided by the individual school. Each school planned its own curriculum and published its program of classes and lectures which may or may not have been given. When state board examinations became nationwide it was necessary that there be uniformity of classes in order that all students would have had the same basic course. This could only be done through a national curriculum which would equip nurses to meet conditions that they might find in any type of community or hospital.

The National League of Nursing Education undertook the preparation of such a curriculum, with M. Adelaide Nutting as chairman and Isabel M. Stewart as secretary of the committee. *The Standard Curriculum for Schools of Nursing* was published in 1917 after three years of work by the committee.

In the introduction of this curriculum the committee stated:

The purpose which the committee has had in view is to arrive at some general agreement as to a desirable and workable standard whose main features could be accepted by training schools of good standing throughout the country. In this way it is hoped that we may be able to gradually overcome the wide diversity of standards at present existing in schools of nursing, and at least supply a basis for appraising the value of widely different systems of nursing training.

This curriculum suggested from 585 to 595 hours: 343 to 355 hours of classes during the first year, and 120 hours for each year in the second and third years.

COLLEGIATE SCHOOLS

Collegiate schools of nursing were first developed in the United States. Many of the early nursing graduates had been school teachers before entering a school of nursing. Many had graduated earlier from "female academies," comparable to our present-day high schools. These nurses were interested in placing more emphasis on education and less on service. Johns Hopkins University, Baltimore, when it opened its school of nursing in 1883, demanded and attracted the intellectual type of young woman.

There have been claims and counterclaims as to the first collegiate school of nursing. A definition of a collegiate school at the end of the nineteenth century delineated, of course, a program differing from our present one. If we define a collegiate school as one having autonomy within the university, then the school would be under the control of a university.

Jenny S. Cottle, a graduate of Massachusetts General Hospital School of Nursing, was brought to Iowa City, Iowa, in 1897 to organize a school of nursing. The school was to be under full control of the University of Iowa, functioning specifically under the medical department.

The university catalogue of 1897-98 announced the opening of the school: "Connected with the Medical Department of the University, the School for Nurses offers a two-year course of training to women who desire to enter the nursing profession. The course of instruction comprises practical work in the wards, theoretical work in class and lecture rooms and a complete course in invalid cooking. The University catalogue of 1899-1900 announced the addition to the curriculum of courses in dietetics, hospital administration, ward management, and massage.

The second school of nursing to be under full control of a university was that at the University of Texas. This school began as the John Sealey Hospital School for Nurses, and was acquired by the University of Texas. When the Board of Ladies found that it could no longer support the school, the regents of the university adopted the nursing school as one of the regular schools of the medical department. It did not function, however, as a regular department of the university until recent years.

In 1909 the University of Minnesota School of Nursing was opened under the leadership of Dr. Richard Olding Beard, who had long been interested in nursing education. This was the first basic program in nursing education to be conducted and controlled by a university on sound principles of education. Students paid tuition for the freshman course and were responsible for finding their own living quarters.

The first educational program for graduate nurses was established as a one-year course in hospital economics in 1899 at Teachers' College, Columbia University. In 1907 a chair of nursing was founded there by Mrs. Helen Hartley Jenkins with an endowment of $200,000. Miss Adelaide Nutting, a graduate of the first class of the Johns Hopkins School of Nursing, was called to fill this position. She became the first nurse in the world to hold a professorship in a university.

PRIVATE DUTY NURSING

When the two-year course was completed, the student became the by-product of the school. The students did all the work, with the senior student assuming head-nurse duties. There was no position for the graduate in the school or community. Because she already had experience in private duty she became a private duty nurse. She registered for duty at the hospital or the local drugstore, packed her bag, and waited for a call.

STAFF NURSING

The "depression" which struck in 1929 and lasted nearly a decade had a beneficial long-range influence on nursing. Because the patient census was greatly reduced, hospitals had difficulty remaining open. Most graduates had been doing private duty for the previous half century, but few sick persons could afford their services in the depression years. These nurses, therefore, were employed by hospitals at a minimum salary plus maintenance.

Another compelling force was at work at the same time: a fast-growing consciousness of the national need for healthful living. This idea of preventive medicine was sponsored by doctors, especially those interested in public health and sanitation. To carry out medicine's objective would require teachers, many teachers. The problem was whether this should be done by nurses or by women with specialized education. The Rockefeller Foundation, 1919-1923, financed a project for the *Study of Nursing Education,* popularly known as the Goldmark Report because the investigation had been made by Josephine Goldmark. This report revealed that most nursing schools were shockingly inadequate in providing laboratories, libraries, demonstration rooms, instructors, and qualified head nurses.

The Goldmark Report stimulated the National League of Nursing Education to undertake another survey which the League hoped would lead to actual grading of schools. Although this survey was carried on for eight years it did not result in a compelling reform; hospital schools faced with expensive improvements decided to close their schools. During the decade between 1920 and 1930 more than 1100 schools closed; and by 1940 a total of 1700 schools had been discontinued. The closing of hospital schools made the hospitals dependent on registered nurses to make up their staffs—although the salaries were low. The closures stabilized the nursing service, and in the hospitals with schools it permitted students to attend all classes because there were staff nurses to take over when students went to class.

STATE REGISTRATION AND ACCREDITATION OF SCHOOLS

There were no standards, no nurse practice acts, in the early days of nursing —each school was a law unto itself. When the Society of Superintendents of Training Schools was organized in Chicago in 1893 during the Columbia Exposition, it began to work for improved conditions in nursing education and nursing service.

By 1900 the organization of state associations was also encouraged. The first objective of these associations was to secure registration laws to protect the nurse and the public. This could be accomplished only by legislative action. At that time women could not vote. In some states women could not even legally hold office. The privately owned hospitals bitterly opposed nurse registration because they knew that it would raise standards of nursing and nursing education.

The first state to carry a registration bill through successfully was North Carolina. The state association was formed in 1902 and the bill was presented a year later. This bill required only the presentation of a diploma from a reputable general hospital, either public or private or from a hospital for mental patients, for a nurse to be permitted to register.

State registration for nurses is one of the most exciting and dramatic accomplishments of modern nursing. Much of the success was due to the leadership of Adda Eldridge, from St. Luke's Hospital School of Nursing in Chicago, a former president of the American Nurses' Association, and to Sophia Palmer, former editor of *The American Journal of Nursing*, whose editorials were a constant stimulus to graduate nurses.

With state registration well under way, the state associations and the League for Nursing began to work for state accreditation of schools. By 1900 state accreditation of schools had become general. The state set minimum requirements which the school had to meet in order for their graduates to be eligible to take state board examinations. By 1930, more than 1100 schools had closed because they could not meet these requirements.

STATE BOARD EXAMINATIONS

Between 1888 and 1893 most of the New York hospitals had established nursing schools. About 1896 these schools adopted the practice of final examinations for their graduates; these were the forerunners of state examinations.

The same pattern is seen in all of the states: state associations were formed, state registration was secured, and registration was followed by board examinations.

The scope of the early examinations was quite general. Some of the better schools had considerable classroom work and clinical teaching, while many others provided little or none of the preparation. If the nurses were needed on the division, no arrangements were made for them to be relieved for class.

In most states the association set up a board of examiners, usually composed of nurses. The department of the state responsible for registration would announce the date of examination for nurse registration. Nurses who had already graduated were granted state board status under a waiver.

These early examinations were permissive and many graduates did not trouble themselves to write a licensing examination. But paradoxically the permissiveness became compulsory through public opinion; the graduate was expected to have passed her examination and become a registered nurse. Registration became a requirement for civil service positions, general duty nursing, private duty in hospitals, public health, industry, and membership in nursing organizations. The change in nursing from the apprentice type of 1900 to the accredited school and curriculum of today would never have developed had there been no registration laws. State examination and registration is the nurse's greatest professional and legal protection.

These examinations were both written and practical. The practical part consisted of an actual demonstration of a procedure. As classes became larger it was difficult to conduct examinations and the day previously devoted to this was eliminated. The written part of the examination consisted of essay-type questions which took much time to grade.

By 1930 the objective-type question had become popular in all fields of education. With the advent of World War II, there was a shortage of nurses who could teach, although there was an increased number of students, and a conference of state board examiners requested that some method be devised for preparing, administering, and scoring papers quickly and accurately. In 1944 the State Board Test Pool of the Committee on Measurements and Educational Guidance of the National League of Nursing Education began using examination papers that could be graded by machine. This method of examination is now used in all of the states.

MEN NURSES

". . . in the early Christian period, and for centuries thereafter, men of the priestly class, or belonging to military or religious orders, have been responsible for at least half of the nursing service through medieval times up to a very recent period."[1]

Although a relatively large number of schools admit men students, it was not until World War II that men themselves, who had served as medical

---

[1] Adelaide Nutting and Lavinia L. Dock, *A History of Nursing*, Vol. I (New York, G. P. Putnam's Sons, 1935), p. 101.

corpsmen, realized the personal satisfaction derived from the care of the sick.

It is believed that the first nursing school for men in America was the School for Male Nurses, connected with the New York Training School for Nurses on Welfare Island. This school closed in 1903. One hundred and forty men had graduated from it but most of them later became doctors.

The Mills Training School for Male Nurses was established in 1888 in connection with Bellevue Hospital. This school was made possible by a gift to the City of New York by the philanthropist, Darius Ogden Mills, for the express purpose of educating men nurses.

Since 1929 the Mills and Bellevue schools have been under the direction of one faculty, but retain their separate identities as schools. In 1942 these two schools became associated with New York University as the Division of Nursing of the College of Medicine.

Following the crusades which ended in 1292, a great many religious and communal organizations were formed for both men and women. These were semi-monastic lay associations whose members did not take vows but who were governed by the rule to live a chaste life and do good works as long as they remained a part of the community.

Groups of men who lived together in brotherhoods were known as Beghards. In using this term some were descriptively known as Bread Beghards because they would accept bread as payment for burying the dead. These brothers were found in the Netherlands, Flanders, and in cities along the Rhine. Eventually their monasteries were centered in Aachen and Cologne. By 1318 there were three groups of Beghards in Cologne. One group, the Poor Beghards, was given the protection of the city council because it was to the city's benefit to have a group to care for the sick poor and to bury the dead.

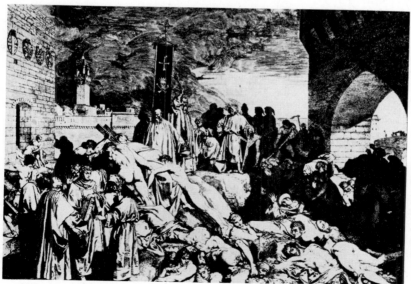

Plague of Florence in the 14th Century is described by Boccaccio.
Engraved by Sabaleth. (Bettmann Archive.)

By the middle of the fourteenth century the Poor Brothers were well organized to grapple with the most devastating scourge in all history. ''In the epidemic of the Black Death—bubonic plague—which razed Europe from 1348 to 1350 and in succeeding outbreaks which occurred locally almost yearly for the rest of the century, destroyed an estimated fourth of the population . . . In their unyielding devotion to the plague-stricken many of the Brothers forfeited their lives . . . for during the pestilence the Brothers could be depended upon to render support and remedy even when the disease inspired such dread that relatives and friends fled the sick in horror.''[2]

In April 1841, the Poor Brothers received papal approval and protection from the Inquisition. Saint Alexius was chosen as the patron saint of this society dedicated to the care of the sick, the burying of the dead, and other works of charity.

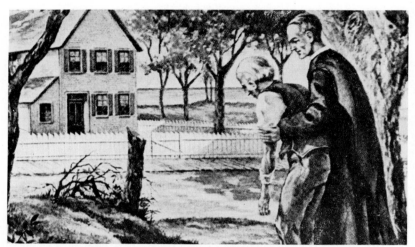

Brother Bonaventure assisting the first patient into the original Alexian Brothers Hospital, Chicago. (Courtesy of Brother Maurice, Director of Nursing, Alexian Brothers Hospital School of Nursing, Chicago.)

The Congregation of the Alexian Brothers established its first hospital for men and boys in Chicago in June, 1866. This was under the direction of Brother Bonaventure Thelen, who had been sent from the Alexian Brothers of Aachen, Germany, to establish a branch house in the United States. Three years later the Alexian Brothers Hospital in St. Louis was officially dedicated. Although men had attended to the wounded on the battle fields of the Civil War, the idea of men nursing professionally in a hospital was novel to the inhabitants of Chicago. The devotion of the Brothers during the cholera epidemic of 1866 and the well-ordered way in which they conducted their hospital gradually obliterated all distrust and prejudice.

---

[2] Ignatius Wiegers, *Of Valiant Men: A Chronicle of the Congregation of the Alexian Brothers*, ed. and rev. by Daniel Ogden, C.E.A. (Gresham, Wis., Novitiate Press, 1951), p. 4.

In February of 1894, a committee of staff doctors of the Alexian Brothers Hospital of Chicago initiated a series of lectures for the Brothers. This was the beginning of the Alexian Brothers Hospital School of Nursing; the first secular students were graduated in 1942. In 1949 the Alexian Brothers School at St. Louis was consolidated with the Chicago school and became affiliated with De Paul University.

In 1955 the Congregation of the Alexian Brothers was asked to operate the newly erected hospital at the internationally famous Boys Town, outside of Omaha, Neb.

There are now many schools admitting men students. Positions in public health, sanitation, and administration are available to men nurses. The number of men in nursing has doubled during the past decade. Today men nurses are serving in South Africa, South America, Dutch West Indies, and as medical missionaries at Sudan Interior Mission in Addis Ababa. They serve wherever they are needed—in any remote corner of the earth.[3]

NURSING PUBLICATIONS

Textbooks. The early nursing textbooks were written by doctors. The books were erudite and scholarly but they did not contain information on nursing care. Miss Nightingale's *Notes on Nursing* was probably the first textbook to be published. The first nursing textbook published in America was written in 1885 by Mrs. Clara Weeks Shaw, a graduate of New York Hospital School of Nursing. Diana Kimber of City Hospital, New York, prepared the first textbook on anatomy and physiology for nurses in 1892. Lavinia L. Dock, a graduate of Bellevue in 1886, wrote the first pharmacology textbook for nurses while on night duty at Bellevue in 1890. The first microbiology textbook for nurses was written by Mary Ried. Amy Pope and Anna Maxwell wrote *Practical Nursing*, which was a popular textbook for twenty-five years. It was a veritable encyclopedia of nursing, concerning professional ethics, bacteriology, care and comfort of the patient, baths and packs, catheterization, bandaging, symptoms, and physical signs, operating room technic, and emergencies. This book was originally published in 1907, continued through four editions, and was translated into Spanish.

Magazines. Magazines are divided into two classes—official and commercial. An official magazine is one that is controlled and owned by the organization sponsoring it and is therefore known as the official organ of that organization. Commercial magazines are those published by private individuals.

The first magazine edited by and for nurses was a commercial publication called *The Trained Nurse*. Margaret Elliot Francis Sirch was its first editor. *The Trained Nurse* was the first and only nursing magazine to be published in the United States until *The American Journal of Nursing* came on the scene in 1900. It was in the pages of *The Trained Nurse* that the early nurse pioneers gave expression to their plans and reached the entire nursing group.

---

[3] Allen Rankin, ''Mr. R.N. Is Wanted on the Nursing Team,'' *The Modern Hospital*, Vol. 93 (Dec., 1959), pp. 71-72, 144.

The two national nursing organizations had a natural desire for self-expression through their own official organ. Consequently, in 1900 *The American Journal of Nursing* began publication with Sophia Palmer as editor. Thirty-five years later the Journal published the ''Story of The American Journal of Nursing'' in which it stated:

Several plans were suggested for financing the new magazine, but it was finally decided to form a joint stock company and to sell shares at $100 each. The shares in the joint stock company were sold only to nurses, so that from the very first the JOURNAL has always been owned and controlled by members of the nursing profession. This is not just a happy accident but was the intention and careful plan of the women who were responsible from the first. . . .

The nurses who planned the JOURNAL in the beginning had in mind three functions which it would carry on for the members of their group. It would be a continuous record of nursing events; a means of communication between scattered groups of nurses; and one means of interpreting nursing to the public.[4]

Around 1900 the Cleveland Visiting Nurse Association began to publish its official report as a quarterly bulletin. By 1911 it had become a national publication, the only one of its kind. At the epoch-making biennial in Chicago, 1912, this bulletin became the official publication of the National Organization for Public Health Nursing. For forty years *Public Health Nursing*, with its clean blue and white cover, was the indispensable publication of the active public health nurse. With the reorganization of the national nursing associations in June, 1952, the National Organization for Public Health Nursing became one of the departments of the National League for Nursing. Its official publication was therefore absorbed by *Nursing Outlook* (first issued in January, 1953), from which the public health nurse benefits because of other articles concerning her field of interest.

Nursing Research began publication in June, 1952. Nurses have been so busy getting their jobs done that there has been little time for research. But nurses are aware of the need for research not only to enable them to qualify as a profession, but also as a major step in planning for the future. *Nursing Research* was published to serve two purposes: ''. . . to inform members of the nursing profession and allied professions of the results of scientific studies in nursing, and to stimulate research in nursing.''[5]

REFERENCES

AMERICAN SOCIETY OF SUPERINTENDENTS OF TRAINING SCHOOLS FOR NURSES, *Eighteenth Annual Report*, 1912.

A CENTURY OF NURSING. New York, G. P. Putnam's Sons, 1916. Reproduced in 1950 with permission of the State Charities Aid Association, New York, and the Bellevue School of Nursing Board of Managers.

[4] *The Story of The American Journal of Nursing* (New York, The American Journal of Nursing Company, 1935), pp. 3-16.

[5] Editorial: ''A Cooperative Venture,'' *Nursing Research*, Vol. 1 (June, 1952), p. 5.

BROWN, AMY F.: *Curriculum Development*. Philadelphia, W. B. Saunders Co., 1960.

CHAYER, MARY E.: The trail of the nursing textbook. *Amer. J. Nurs.* 50:606 (Oct.) 1950.

DEWITT, KATHERINE, and MUNSON, HELEN W.: The Journal's first fifty years. *Amer. J. Nurs.* 50:590 (Oct.) 1950.

DOLAN, JOSEPHINE A.: *Goodnow's History of Nursing*, 10th ed. Philadelphia, W. B. Saunders Co., 1958.

FILLMORE, ANNA: Scene—U.S.A., 1900. *Amer. J. Nurs.* 41:913 (Aug.) 1941.

"FROM THE JOURNAL FIFTY YEARS AGO." *Amer. J. Nurs.* 50:604 (Oct.) 1950.

McMANUS, R. LOUISE: The state board test pool. *Amer. J. Nurs.* 44:380 (Apr.) 1944.

"MRS. CLARA WEEKS SHAW." *Amer. J. Nurs.* 40:356 (Mar.) 1940.

MUNSON, HELEN W.: *The Story of the National League of Nursing Education*. Philadelphia, W. B. Saunders Co., 1934.

PARSONS, SARA E.: *History of Massachusetts General Hospital Training School for Nurses*. Boston, Whitcomb and Barrows, 1922.

ROBERTS, MARY M.: *American Nursing: History and Interpretation*. New York, The Macmillan Co., 1954.

STEWART, ISABEL M.: A half-century of nursing education. *Amer. J. Nurs.* 50:617 (Oct.) 1950.

WIEGERS, IGNATIUS: *Of Valiant Men: A Chronicle of the Congregation of the Alexian Brothers*, ed. and rev. by Daniel Ogden, C. F. A., Bresham, Wis., Novitiate Press, 1957.

CHAPTER 11

Nursing Organizations

Following the Civil War, industry attracted people to the cities. The American middle-class was still a minority. In the cities, people were either wealthy or poor; they lived close enough together to talk things over and to pool their opinions. Thus the latter half of the nineteenth century saw the beginning of numerous types of organizations for both men and women.

BIRTH OF NURSING ORGANIZATIONS

Mrs. Edith Gordon Fenwick of England may be given credit as the mother of nursing organizations. Admittedly, the time was ripe for beginning such organizations in both England and the United States, but leadership was needed, and Mrs. Fenwick supplied it. Before her marriage, Edith Gordon, an English girl from a wealthy and influential family, had graduated from the Manchester Hospital and had been director of nurses of St. Bartholomew's Hospital, a famous old hospital built by the King's jester in 1123. She married Dr. Bedford Fenwick in 1887.

Mrs. Fenwick had real talent for organization and sharing responsibility among a large number of persons. She was also aware of how much could be accomplished for nursing by the formation of a national organization. Although her beauty, graciousness, and social prestige were valuable assets, it was her initiative, courage, and boundless enthusiasm that helped to establish, in 1887, the British Nurses' Association, the first national organization for nurses. This was the beginning of professional freedom for nurses.

The World's Fair, held in Chicago in 1893, provided an excellent opportunity for organizational meetings of every kind. The International Congress of Charities, Correction, and Philanthropy held their meetings at the fair in June, 1893. Dr. Henry Hurd, administrator of Johns Hopkins Hospital, was secretary of this congress and was also responsible for the program on hospitals, nursing, first aid, and dispensaries. In 1892 Mrs. Fenwick came to the United States to arrange for a nursing exhibit at the fair, and during these preparations she was the guest of Isabel Hampton, director of nurses at Johns Hopkins Hospital. Together they planned the nursing exhibits and programs.

Many nurses attended this fair; they visited the nursing booth on the midway and listened to lectures on hospitals, nursing, and first aid. Miss Hampton suggested that a meeting of the directors of nursing be held before the congress adjourned.

On June 13, 1893, some twenty superintendents met in the sitting-room of St. Luke's Hospital at the invitation of Katherine Lett, director of nurses. At this meeting a temporary organization was formed with Anna L. Alston as chairman. It was decided that a proper organizational meeting be held in New York in January of 1894. This would allow time for studying other organizations and becoming acquainted with the legal machinery necessary for a national organization. The name of the society was agreed upon—The American Society of Superintendents of Training Schools for Nurses. In 1912 this long name was changed to the National League of Nursing Education and again in 1952 to the National League for Nursing (referred to as the NLN).

At the meeting in 1894, the foremost interest of the members was education in general, a uniform curriculum, regular entrance time for classes, a reduction of the twelve-hour working day and making sure that the students would have some preliminary instruction before they began their experience with patients.

AMERICAN NURSES' ASSOCIATION

The Society of Superintendents of Training Schools for Nurses was an exclusive organization because it was limited to directors of nurses. Because these members were heads of schools their basic interest was education, but they were concerned also with the problems of nursing as a whole. It had been twenty years since nursing schools were first established and there were a good many graduate nurses, most of whom were doing private duty nursing. The Society of Nurse Superintendents felt that there should also be a national organization to which all nurses could belong. There already were alumnae associations, whose units would logically make up a national association.

With an objective to include all nurses, the Society of Superintendents began working toward such an organization. At its meeting in 1896, a committee of seven members was appointed to select seven others to form a nucleus of a convention to prepare a constitution. The latter seven were to be selected from members of the oldest alumnae associations and who were not holding hospital positions.

Lavinia Lloyd Dock,[1] endowed with one of the keenest and most practical minds in modern nursing, made a careful study of the organizational machinery of the American Medical Association and other national groups having local units. Miss Dock read her paper at the meeting of the Society of Nurse Superintendents in 1896 in which she outlined the principles on which the American Nurses' Association was founded and which remain the basis of the organization today:

The most striking characteristic of all alike may be said to . . . a systematic division and subdivision of work and responsibility. The central bodies . . . lay down principles; keep an outlook over the whole country; support ideal standards. . . . The state organizations take up each one its share of the actual burden of the whole. They are working bodies . . . while in the small component parts, the twigs, be they railroad divisions, parishes, alumnae associations, county societies, or what not, all the close individual work must be done, which is of all the most important.[2]

The nucleus of seven members of the Society of Nurse Superintendents and the alumnae delegates began laying the plans for the formation of a national association of graduate nurses.[3] The delegates met at Manhattan Beach, New York, in September, 1896, and organized the Nurses' Associated Alumnae of the United States and Canada[4] with Mrs. Isabel Hampton Robb as president. The name of this organization was changed in 1911 to the American Nurses' Association.

The over-all purposes of the American Nurses' Association today, as it was in 1896, are "to foster high standards of nurse practice and to promote the welfare of nurses to the end that all people may have better nursing care."[5]

The American Nurses' Association has developed and carried out many projects to promote the welfare of nurses; among these projects are the eight-hour day, economic security, malpractice insurance, legislation, elimination of race discrimination, and extension of federal social security. None of these came easily. They represent careful planning, work time, and a dedicated interest on the part of hundreds of nurses. This concern can be seen in the present national effort to bring about legislation to increase social security benefits to the disabled and aging who are in need of hospitalization and who are unable to pay the high hospital costs.

---

[1] Miss Dock died in 1956 at the age of 98. Her contribution to nursing has been valuable and lasting in the fields of organization, writing, legislation, and executive action.

[2] Lavinia L. Dock, "A National Association for Nurses and Its Legal Organization," *Third Annual Report of the American Society of Superintendents of Training Schools for Nurses, 1896*, p. 42.

[3] Nurse registration was then unknown.

[4] The Canadian nurses formed their own dominion association in 1908.

[5] "Platform of the American Nurses' Association," *The American Journal of Nursing*, Vol. 52 (Aug., 1952), p. 93.

NURSES' RELIEF FUND

The history of the Nurses' Relief Fund is given in considerable detail here in order to give the student a picture of the manner in which the American Nurses' Association works for the welfare of the individual nurses.

At the time of the organization of the American Nurses' Association it was not unusual for two or even three members of a nursing class to develop active tuberculosis before they had been able to provide for themselves. In those days there were no income-protection policies or hospital insurance.

At the national convention held in Buffalo, New York, in 1911, A.N.A. President, Jane A. Delano, presented the subject of relief for disabled members to the open meeting. It was proposed that a fund be accumulated and held by the American Nurses' Association for the purpose of assisting needy members. Sophia Palmer, then editor of *The American Journal of Nursing*, described vividly the response to this proposal:

... Immediately nurses from all parts of the room were on their feet, all eager to be heard, and in fifteen minutes nearly $1800 was pledged with an enthusiasm which showed how strongly the members felt the need of a fund to draw from for disabled members. ... [6]

We can get an idea of the number of nurses who have been helped by this fund by realizing that in a ten-year period nearly a quarter of a million dollars was paid out for sick relief although no beneficiary received more than $20 a month nor less than $5.

Because this fund was national in scope, it was impossible to investigate each individual request. On a national basis, social workers could not get the most elementary information, even from district sources.

The subject was thoroughly discussed at the 1930 national convention in Milwaukee, Wis., and two years later it was decided to allocate the residue of the relief funds on a per capita basis to each state—the Nurses' Relief Fund then became a state and district responsibility.

THE INTERNATIONAL COUNCIL OF NURSES

The Columbia Exposition held in Chicago in 1893 was the birthplace of the National League of Nursing Education. It was also the place where the idea for an international organization for nurses originated. The International Council of Women was beginning its work about this time and its importance was being recognized. In 1899 this international organization held its quinquennial meeting in London. Mrs. Fenwick set about to find nurses from the United States who might be attending this council. She broached the subject at a meeting of the Matron's Council of Great Britain and Ireland, which received the idea favorably. The council appointed a provisional committee to work out a plan of organization. This committee included nurse

---

[6] Editorial Comment: ''Meeting of the Two National Societies in Boston,'' *The American Journal of Nursing*, Vol. 11 (July, 1911), p. 772.

representatives from nine countries. A constitution was drafted, and when the provisional committee convened in London in 1900 the constitution was adopted, thus bringing into existence the International Council of Nurses.

The constitution of the ICN, with only slight modifications, stood until 1925, when Clara D. Noyes, an American nurse, accomplished the difficult task of revising it to meet better the demands of a greatly increased membership. The objectives stated in the preamble of the original constitution still stand as foundation principles of the International Council of Nurses:

We, nurses, of all nations, sincerely believing that best good of our Profession will be advanced by greater unity of thought, sympathy, and purpose, do hereby band ourselves in a confederation of workers to further the efficient care of the sick, and to secure the honour and the interests of the Nursing Profession.[7]

Membership. The national nursing association from each member-country is considered to be a member of the ICN. In the United States, the American Nurses' Association is the member. When the organization was formed in 1900 few countries had an association that was national in scope. (The American Nurses' Association was only three years old.) For this reason the early membership included individual members, known as councillors who returned to their countries to work for the establishment of national associations. As such an association was formed, councillors withdrew as individual representatives and were replaced by the nursing associations of their respective countries.

The history of the ICN is really a history of professional emancipation for nurses throughout the world and the task is not yet finished. In countries where nursing is growing and where individual nurses are anxious to divorce nursing from servitude, the council is still looked to for guidance and support in nursing legislation and promoting public interest in the educational, professional, and economic status of nursing.

NATIONAL ORGANIZATION FOR PUBLIC HEALTH NURSING

Nonoffical or private agencies initiated and developed public health nursing for the purpose of furnishing care to the sick poor in their homes on a visit basis.

This form of nursing appeared first in Liverpool, England, in 1858, sponsored by a private citizen, William Rathbone. The idea spread until an organized district nursing association developed in other cities throughout England. In 1877 the New York City Mission first sent trained nurses to care for the sick poor in their homes. Finally, in 1885 and 1886, the first visiting nurse associations in the United States were developed at Buffalo, Boston, and Philadelphia.

The early visiting nursing was a generalized service; it slowly became specialized. At first the visiting nurses cared mainly for patients with tubercu-

---

[7] Mary M. Roberts, *American Nursing: History and Interpretation* (New York, The Macmillan Co., 1954), p. 80.

losis or other communicable diseases. Then one day in New York City an intelligent twelve-year-old boy was refused admission to school because of an untreated skin disease. Lillian D. Wald, an 1891 graduate of the New York Hospital, went to the health authorities to protest the wastefulness of medical inspection of school children without a follow-up service. She offered the services of a nurse from the Henry Street Settlement for one month. The result of her experiment was so convincing that enough money was appropriated to pay the salaries of twelve school nurses.

Industrial nursing was first started in Vermont in 1895 by a marble company interested in the welfare of its workers and their families. Since that time the nurse has become an essential part of industrial organizations.

In 1909 the Metropolitan Life Insurance Company had a nursing service for its industrial policy holders. The company's actuaries soon proved the value of nursing service and within three years the company had made contracts with 400 visiting nurse associations in the United States and Canada to care for its policy holders.

These new nursing services had grown too rapidly for public health policies to be planned and standardized, much as nursing schools had been twenty years earlier. Mary Sewall Gardner, who had been present for the organizational meeting of the National Organization for Public Health Nursing, described the progress of the public health movement in *Katharine Kent:*

. . . After having lived an obscure and rather limited existence for a good many years, public health nursing has leaped out of its obscurity and become alarmingly popular. As a result several things are happening. Any number of new visiting nurse associations are being started up. Sometimes they are well and wisely organized and administered, but this is by no means always the case. Frequently the organizers haven't a ghost of an idea what is involved. If they are fortunate enough to get hold of the right nurse, they go along fairly well. . . . Sometimes the organizers are mere infants. A group of girls . . . will be seized with charitable yearnings. They raise the money and engage a nurse, preferably a young and pretty one, wearing a becoming uniform. Just as her patients are beginning to depend upon her . . . the interest flits to something else . . . the patients find themselves without a nurse because the nurse finds herself without a salary.[8]

Early in 1912 a small group of public health nurses suggested to The American Society of Superintendents of Training Schools for Nurses (now the National League for Nursing) and the Nurses' Associated Alumnae (now the American Nurses' Association) that plans be made for an organization of public health nurses that would be national in scope. A committee was appointed and wrote letters to some 800 agencies concerned with public health in the United States, asking that they send delegates to a meeting of the two national organizations for the purpose of forming a national public health organization.

The meeting was held in Chicago on June 6, 1912. It was so well attended that twice it was necessary to move to a larger room. It was at this memorable

---

[8] Mary Sewall Gardner, *Katherine Kent* (New York, The Macmillian Co., 1946), p. 114.

meeting that The Society of Superintendents of Training Schools for Nurses changed its name to the National League of Nursing Education (now the National League for Nursing), and the Associated Alumnae of the United States changed its name to the American Nurses' Association.

In the two parent organizations only nurses were eligible for membership. But the public health nurses wanted to invite members of their boards to join the profession in working for a common cause. Alma C. Haupt, writing in *Public Health Nursing,* January, 1945, recalled this meeting:

And I remember how the A.N.A. members, meeting in the other room, were rather scandalized at what these radical youngsters were doing and they weren't quite certain whether to recognize this mongrel child we were giving birth to. It was Jane Delano, regal and white haired as she was, who succeeded in persuading the A.N.A. that we were safe, and who came in to give us her blessing.

Great care was taken in the selection of a name for this organization. The name finally decided upon was National Organization for Public Health Nursing (NOPHN). Those founding nurses always emphasized the preposition *for* and that it was for public health nursing and not public health nurses.

THE MODERN STRUCTURE OF ORGANIZED NURSING

Nursing had two major groups: the National League of Nursing Education and the American Nurses' Association. In addition to these organizations, five special groups gradually evolved: National Association of Colored Graduate Nurses,[9] 1908; National Organization of Public Health Nursing, 1912; American Association of Nurse Anesthetists, 1931; Association of Collegiate Schools of Nursing, 1933; and American Association of Industrial Nurses, Inc., 1942.

Nurses tended to become absorbed in their particular groups, limiting their interests as a whole.

In 1946 plans were considered for combining all nursing organizations into one over-all plan. Exhaustive studies were made; specialists in social studies were employed; and studies of other organizations were made. Perhaps the most crucial point was whether the single organization should be a professional organization or one which would include lay members.

Finally, in 1952, two organizations were formed: the American Nurses' Association with only nurses as members, and the National League for Nursing, which has both nurses and lay members. These two companion organizations have a coordinating council which provides for teamwork between them. When the reorganization was completed the National Association of Industrial Nurses, Inc., remained as a separate specialized group.

---

[9] This association was absorbed in the American Nurses' Association in 1951.

WORLD HEALTH ORGANIZATION

The United Nations Organization was founded in San Francisco in 1945. At this meeting, delegates from two such widely separated countries as Brazil and China suggested that the United Nations work toward setting up an international health program. Delegates were enthusiastic about such a program: ''The conferences revealed again and again the depth of suffering of European and Asiatic peoples during the War [World War II], the present insecurity of many governments in all corners of the world, and the ever-present fear of near-starvation or, at best, the malnutrition of vast populations, particularly children, engendered by our present uneven distribution of the world's food supply.''[10]

The following year (June, 1946), delegates of sixty-one nations met as the Henry Hudson Hotel in New York City and prepared a constitution for the World Health Organization within the United Nations.

The only nurse in this great assembly was Mrs. Elmira Bears Wickenden,[11] a member of the United Nations delegation. Surgeon General Thomas Parran of the United States Public Health Service was chairman of the United Nations delegation, and it was due to his foresight that nursing was established as part of the international health program. Mrs. Wickenden, as a nurse advisor, had all the rights and privileges of the advisors of medicine and pharmacy.

During the month-long session of this meeting, Dr. Parran gave several informal dinners for the delegates of other countries and to one of these dinners he invited Mrs. Wickenden. At the dinner Dr. Parran described in detail the work and services of United States nurses, then he gave Mrs. Wickenden an opportunity to make a plea that nurses be included in the delegations appointed to represent the permanent structure of a world health organization. She was warmly received and many of the delegates promised to include nurses in their health delegations in the future. Both Dr. Parran and Mrs. Wickenden were aware that unless there was nurse participation included in the initial organization, nursing would never have representation in the World Health Organization.

The preamble to the constitution of the World Health Organization is evidence of the sincerity of these delegations:

The enjoyment of the highest attainable standard of health is one of the fundamental rights of every human being without discrimination of race, religion, political belief, economic or social condition.

---

[10] Elmira B. Wickenden, ''A Magna Carta for Health,'' *The American Journal of Nursing,* Vol. 46 (Sept., 1946), pp. 613-14.

[11] Mrs. Wickenden was appointed as advisor-delegate by President Harry S. Truman. She was well qualified for this position. She had served overseas with the American Red Cross during World War I and remained as chief nurse for Northern France and Belgium for the Hoover Commission for Relief. She was executive secretary of the National Nursing Council at the time of her appointment to the American delegation of the World Health Organization.

All of this sounded lofty and idealistic, and to put it into practice was difficult. In most countries, nursing was at an early stage or nonexistent. By 1950 the delegations realized that nurses and nursing were essential in order to carry out the objectives of the organization; therefore, the delegations, in preparing the agenda for the 1951 meeting, voted to consider nursing as a special subject and to formulate plans to encourage and stimulate the education of nurses.

It is interesting to follow the development of nursing in such an international organization: The first meeting, in 1946, was attended by only one nurse, Mrs. Wickenden; at the second meeting in Geneva, Mrs. Lucile Petry Leone was present. Later three or four nurses attended; then in 1956 nursing was chosen as the main topic of the assembly and twenty-one countries included nurses in their delegations. Now the inclusion of nurses in the World Health Organization is taken for granted.

History again repeats itself: In 1873 nurses were neither needed nor desired; now they are indispensable and their use is an indication of the degree of civilization attained by any country.

REFERENCES

AGLER, GEORGE W.: LILLIAN D. WALD: An artist in the joy of living. *Amer. J. Nurs.* 60:354 (Mar.) 1960.

"BIENNIAL HIGHLIGHTS." *Amer. J. Nurs.* 52:824 (July) 1952.

DIETZ, LENA D.: *Professional Adjustments II*, 5th ed. Philadelphia, F. A. DAVIS CO., 1959.

DOLAN, JOSEPHINE A.: *Goodnow's Nursing History*, 10th ed. Philadelphia, W. B. Saunders Co., 1958.

DUFFAS, R. L.: *Lillian Wald-Neighbor and Crusader*. New York, The Macmillan Co., 1938.

"FORTY NATIONS AND ONE WORLD." *Amer. J. Nurs.* 47:437 (Apr.) 1947.

HAUPT, ALMA C.: Thirty years of pioneering in public health nursing. *Amer. J. Nurs.* 39:619 (June) 1939.

HUBBARD, RUTH W.: Public health nursing: 1900-1950. *Amer. J. Nurs.* 50:608 (Oct.) 1950.

JAMIESON, ELIZABETH M., SEWALL, MARY and GJERTSON, LUCILLE S.: *Trends in Nursing History*, 5th ed. Philadelphia, W. B. Saunders Co., 1959.

MARKOFF, ADA S.: Industrial nursing begins in Vermont. *Public Health Nurs.* 37:125 (Mar.) 1945.

ROBERTS, MARY M.: American Nursing: History and Interpretation. New York, The Macmillan Co., 1954.

THE STORY OF THE AMERICAN JOURNAL OF NURSING COMPANY, 1900-1950. New York, American Journal of Nursing Company, 1950.

WICKENDEN, ELMIRA B.: A magna carta for health. *Amer. J. Nurs.* 46:613 (Sept.) 1946.

CHAPTER 12

Early American Wars

THE REVOLUTIONARY WAR, 1775-1781

The British colonists in North America gained their independence by the Revolutionary War. Tired of the tyrannies and feuds of Europe, their ancestors had sought liberty in the New World, establishing the first permanent settlement at Jamestown, Virginia. Gradually other groups of colonists arrived, and each in its own way conquered the wilderness, subdued the Indians, and developed a standard of living that was generally better than the life these colonists had known in Europe.

As the colonists became more self-reliant and self-sufficient their desire for independence increased. They developed a tradition of self-government which made them resent any infringement England made on their home rule. And as the British tried to enforce the policy of mercantilism, they placed trade restrictions on the colonies which aggravated the discontentment of the settlers. The causes of the American Revolution were complex, but these were the three basic factors underlying the revolt.

The British colonists, who did not call themselves Americans until 1774, had become ready and anxious to turn their backs on Europe. Perhaps Patrick Henry more than anyone else brought about greater unity of thought among the colonists. His famous statement made in September 1774 helped to crystallize their convictions: ''The distinctions between Virginians, Pennsylvanians, New Yorkers, and New Englanders are no more. I am not a Virginian but an American.'' The clash between the colonies and the mother country became inevitable.

When the Revolutionary War finally broke out—April 19, 1775—the colonies were poorly prepared; there was no central government, no navy, no army. There was not even a commander-in-chief until July 3, 1775, when George Washington was appointed. Upon organizing the affairs of his great office, he found himself presiding over thirteen weak states. In June, 1776, word reached America that King George III had arranged to hire 20,000 troops from the German province of Hesse to subdue the Americans. This aroused such feeling among the colonists that a resolution of independence was prepared and on July 4, 1776, it was ratified by twelve of the thirteen colonies, New York being the only one to hold off.[1]

In preparing for the war, the Americans had made no plans for the care of the wounded. Medical practice during that period was crude and cruel; little thought was given to the plight of the wounded unless he was an officer. There was no anesthesia (ether was discovered in 1842), opium was used by mouth (morphine was isolated in 1806), but rum and whisky were available. Malaria was endemic; although quinine was known, it was much too expensive for the common soldier.

There were only nine hospitals throughout the colonies, and six of these were almshouses with only infirmaries for the acutely ill. There were no nurses in the colonies, although the Canadian hospitals were staffed with competent nurses.[2] Army sanitation was unknown; flies and mosquitoes carried dysentery and malaria. The records of the military hospital at Sunbury, Pa., reported that about four-tenths of the patients were wounded; three-tenths suffered from dysentery; and one-tenth had rheumatism. Lack of proper food and shelter crippled the army as much as did the fire of the enemy.

Pennsylvania, especially the eastern portion, bore much of the brunt of the Revolution. After the first year of war the enthusiasm died down, and New England and the southern colonies were inclined to let Pennsylvania and the British fight it out. The Pennsylvania Dutch country was almost untouched by the war but it was used as the arsenal, the commissariat, and the hospital of the Continental Army. It was the source of supplies for Washington's men during the darkest days of the Revolution; because of these facilities he chose to camp at Valley Forge. In the valley were forges, furnaces, and foundries to smelt the ore and to cast cannon and balls. Here also were gun-shops; sulfur, charcoal, and potassium nitrate to make gunpowder; the horses and wagons that gave the American Army its mobility.

The Moravian settlement at Lititz, Pennsylvania, was used as a hospital

---

[1] Visitors to Williamsburg, Virginia, are awed and humble when viewing on the broad screen the movie ''Birth of a Patriot,'' shown daily in the museum building.

[2] During Gen. Benedict Arnold's expedition against Quebec in the winter of 1775, scarlet fever and smallpox broke out and in some regiments one-fourth to one-third of the men died. The wounded and ill from both sides were given kindly care by the Ursuline nuns.

center. The first patients, approximately eighty in number, reached Lititz on December 19, 1777, and were cared for in the Single Brethren House. The following day fifteen wagons arrived carrying men who suffered from putrid fever (in the humours), which caused half of these men to die.

Few of the Army hospitals had beds or blankets, and none had medicines or nurses. Colonel Anthony Wayne, writing to General Horatio Gates in December, 1776, said, "Our hospital, or rather house of carnage, beggars all description and shocks humanity to visit. The cause is obvious; no medicine or regimen on the ground suitable for the sick; no beds or straw to lay on; no covering to keep them warm other than their own thin wretched clothing."

Antisepsis was unknown at that time—cleanliness during a difficult operation was not considered to be important. Putrefaction and pain were taken for granted, and many soldiers who somehow managed to survive never did regain their health.

Visitors to Valley Forge can still see the small log cabins that were used as field hospitals by General Washington during the winter of 1777. Each cabin contains two double and four single bunks, a table, and a fireplace. A nearby stone school house, built by William Penn's daughter, was used as an operating room.

Although there were no trained nurses, records indicate that a few nurses were employed to care for soldiers. "A Congressional resolution dated July 17, 1775, includes 'one nurse to every ten sick' in the personnel for military hospitals. They were to be paid 'one fifteenth of a dollar per day or two dollars per month.' The service could only have been that which one neighbor might give another."[3]

THE CIVIL WAR, 1861-1865

In the seventy-eight years between the end of the Revolutionary War and the start of the Civil War, 1200 officers had been trained at West Point, but none had ever served with large forces. Both the Union and the Confederacy were as unprepared for waging a war as had been General Washington eighty-five years before.

Actually, neither the North nor the South expected the war to last more than three months. President Jefferson Davis declared, "Let us lick the Yankees twice and the War will be over in three months." And when President Lincoln called for 75,000 volunteers for the Union Army he asked them to serve only ninety days. President Lincoln did not even have anyone with enough experience to place in charge of such a force. The War Department had made no provision for moving, equipping, or supplying an army; nor were there any plans for sanitation and care of the sick and wounded.

At the outbreak of the war there were fewer than 150 hospitals in the country and no schools of nursing to train the nurses who would be needed in the conflict. Communicable diseases were rife; ideas of sanitation were just

---

[3] Mary M. Roberts, *American Nursing: History and Interpretation* (New York, The Macmillan Co., 1954), p. 9.

being formed and were still unknown to military medicine. Within six months 30 per cent of the soldiers were suffering from malaria, typhoid fever, small-pox, and dysentery. The greatest cause of death was typhoid fever; malaria took a heavy toll of the Union soldiers fighting in the hot South. The first military hospitals used to care for these men were mostly converted barns and tobacco warehouses.

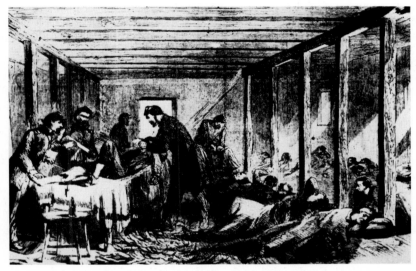

Interior of the hospital on the battlefield of Williamsburg, 1862. One of the earliest pictorial representations of the use of ether in wartime. President Grant assigned Dr. Morton, the first to publicize the use of ether as an anesthetic, to organize courses teaching the use of the drug. (Bettmann Archive.)

Although medicine made great strides during the nineteenth century, bacteriology and sanitation were still to be developed. Ether had been discovered in 1846 and chloroform had been discovered in 1847, but they had not come into general use. Many surgeons would not administer anesthetics, claiming that the excitement of the soldier was sufficient to carry him through, anesthetics given to men in shock only add to depression, and anesthetics predisposed to bleeding and retarded healing. In addition to these problems, transportation difficulties were such that dressings and drugs seldom arrived at the military hospitals when they were most needed.

During the war, maggot therapy was used empirically. Neglected wounds often became covered with maggots. The Surgeon General advised his medical corps to use common elder or calomel to rid the wounds of these larvae, but some surgeons realized that the maggots destroyed the necrotic tissue and left the wound in a healthy condition. Then it was recalled that maggot therapy had been used in the Napoleonic Wars. (There was a revival of maggot therapy in the United States during the 1920's.)

Because of his astute powers of observation and his ability to interpret and report observations made in military hospitals during the Civil War, the reactions of Walt Whitman are particularly interesting. One of America's greatest writers, Mr. Whitman had direct contact with hospitals during the war. He had gone to Washington in search of his younger brother, wounded at Fredericksburg; he remained in Washington to work as a war correspondent and government clerk. Whitman spent every spare minute in the military hospitals as an unofficial nurse and comforter of the sick and wounded.

He often used his own means to help sick soldiers, and partly as a result of these labors, he was stricken with paralysis and lived as an invalid for nineteen years.

His daily work among the men of both Union and Confederate armies made a profound impression on the great poet, as can be seen in his poems, "The Wound Dresser," "Drum Taps," and the universally loved "When Lilacs Last in the Dooryard Bloomed." In writing to some of his New York friends on March 19, 1863, Whitman reported:

Dear Nat, and Fred Gray:

Since I left New York, I was down in the Army of the Potomac in front with my brother a good part of the winter, commencing time of the battle of Fredericksburgh—have seen war-life, the real article—folded myself in a blanket, lying down in the mud with composure—relished salt pork & hard tack—have been on the battle field among the wounded, the faint, and the bleeding, to give them nourishment—have gone over with a flag of truce the next day to help direct the burial of the dead—have struck up a tremendous friendship with a young Mississippi Captain, (about 19) that we took prisoner badly wounded at Fredericksburgh—and he followed me here, is in Emory Hospital here, minus a leg—he wears a Confederate uniform, proud as the devil—I met him first at Falmouth, in the Lacy house, middle of December last, his leg was cut off, and cheered him up—poor boy, he has suffered a great deal, and still suffers—his eyes bright as a hawk, but face pale, sometimes when I lean over to say I am going, he puts his arm around my neck, draws my face down, etc. (quite a scene for the New Bowery). . . .

During January came up hither, took a lodging room here, did the 37th Congress, especially the night sessions the last three weeks, explored the Capitol then, meandering the gorgeous painted interminable senate corridors, getting lost in them, (a new sensation, rich & strong, that endless painted interior at night,) got very much interested in some particular cases in Hospitals here, go now steadily to more or less of said Hospitals by day or night . . .

These Hospitals, so different from all others, these thousands, and tens and twenties of thousands of American young men, badly wounded, all sorts of wounds, operated on, pallid with diphtheria, languishing, dying with fever, pneumonia, &c. open a new world somehow to me, giving closer insights, new things, exploring deeper mines than any yet, showing our humanity. (I sometimes put myself in fancy in the cot, with typhoid, or under the knife) tried by terrible, fearfulest tests, probed deepest, the living soul's, the body's

*tragedies, bursting the petty bounds of art. To these, what are your dramas
and poems, even the oldest and tearfulest? Not old Greek mighty ones, where
man contends with fate, and always yields; not Virgil showing Dante on and
on among the agonized and damned, approach that here I see and take part
in. For here I see, not at intervals, but quite always, how certain man, our
American man, how he holds himself cool and unquestioned master above all
pains and bloody mutilations. It is immense, the best thing of all, nourishes
me of all men. This then, what frightened us all so long! Why it is put
to flight with ignominy, a mere stuffed scarecrow of the fields.*

*O death where is thy sting? O grave where is thy victory? etc. In the Patent
Office, as I stood there one night, just off the cot-side of a dying soldier, in a
large ward that had received the worst cases of 2d Bull Run, Antietam and
Fredericksburgh, the surgeon, Dr. Stone, (Horatio Stone, the sculptor,) told
me, of all who had died in that crowded ward the past six months, he had
still to find the first man or boy who had met the approach of death with a
single tremor or unmanly fear. . . .*[4]

These observations throw some light on the much discussed question, What
is it that makes the American a good soldier? Walt Whitman saw something
in the military hospitals of the capital that convinced him that the Union
would stand the test. This something, as he expressed in his letter to the
Gray brothers, was ''how certain man, our American man, holds himself cool
and unquestioned master above all pains and mutilations.'' As an untrained
nurse, he noted ''that even moving around among the men, or through the
ward, of a hearty, healthy, clean, strong, generous-souled person . . . does
immense good.''

There were no trained nurses serving in the Civil War, but there were
many ''generous-souled'' persons who did much to comfort the sick and
wounded.

Nursing. The majority of women had lived in domestic seclusion since
the Fall of Rome. Women's place, it was believed, was in the home and the
social mold was such that she stayed in the home. In the South many large
southern homes were turned into private hospitals; the woman of the house
became nurse, administrator, and assistant to the medical staff. One such
hospital was established in Richmond, Virginia, under the supervision of
Louise Thompkins. Later an order placed all private hospitals under government control. Miss Thompkins disapproved of such an order and applied to
Pres. Jefferson Davis who appointed her to the rank of captain, making her
the only woman to hold a commission in the Confederate Army.

While the whole idea of war is abhorrent, the Civil War did offer opportunities for liberalizing women's legal and social freedom which today's
women take for granted. Dorothea Lynde Dix, at the outbreak of the war,
was perhaps the best known woman in political circles in the country. Because

---

[4] Together with a letter by Mark Twain, this letter appeared in the feature ''Two Civil
War Letters,'' *American Heritage*, Vol. VIII (New York, American Heritage Publishing
Co., 1957), pp. 63-64.

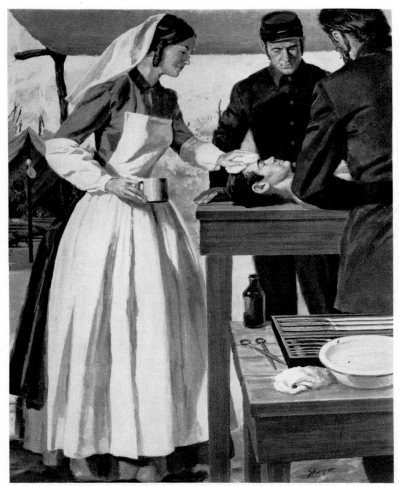

American nurses, without formal nursing education, assisted the military surgeons and cared for both Confederate and Union men near the battle areas.

of her records in humanitarian endeavors she was appointed Superintendent of Women Nurses in June, 1861, the first woman to be placed in charge of nursing forces in the United States. She was, however, unpopular with Army surgeons and nurses: Women from all parts of the country volunteered their services but Miss Dix preferred older, plain-featured women. She could not be convinced that young and lovely women could give conscientious care to the sick and wounded. Some that were refused applied directly to the Secretary of War and were accepted. Many young women went to camp with their husbands and remained to work in military hospitals.

The hospitals established by religious orders also cared for the injured.

In fact, the Roman Catholic sisterhoods provided most of the nursing care for both the North and the South. They nursed the sick and comforted the dying and justly earned the title Angels of the Battlefields. First the Sisters of Charity, founded by Mother Seton, and later other orders, had established hospitals in various parts of the country. The Sisters of Mercy had flourishing hospitals in Pittsburgh, Pennsylvania, and Chicago, Illinois; the Ursuline nuns had come to New Orleans under French occupation in 1739. By the time war was declared the sisterhoods had become well established.

No one nurse stands out from the Civil War as Florence Nightingale did from the Crimean War, but Mother Angela's work in the Union Army is comparable to that of Miss Nightingale. Mother Angela (Elisa Maria Gillespie) was director of St. Mary's Academy, Notre Dame University, in South Bend, Indiana, when war was declared. She at once organized a large group of sisters and hurried to the front where the need was most urgent; there she established field hospitals staffed by the Sisters of the Holy Cross.

During the first year of the war, supplies were inadequate and provisions for the nurses who cared for the sick were entirely lacking. Mother Angela had powerful influence in Washington because of her family connections and because of her work among the wounded. There were times when even generals could not obtain the necessary supplies—then Mother Angela would make a hurried trip to Washington and the necessary supplies were provided.

When the war broke out Mother Angela was forty-one and the work and strain of four years had sapped her strength. Yet in spite of this she devoted her remaining years to the founding of hospitals, orphanages, schools, and welfare institutions that still stand as monuments to this great woman.

Nursing throughout the Civil War was provided, in large part, by 2000 women whose only experience had been caring for their families. These dedicated women worked in both Union and Confederate hospitals.

Clara Barton, who has been immortalized as the founder of the American Red Cross, did actual nursing, although her greatest contribution was securing supplies, identifying the severely wounded and dead, and the establishment of the first national cemetery. Miss Barton, at her own expense, during the years 1865-1867 conducted a search for 80,000 missing men.

Louisa May Alcott, famed author of *Little Women*, was also a nurse in the Civil War. She described her work in *Hospital Sketches:*

My three days experience had begun with a death, and, owing to the defalcation of another nurse, a somewhat abrupt plunge into the superintendence of a ward containing forty beds, where I spent my shining hours washing faces, serving rations, giving medicine, and sitting in a very hard chair, with pneumonia on one side, diphtheria on the other, five typhoids on the opposite, and a dozen dilapidated patriots hopping, lying, and lounging about, all staring more or less at the new 'nuss' who suffered untold agonies . . . and blundered through her trying labors with a Spartan firmness. . . .[5]

Perhaps the most colorful of the lay nurses of the North was Mother Mary Bickerdyke who, as Mary Ann Ball of Galesburg, Illinois, had answered

---

[5] Louisa M. Alcott, *Hospital Sketches* (Boston, Roberts Bros., 1885), p. 28.

President Lincoln's call for nurse volunteers. Dr. J. J. Woodward, a surgeon of the 22nd Illinois Infantry, described Mother Bickerdyke in 1861: "A large heavy woman of forty-five years; strong as a man, muscles of iron, nerves of finest steel; sensitive, but self-reliant, kind and tender; seeking all for others, nothing for herself."[6]

The midwest was of strategic importance to the Union armies. The two points of greatest importance were Cairo, Illinois—where the Ohio joins the Mississippi—and Memphis, Tennessee—an important railroad center and river port. Soldiers sent to Cairo lacked proper commanders or physicians and the camp soon became a camp of sick recruits. This was the situation which faced Mother Bickerdyke on her first assignment which she proceeded to remedy with system and efficiency.

She cared for the wounded of nineteen hard-fought battles. Victor Robinson said concerning the battle of Fort Donaldson:

Mother amazed all who beheld her. She was commissariat, diet-kitchen, ambulance service, and nursing staff. . . . Blood-stiffened uniforms were removed and out of magic cabinets appeared clean, hospital garments. The frozen mire of the battleground was washed from bodies which never thought to rest in bed again, and hardened filth was sponged from clotted wounds. From everywhere in the boat came the incessant cry Mother! Mother! Mother! Mother!—and Mother was everywhere. A volunteer surgeon on the boat spoke for all when he said, "I never saw anything like her. To every man she turned with a heavenly tenderness, as if he were indeed her son."[7]

Her philosophy in caring for the sick was cleanliness and good food. The hospitals at Cairo and Memphis received food supplies from the government and the Sanitary Commission, but milk and eggs were brought from local merchants who charged exorbitant prices. Mother took a month's furlough and went north. In Chicago she met Jacob Strawn, the cattle king of Jacksonville, Illinois, and said, "I want cows," and from the Chicago Sanitary Commission she asked for chickens. She returned in triumph to Memphis with a hundred cows and a thousand chickens so that her boys could have fresh milk and eggs.

Mother Bickerdyke's natural gentleness turned into violent rage when she found the sick neglected or subject to injustice. Her clashes with Army officials and surgeons were quite dramatic. Once a surgeon who neglected the men assigned to him appeared at noon yawning from a night's debauch. Mother saw that he was given a dishonorable discharge. The surgeon appealed to General William T. Sherman who, upon learning who had accused the surgeon, said, "Then you are indeed out. She ranks me. There is nothing for you to do but to bring your case before President Lincoln."

Meanwhile, the Confederate Army had little or no training in military medicine, surgery, or sanitation, yet it was responsible for caring for more than three million persons in an invaded and blockaded country. According

---

[6] Beverly Maureen Thomann, Ripon, Wisconsin. Thesis on "Mary A. Bickerdyke," written while at Knox College, Galesburg, Illinois.

[7] Victor M. Robinson, *White Caps* (Philadelphia, J. B. Lippincott Co., 1946), pp. 187-188.

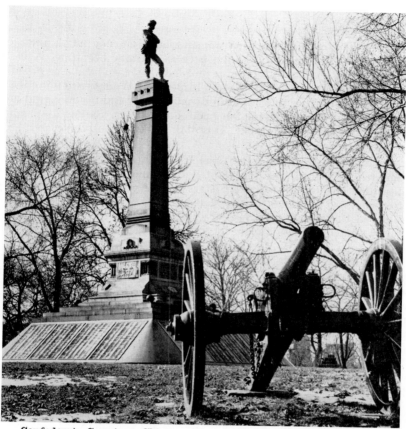

Confederate Cemetery, Chicago. Five thousand soldiers were buried in trenches here. They were prisoners of war in the Douglas Prison Camp, brought to Chicago from the battles of Shiloh and Vicksburg. (Courtesy of the ''South Town Economist,'' Chicago.)

to Joseph Jones of Georgia, a military hygienist, one-third of the 600,000 Confederate soldiers were either killed outright or died of disease.

From the standpoint of medical supplies the Confederacy was markedly unprepared for war. Chloroform, the magic fluid of the military surgeon, had to pass through the tightest blockade of the southern ports. It is interesting to note the medical substitutes that became common practice: the common Jamestown or Jimson weed was substituted for belladonna; colchicum was unavailable, so Indian poke juice was used when neither opium nor morphine could be obtained. American hemlock was used; and wild cherry and black root was used instead of digitalis.[8] Quinine was the prize item of the blockade runners and brought fabulous prices.

[8] For a description of pharmaceutical laboratories of the Confederacy see H. H. Cunningham, *Doctors in Gray* (Baton Rouge, La., Louisiana State University Press, 1958), Chap. 8.

To outwit the blockade, southern women would journey north and smuggle large quantities of quinine and opium back to military hospitals. A beautiful doll, for example, stuffed with quinine and listed as a gift for a crippled child, easily passed a sympathetic blockade inspector. Women would open their traveling bags for inspection, knowing that bags of opium and quinine were sewed among the many layers of hooped skirts. Mrs. Sallie Chapman Law, sponsor of the Southern Mothers' Hospital, was especially successful in her smuggling activities.

An outstanding southern nurse was Mrs. Ella King Newsom, known as the Florence Nightingale of the Confederate Army. She received intensive training from the medical staff and Sisters of Mercy at Memphis City Hospital. Mrs. Newsom was a woman of unusual organizational and executive ability who followed the retreating army, erecting and administering hospitals that were noted for cleanliness and good treatment.

The United States Sanitary Commission. The Army Medical Department entered the war unprepared. Its chief, Colonel Thomas Lawson, a veteran of the war of 1812, was still in command because there was no retirement law. He considered the purchase of medical books an extravagance and he is reported to have flown into a rage on learning that one Army post had two sets of surgical instruments.

The public demanded that something be done lest the sanitary horrors of the Crimean War of eight years before be repeated during the war in America. A group of New York women, led by Louisa Lee Schuyler and Dr. Elizabeth Blackwell, organized the Women's Central Association of Relief. Two other organizations, the Lint and Bandage Association and the Physicians and Surgeons of the Hospitals of New York, were also formed. Representatives of these groups went to Washington and formally requested that the Secretary of War appoint a sanitary commission. President Lincoln could see no special advantage in such an organization, and the senior surgeon considered the representatives a nuisance. In June, however, the War Department yielded to public demand, but with the understanding that the commission would never meddle with the regular troops. It was to work entirely as a volunteer organization.

The commission helped to get food and medical supplies to the Union Army and investigated conditions—especially sanitation, fresh water, and adequate diets—in military camps and hospitals. Fresh fruits and vegetables were supplied to prevent scurvy. Box-cars fitted with swinging beds to transport the wounded, and hospital steamboats operated on the Ohio and lower Mississippi rivers. The commission also organized local groups to make surgical dressings.

As the war continued the commission located missing men and reported the conditions of the wounded to their relatives. When the troops were demobilized at the end of the war the commission assisted men in returning to their homes.

Relief Societies of the South. Soldiers' aid and relief societies were organized early in the war. In some areas of the South each county had such associations. They collected linen, hospital shirts, lint, bandages, and food, all of which were supplied to purveyors who transported them to the nearest hospital. These relief societies were seldom organized on a statewide basis, although state aid societies were formed in Georgia, Alabama, Louisiana, and South Carolina. The funds of all of these societies were supplemented by state aid from the Confederacy.

The only relief society organized on a Confederacy-wide basis was the Association for the Relief of Maimed Soldiers whose objective was "to supply artificial limbs for all officers, soldiers, and seamen who have been maimed in the service of their country."

Prison Camps. A century of time has not softened the bitterness and disgrace felt about the cruelty of the prison camps maintained during the Civil War by the Union and the Confederacy.

Mackinlay Kantor, in his book, *Andersonville*, presented an authentic account of the Confederate prison at Andersonville, Georgia. It took him twenty years to collect data from reliable sources in order to bring to the American public an accurate story of this prison.

Northern camps were equally inhuman and merciless. Camps for the midwest were located in Illinois at Rock Island and Chicago. The camp for captured Southern officers was on an island in Lake Erie. The Chicago camp —called Camp Douglas because it was on the property of Senator Stephen A. Douglas—was used for the common soldier and covered sixty acres.

Conditions at Camp Douglas were comparable to those of Andersonville, but although no recent popular book has been written about these conditions *The Autobiography of Sir Henry Morton Stanley,* published in 1909, gave an eyewitness account of conditions at the camp. Stanley was captured at the battle of Shiloh in 1862 and was shipped with thousands of other Confederate prisoners to Chicago. Sir Henry Stanley wrote:

Our buildings swarmed with vermin, the dust-sweepings were alive with them. The men began to suffer from bilious disorders; dysentery and typhus began to rage. Day after day my company steadily diminished; and every morning I had to see them carried in their blankets to the hospital from whence none ever returned. . . .

Every morning the wagons came to the hospital and deadhouse, to take away the bodies; and I saw the corpses rolled in their blankets, taken to the vehicles, and piled one upon another, as the New Zealand frozen-mutton carcasses are carted from the docks. . . . It was the age that was brutally senseless, and heedlessly cruel. It was lavish and wasteful of life. . . . [9]

The annual meeting of the Civil War Round Table, a national organization, was held in October, 1959. At this meeting Timothy J. O'Connor, an ardent student of the Civil War said, "The conditions under which they died are

[9] Sir Henry Morton Stanley, *The Autobiography of Sir Henry Morton Stanley* (Boston and New York, Houghton Mifflin Co., 1909), pp. 208-211.

almost too horrible to believe today. Imagine these young Southern boys brought up from the Deep South with only a thin homespun or cotton uniform, required to face the rigors of the bitter cold winters on the shore of Lake Michigan with no heat, few blankets, and nothing to prevent the ravages of pneumonia and influenza.''

Postwar Nursing Leader. While the prison camps of the Civil War were stunning examples of ''man's inhumanity to man,'' and there were further examples of revengeful cruelty following the war, there was again evidence of man's good nature in the activities of such persons as St. Frances Xavier Cabrini.

Following the reconstruction period after the American Civil War, the United States embarked on an industrial expansion greater than the world had ever known. Iron ore was plentiful, coal was cheap, and the process for making steel had been improved. New factories were springing up everywhere and there was a need for cheap labor. The people of Italy, land-poor and hungry, were glad to fill the need. Immigration to the United States increased rapidly until by 1900 more than 20,000 Italians were entering each year; by 1910 there were 4,000,000 Italian immigrants living in the United States. Large numbers of Italians also took up residence in Brazil, Argentina, and other Latin American countries.

The newcomers were for the most part illiterate and desperately poor. Beset with language difficulties, as well as the hostility of many already established Americans, the Italians were able to find only jobs requiring heavy labor. Their work in railroad construction, mills, and factories often led to accidents and death. Both Pope Leo XIII and the Italian government were concerned about the conditions of Italians in the United States. When St. Frances Xavier Cabrini (1850-1917 A.D.), foundress of the Institute of Missionary Sisters of the Sacred Heart in Italy, asked for permission to open a mission school in China, the Pope directed her instead to the United States.

Mother Cabrini arrived in New York City in 1889 and promptly opened an orphanage for Italian children. She was a born ruler and an extraordinarily able woman; she founded schools in New York and, in 1892, opened Columbus Hospital, which accommodated Italian patients and was staffed by Italian nuns.

Through her initiative, schools, orphanages, and hospitals were opened in New Orleans, Denver and Seattle. In 1904 a second Columbus Hospital—this one in Chicago—was opened. Mother Cabrini did not limit her efforts to the United States, for she also helped provide education and hospital care for immigrant Italians in Panama, Brazil, and Argentina. Her work spread to Spain, France, and to her native Italy. In all, Mother Cabrini founded 67 institutions before her death in Chicago in 1917. She was canonized a saint in 1946.

THE SPANISH-AMERICAN WAR, 1898-1899

The Spanish-American War, although lasting only nine months, had far-reaching effects both on nursing and medicine.

While there had been serious rumors of war with Spain for three years, neither the American government nor the American Red Cross, which had been established in 1881, had organized a committee for war service. Indeed, the American Red Cross was prepared only to give relief in times of disaster and natural calamities, for at the time of its formation, the nation had believed there would be no more wars.

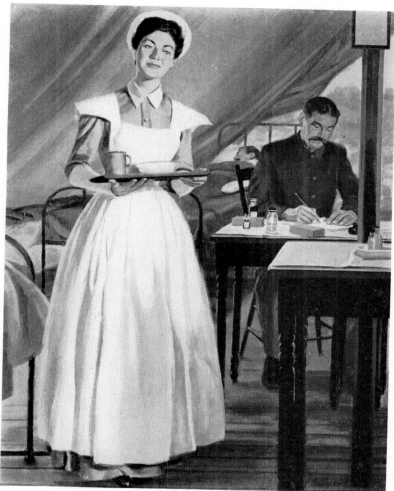

An American nurse in a field hospital in the Philippines
during the Spanish-American War.

The American Nurses' Association, organized in 1896, had a membership of 2000 graduate nurses in 1898. By February of that year, while the American press was giving wide coverage to the likelihood of war, the Army and Navy Departments began to receive applications from nurses offering their services in case of war.

When war did erupt, the Army and Navy were reluctant to use women nurses—there were few casualties, and these could be cared for by regular corpsmen. But the picture changed by June: Because of poor military sanitation, a typhoid epidemic was lashing throughout the American forces and yellow fever was taking a heavy toll of lives in Cuba. Nurses were urgently needed and welcomed by the Army and the Red Cross. They enrolled in the Red Cross and in the Army, although neither service was organized to place or house these nurses.

In the midst of this confusion Dr. Anita Newcomb McGee became the official head of nurses employed by the Army; these nurses later developed into the Army Nurse Corps. Dr. McGee occupied a high social and scientific position in Washington, D. C., and was a personal friend of Dr. George Sternberg, Surgeon General of the Army. As Vice-president General of the Daughters of the American Revolution, Dr. McGee had suggested that this organization form a Hospital Corps Committee. The Committee was formed and Dr. McGee was named chairman. Two weeks after hostilities began she offered the services of this committee to Dr. Sternberg who accepted them.

During the war, yellow fever became epidemic and required a different type of nurse. Since the cause of yellow fever was unknown it was impossible to know how to protect the nurse against the disease, although it appeared that once a person contracted and overcame the disease he developed an immunity to it. Therefore, a hundred women, mostly untrained but who had recovered from yellow fever, were employed to care for yellow-fever patients.

For twenty years Dr. Carlos Findlay, a Cuban physician, had strongly championed the idea that yellow fever was transmitted by the Aedes mosquito. Acting upon this suggestion, the United States Army Commission conducted experiments using human volunteers from the Army.

One of these volunteers was Clara Louise Maass, a graduate of Newark German Hospital Training School for Nurses, Newark, N. J. Miss Maass had been one of the first nurses to volunteer for the war and was assigned as contract nurse in Army camps in the United States and Cuba. Later the government issued an appeal for nurses in Manila where Miss Maass was assigned to the Field Reserve Hospital. By that time the war was over but the hospital was filled with men ill from typhoid, smallpox, and yellow fever. She cared for the men and remained in excellent health. In 1901 she returned to Cuba and was assigned to Las Animos Hospital where extensive research on the cause of yellow fever was being conducted. Miss Maass was interested in these experiments and volunteered to be bitten by a mosquito. This was not foolish bravado, for she had worked with yellow-fever patients for three years and had remained well, although she doubtless had been bitten by mosquitoes many times. She volunteered in June, 1901, and developed a slight attack of yellow fever, but this evidence was not conclusive. In August she volunteered again; this time she had yellow fever in a most virulent form and died ten days after the inoculation—a heroine to scientific investigation.

The confusion and bitterness of the war had made the government, the American Red Cross, and the American Nurses' Association aware that there should be a permanent, efficient army nursing service. In December, 1898, women of national distinction who had been active in war work, prominent nurses, and the faithful, politically influential Dr. McGee formed a Committee to Secure by Act of Congress the Employment of Women Nurses in the Hospital Service of the United States Army. The committee set about to prepare, in only two months, a bill to be introduced into Congress, where women had no vote. The bill failed to pass but the committee worked through 1900 and presented their bill to Congress in January, 1901. It was passed and signed one month later. Mrs. Dita H. Kinney became the head of the new Army Nurse Corps.

In the preparation of this bill Dr. McGee had discussed the subject of rank for Army nurses with the Surgeon General, but he was sternly opposed to such an innovation.

The Navy Nurse Corps was organized in 1901 and a bill recognizing it was introduced in Congress in 1903, but the final passage of the bill did not occur until 1908. Once again Dr. McGee helped in framing the bill and used her political influence to convince legislators of the benefits of such a corps in the Navy.

More than 1600 nurses served during the Spanish-American War. Of these there were ten fatalities, eight from typhoid fever. During the short duration of the war women nurses conclusively proved their worth, and it was their work that had an extremely important influence on further development of nursing.

REFERENCES

Revolutionary War:

BOLTON, CHARLES K.: *The Private Soldier Under Washington.* New York, Charles Scribner's Sons, 1902.

"DOCTORS OF THE REVOLUTIONARY WAR." *Today's Health* 39:24 (July) 1961. (Reprinted from *Spectrum Medical Journal,* published and copyrighted by Pfizer Laboratories.)

DOYLE, ANN: Nursing by religious orders in the United States, Part I. *Amer. J. Nurs.* 29:775 (July) 1929.

DUNCAN, LOUISE C.: *Medical Men in the American Revolution,* 1775-1783. Carlisle Barracks, Pa., Medical Field Service School, 1931.

DUNLOP, RICHARD: The doctor was a rebel. *Today's Health* 39:28 (July) 1961.

HARLOW, RALPH V.: *The United States from Wilderness to World Power.* New York, Henry Holt and Co., 1954, Ch. 1-12.

HURD-MEAD, KATE CAMPBELL: *A History of Women in Medicine.* Haddam, Connecticut, Haddam Press, 1938.

KLEES, Frederic: *The Pennsylvania Dutch.* New York, The Macmillan Co., 1950.

"TWELFTH CENTURY PHYSICIAN." J.A.M.A. 177:26 (July 8) 1961.

VATH, WILLIAM: Why George Washington never smiled. *Today's Health* 38:40 (Feb.) 1961.

Civil War:

ADAMS, GEORGE W.: *Doctors in Blue: The Medical History of the Union Army in the Civil War.* New York, Henry Schuman, Inc., 1952.

ALCOTT, LOUISA M.: *Hospital Sketches.* Cambridge, Mass., University Press, 1869.

BAKER, NINA B.: *Cyclone in Calico: The Story of Mother Bickerdyke.* Boston, Little, Brown and Co., 1952.

BETTMANN, OTTO: *Pictorial History of Medicine.* Springfield Ill., Charles C Thomas, 1956.

CUNNINGHAM, H. H.: *Doctors in Gray.* Baton Rouge, La., Louisiana State University Press, 1958.

DOCK, LAVINIA L., *et al.: History of American Red Cross Nursing.* New York, The Macmillan Co., 1922, Ch. 2.

HARLOW, RALPH V.: *The United States from Wilderness to World Power.* New York, Henry Holt and Co., 1953, Ch. 21-24.

JOLLY, ELLEN R.: *Nuns of the Battlefield.* Providence, R. I., Providence Visitor Press, 1929.

KANTOR, MACKINLAY: *Andersonville.* New York, World Publishing Co., 1955.

LIVERMORE, MARY A.: *My Story of the War: A Woman's Narrative of Four Years' Experience as a Nurse in the Union Army.* Hartford, Conn., A. D. Worthington Co., 1888.

LOWENFELD, WALTER: *Walt Whitman's Civil War.* New York, Alfred A. Knopf, Inc., 1960.

NUTTING, M. ADELAIDE, and DOCK, LAVINIA L.: *A History of Nursing.* New York, G. P. Putnam's Sons, 1935.

OATES, LOUISE: Civil War nurses. *Amer. J. Nurs.* 28:207 (Mar.) 1928.

TIFFANY, FRANCIS: *Life of Dorothea Lynde Dix.* Boston, Houghton Mifflin Co., 1890. Reprinted, 1934.

WALSH, JAMES JOSEPH: *These Splendid Sisters.* New York, J. H. Sears and Co., 1927.

WHITMAN, WALT: Civil War Letter. *American Heritage, Vol. VIII* (New York. American Heritage Publishing Co., 1957), pp. 63-64.

WILLIAMS, BLANCHE C.: *Clara Barton, Daughter of Destiny.* Philadelphia, J. B. Lippincott Co., 1941.

Spanish-American War:

"CLARA LOUISE MAASS." *Amer. J. Nurs.* 50:343 (June) 1950.

FLIKKE, JULIA O.: *Nurses in Action, A Story of the Army Nurse Corps.* Philadelphia, J. B. Lippincott Co., 1943.

GUINTHER, LEOPOLDINE: A nurse among the heroes of the yellow-fever conquest. *Amer. J. Nurs.* 32:173 (Feb.) 1932.

CHAPTER 13

The Two World Wars

WORLD WAR I, 1917-1918

Three weeks after President Woodrow Wilson signed a declaration of war with Germany and its allies on April 9, 1917, representatives of three national nursing organizations assembled in convention in Philadelphia, Pa. In a solemn, tense atmosphere they drafted the following resolution and sent it to President Wilson:

. . . We pledge our best to the nation wherever called upon to render it, either in home or foreign field, in the daily routine of civil or military hospital, or in the equally great effort to conserve, protect and strengthen the health and endurance of the citizen population, the men, women and children at home in our land.[1]

This was the nurses' pledge of allegiance to their country. Things happened quickly. During the course of that convention chief nurses of three base hospitals received instructions from the War Department to mobilize their units at once.

---

[1] "Editorial Comment, The Philadelphia Meetings," *The American Journal of Nursing,* Vol. 17 (June, 1917), pp. 761-65.

144

Like any other soldier, American nurses responded to the call. Within six weeks after war was declared, six base hospitals moved across the Atlantic Ocean, in which submarines were ploughing. American nurses were on the march to participate in "The War To End War." Along with the soldiers, the nurses entered the tragedy singing "And we won't come back till it's over over there."

But the mood of the singing soldiers with the wooden guns soon changed. Hospitals called "gangrene tents" started filling too fast with too many of their buddies. And there were no miracle drugs in that war—no sulfa, no penicillin—only morphine sulfate to help ease the pain. And there was one hazard that was nonexistent in World War II: poison gas (called "mustard gas" by British soldiers). This gas, present everywhere, produced such conditions as swollen eyes, shortness of breath, and inflammatory conditions of the body.

In the early part of the war there was only a handful of nurses available. The American Red Cross had the only available roster of nurses, consisting of 8000. The great allied offensive began four months after war was declared. And as the need for fighting men increased so did the need for nurses. In July, 1918, the Surgeon General of the Army called for 1000 nurses a week for eight weeks, and the nurses responded generously.

Although members of the three national nursing organizations had assembled in convention in Philadelphia to draft resolutions indicating the readiness of American nurses to serve in the war, they failed to design a wartime action program. Within a month, Miss Adelaide Nutting, dean of American nurses, called an informal meeting to organize a National Emergency Committee on Nursing. This Committee, within a short time, became the Committee on Nursing of the General Medical Board of the Council of National Defense. The purposes of the committee on nursing were:

To ascertain through a census the real nursing resources of the country; to find an effective way of making them readily available for service where needed; to increase the supply of pupils in training schools for nurses; to conduct a serious educational campaign with that end in view; to secure co-operation from hospitals in enlarging their training schools and teaching forces; to consider and advise upon problems of nursing as they may, from time to time, arise during the war.[2]

Despite the efforts of the committee to promote the interests of nursing and hospitals, some of the hospitals felt they were not consulted by the committee. This feeling introduced a somewhat difficult situation.

Both the Red Cross and the committee on nursing were urged to set up short courses in nursing but Miss Nutting and members of her committee realized that such a plan would have disastrous effects on both war and postwar health programs. They held steadfastly to the views that nursing no longer consisted of routine care, comfort, and custards; it required a scientific background and skills unknown in the Civil War and the Spanish-

---

[2] Mary M. Roberts, *American Nursing: History and Interpretation* (New York, The Macmillan Co., 1954), p. 131.

American War. To meet the nation's demands, three major projects were developed. Some nursing courses were shortened, the Army School of Nursing was established, and the Army Nurse Reserve Program was organized.

Mrs. John Wood Blodgett, a trustee of Vassar College, conceived the idea of shortening the nursing course to two years by enrolling college graduates. A twelve-week preliminary course in nursing was offered to graduates of approved colleges. More than 400 graduates of 115 colleges in the United States enrolled for the preliminary course and a high percentage enrolled for the two-year hospital affiliation. Following the signing of the Armistice on November 11, 1918, many of the nursing students left the school; however, 42 per cent remained to complete the course and at mid-century an impressive number could be called distinguished nurses.

Early in 1918 Annie Warburton Goodrich made a survey of nursing in military hospitals and recommended the establishment of a school of nursing by the United States Army. The recommendation was presented to the convention of the American Nurses' Association where it received concentrated attention by the House of Delegates. Approval of such a school was given, yet the Secretary of War, Newton D. Baker, refused to consider such a plan. But Mrs. Frances Payne Bolton, a member of the Committee of the Army Nurse School, was Mr. Baker's neighbor in Cleveland, Ohio. Through her influence, the Secretary granted a hearing to the Surgeon General of the Army, Miss Goodrich, and Mrs. Bolton. As a result of this meeting he gave his approval to the Army Nurse School which was opened in May, 1918. The school received more than 10,000 applications for admission. Assignments to military hospitals were discontinued in December, 1918, but the Army School of Nursing continued until 1931. The Army Nurse Reserve program—a cooperative project of the Women's Committee of the Council of National Defense, the National Association of Collegiate Alumnae, the Army, and the Red Cross—had as their objective the recruitment of 25,000 students for the Army and civilian schools of nursing. Circular letters were sent to high schools and to college graduating classes. Approximately 14,000 eligible candidates applied and there was a substantial waiting list when the Armistice was signed.

War Conditions. World War I was fought principally in trenches. Shrapnel, which was used extensively, caused deep, penetrating wounds that were ready culture for infections. Doctors Alexis Carrel and Henry Dakin devised a solution and an apparatus to irrigate these deep wounds; the solution is now called Dakin's solution.

Nurses were assigned to base hospitals, camp, evacuation, and mobile hospitals, as well as hospital trains. Many of the nurses served with surgical teams close to the front lines; those who served on hospital trains hastened the return of patients to the base hospitals or to hospitals in the United States if the patients had long-term conditions. The nurses who were assigned to base hospitals and camp units worked under the most primitive conditions in rain and mud, but through their own ingenuity they maintained principles of safe nursing.

The care of patients suffering from poison gas was a challenge to the nurse's powers of observation and technical competency. Shock, hemorrhage, and infection were less of a challenge to the nurse since she had had more experience in caring for such conditions.

Influenza Epidemic.   In the fall of 1918 a disease known as Spanish influenza reached pandemic proportions. It was the most destructive epidemic in history; in fact, it ranks with the plague of Justinian and the Black Death as one of the severest holocausts ever encountered. In the United States more than half a million people died. It discriminated against none: Both civilian and military personnel suffered a high morbidity and mortality rate. The disease was characterized by an acute inflammation of the throat and bronchi, with severe prostration, and usually complicated by pneumonia. Mary M. Roberts gives an apt description of this plague:

Transports buried many victims of "flu" at sea. One ship alone landed 2000 soldiers with "flu" and pneumonia at Southampton at a time when casualties from Flanders were pouring into hospitals of the AEF in Britain. . . . The incidence in France, however, was lower than the cantonment hospitals in the U. S., none of which escaped. The census of one 2000-bed hospital rose to 8000 and at a time when 90 of the 300 regular nurses were sick.[3]

Edith Cavell.   Edith Cavell (1865-1915) was an Englishwoman, daughter of the vicar of Swardeston, England. As a young teacher she became governess to four children in Brussels, Belgium, returning after five years to England to study nursing at the London Hospital.

In 1907 Dr. Antoine Depage, appalled by the lack of nursing in Brussels, opened the first school of nursing in Belgium and invited Miss Cavell to return as director of the nursing school *Ecole Belge des Infirmières Diplômées*. Within five years the school was furnishing graduate nurses for three hospitals, three private clinics, twenty-four public schools, and thirteen kindergartens.

When World War I began in July, 1914, Miss Cavell was offered a safe conduct to England but she chose to remain in Brussels which after twelve years was her home. When the city was captured by the Germans in August, 1914, Miss Cavell at once made plans to oppose the enemy. The German commander in charge of Brussels issued a directive that discharged male patients over eighteen years of age were to report at once to the German military police, which usually meant they would be sent to forced labor camps in Germany. To thwart this plan Edith Cavell arranged that when a young man was discharged, either she or the nurse in charge would direct him to the police or to the home of Mme. X, leaving the choice to the patient. If he chose to go to the home of Mme. X, she would hide him until some way was found to spirit him out of the city.

By late winter of 1914 wounded French and British soldiers were being cared for in the hospital and were helped to escape from there. Soon allied soldiers in disguise began coming to the hospital from all parts of Belgium. To befriend and hide these men was perilous work but it had to be done. Miss Cavell helped to organize an underground system whereby, when it was time for the soldiers to leave, guides would take them away in late afternoon or

---

[3] *Ibid.,* pp. 152-53.

at night in groups of four or five, disguised as laborers and carrying forged identification papers. Since the German guards at the border could not speak French, those crossing the border were seldom questioned.

By July, 1915, the Germans had become suspicious and had installed an inspector in the hospital to secure evidence against those involved in the conspiracy. Soon German detectives were added, and within a month the underground organization was crushed, Miss Cavell was imprisoned and held incommunicado, and her assistant, Sister Wilkins, denied all accusations. The police tried to trick Sister Wilkins into confessing that the school had given refuge to the enemy but she maintained that she knew nothing about the presence of these soldiers; although they had sufficient evidence that she was guilty, the police released her.

Miss Cavell made no effort to defend herself, she seemed to have lost interest in self-preservation. She signed a confession although she had not been persecuted or exhaustively questioned by the German police. Her ready answers and admission that she had helped some 200 soldiers to escape made it difficult for her attorney to defend her. During the court-martial she was asked why she had aided the English to escape; she replied that she thought the Germans would have shot them and she believed it was her duty to save their lives. She did not consider her activities to be espionage.

Miss Cavell was court-martialed on October 3, 1915, and was shot at 7:00 A.M. five days later. Before she was led out to the firing range she requested several safety pins, a strange request which was granted. Then she leaned down and carefully pinned her long skirts around her ankles—she did not want her skirts to flare up when she fell.

To the present-day student, the shooting of a woman is a horrible outrage, but this was war and mercy was an unknown word to either the allies or Germans. For as Edith Cavell said to the chaplain who remained with her during those last tragic moments, "I now know that patriotism is not enough; I must have no hatred and no bitterness toward anyone."[4]

Military Rank.   During the American wars nurses had been as essential as men but they had no rank or authority; their station was even below the grade of private. The nurse was responsible for the care of the patients in military hospitals, yet she had no authority to regulate hygienic conditions, care of patients, or the cleanliness of the wards and operating rooms, as is done in civilian hospitals. The American Nurses' Association made a request to the War Department for a definite status and authority for nurses. In reply to this request the War Department issued the following statement:

As regards medical and military matters in connection with the sick, members of the Army Nurse Corps and the Army Nurse Corps Reserve are to be regarded as having authority in matters pertaining to their professional duties (the care of the sick and wounded) in and about military hospitals next after the officers of the Medical Department and are at all times to be obeyed accordingly and to receive the respect due their position.[5]

[4] Helen Judson, *Edith Cavell* (New York, The Macmillan Co., 1941), p. 281.

[5] Lavinia L. Dock, *et al.*, *History of American Red Cross Nursing* (New York, The Macmillan Co., 1922), p. 1065.

But this regulation did not give the nurse authority beyond the person of the patient. Matters such as ventilation, light, temperature, sanitary conditions, and supplies were left up to the corpsmen who had rank.

Early in 1918 bills were introduced in both houses of Congress for commissioned rank for nurses. In April the House Committee on Military Affairs held its first meeting. The objective of the committee was to secure rank:

. . . in order to promote the efficiency of the nursing service of our boys by conferring upon the nurses some outward, visible sign of the authority which is supposed to be in them, a sign by virtue of which their instructions may be promptly carried out in the wards. For at present their authority to give orders is continually disputed by the enlisted men who serve as orderlies and friction and dangerous delays in the execution of orders result. We believe that the insignia of rank will give conclusive notice to all that nurses are officers and that they are to be obeyed.[6]

After conferring with General William C. Gorgas, who was not sympathetic toward commissioned rank for nurses, the legislative sponsors formulated and presented a bill, which provided for relative rank for nurses, as an amendment to the War Department's bill for reorganization. Relative rank was defined as quasi rank: it did not call for a commission; it did not carry the pay, allowances, or emoluments of absolute rank; and it made no attempt to confer the power of command incident to a line officer of similar grade. It did, however, give nurses the authority "as regards medical and sanitary matters and all work in the line of their duties; they shall have and shall be regarded as having authority in and about military hospitals next after the medical officers of the Army. . .''

The bill failed to pass due to the strong opposition of the War Department, but when nurses began to return from foreign service early in 1919, rank for nurses became the foremost issue of the demobilization period. During the summer and fall of 1919, nurses organized their forces with headquarters in Washington, D. C. Sara E. Parsons, nurse educator and war leader, volunteered her services and during the fall and winter of 1919-1920 brought to the attention of congressmen the experiences and privations to which nurses had been needlessly subjected overseas because of lack of rank.

At the time women did not have the right to vote, but their war experience made them aware of their influence with the people at home. They launched a campaign to solicit the aid of congress and used their political support as a weapon in the fight to have the bill giving rank to nurses passed.

This bill was introduced January 9, 1920, and for the next five months nurses and their friends pitted their influence against that of the powerful War Department. Both Houses of Congress passed the bill on May 28, 1920, bestowing relative rank on Army nurses. The bill was signed by President Woodrow Wilson on June 4, 1920.[7]

---

[6] *Ibid.*, p. 1066.

[7] The Canadian nurses in the Boer War (1899-1901) were given relative military rank upon the recommendation of the Surgeon General. Canada was the first country in all history to give military rank to nurses.

Influence of the War on Nursing. Wars cannot be justified but some of the beneficial results of World War I should be enumerated.

The 23,000 nurses who had served under the armed forces and the Red Cross returned home with a desire for change, a desire for a more liberal, independent status for nurses. When they returned home they witnessed radical changes in the American way of life, as well as in their professional practice. The standard of living was rising and a rural society suddenly became an urban society. Smaller homes were being built, with fewer servants being employed in the homes. These developments together with the advances in medicine increased the use of hospitals. This brought a drastic change in the practice of the private duty nurse, for they were now nursing in hospitals rather than in the homes.

The construction of more hospitals meant opening more nursing schools. Yet many of these nursing schools were without qualified nurse instructors. This situation created an imbalance in the types of services expected of nurses and those which they were prepared to render.

The fact that 29 per cent of the young men who were drafted were found to be physically unfit to serve in the armed forces was a shocking revelation, especially since much of their disability could have been prevented. The preventive aspects of their conditions created a tremendous demand for public health nurses. And nursing was not prepared to cope with the situation immediately, since nursing had always been closely allied with traditional medicine and traditional medicine had given little emphasis to public health, hygiene, and preventive medicine.

The important question at the time was how public health nurses could be prepared to carry out the newly expressed need for their services. In an attempt to answer this question a study of public health nurses at work as teachers and administrators was conducted. The findings of this study indicated that public health nurses should first be graduates of a basic course in nursing, then they should pursue special preparation in both the classroom and field work.

Again on the credit side of the war—if it can be said to have such a side— Americans lost much of their isolation and provincialism by learning the cultures of other countries. Two million men and 10,000 nurses, along with the Red Cross personnel, had gone to Europe. For most of them this was their first experience outside the continental United States, and as a result their horizons were greatly widened as had been the case with the Crusaders of the eleventh and thirteenth centuries.

Great, gapping shrapnel wounds gave impetus to surgeons and dentists to develop new methods of treatment. Faces that had lost all semblance of humanity were reconstructed and the art of plastic surgery lost its connotation of vanity and became regarded as reconstructive surgery. Intensive on-the-spot research was done in skin grafting, and orthopedic surgery made great strides. Plaster casts were molded and applied so that badly injured men could be returned safely to the United States.

When the war ended there were at least 33,000 nurses in the Army and another 6000 nurses in the Navy. Of this number about 24,000 had been in actual war service. Their patient census was staggering compared with what these nurses had known in civilian nursing. Forty-nine thousand men were killed in action, 59,000 died of disease, and 237,135 were wounded. Major Julia Stimson said, "Never before had such a thing occurred, the sending across three thousand miles of danger-strewn seas ten thousand soldier-women to be part of a great expeditionary force."

The United States Government gave little recognition to the nurses, but the nurses knew that their work was well done and the gratitude of the men was rewarding. This gratitude was shown in a practical way when the bill for rank for nurses was introduced and passed without nurses being able to cast a single vote.

WORLD WAR II, 1941-1945

At 7:55 A.M., December 7, 1941, a thunderous sound suddenly roared over a nurse's cottage in Pearl Harbor, Hawaii. There was no mistaking what it was. It was the sound of guns and the increasing drone of planes—Japanese bombers. Hastily, Lieutenant Gertrude B. Arnest, chief nurse of the Pearl Harbor Naval Hospital, adjusted her white cap with its two gold stripes indicating her rank and walked resolutely across the shell-furrowed lawn to the hospital. Anti-craft shells fell around her and shrapnel whistled close by. World War II had begun for the United States.

Like Lieutenant Arnest, the other nurses on duty at the Pearl Harbor Hospital and those aboard the hospital ship *Solace* swung into action; within a few hours many of these nurses were boarding transports to care for the wounded who were being transferred to the States. It was this speed in giving care to the wounded that reduced the Army's death rate from 8.1 per cent in World War I to 3.3 per cent in World War II.

As the days wore on and the war picture grew darker, nurses brought into full play all of their creativity and vigor to endure the hardships in the European theater of war, which included North Africa, and in the Pacific theater of operation, which included the East Indies, the Philippines, and the southern Asiatic countries. Nurses helped to create the open-air hospital in the jungle on Bataan, and also the tunnel hospital in Corregidor. In these tunnels they cared for the sick and wounded round the clock until they were driven out by the Japanese or captured. Although the captured nurses were in weakened conditions, they continued to give as much care as possible to their fellow prisoners.

High Moments. Those who escaped imprisonment underwent the tense and exciting experience of being taken to Australia by submarine. Equally exciting was the landing under fire of Army nurses on the beaches of Anzio, Italy, where they dug their own foxholes. Navy nurses were the first white women ever to enter Tinian in the Marianas.

What was nursing like up close to the front lines? Theresa Archard, captain of the Army Nurse Corps and author of *G.I. Nightingale: The Story of an Army Nurse,* gives a realistic picture of nursing in a unit near the front lines in North Africa. This scene could be duplicated in scores of battles in both the European and Pacific theaters of war:

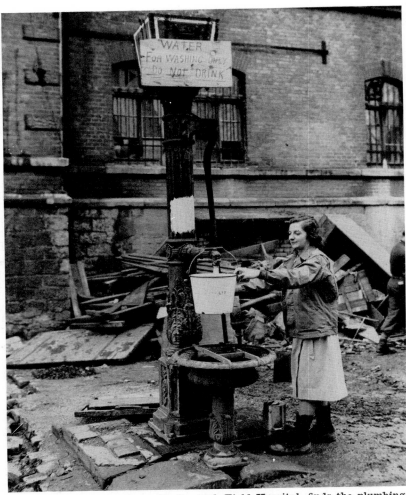

An army nurse, serving with the 10th Field Hospital, finds the plumbing system not always the best as she pumps water from an open pump to be used for washing, February, 1945. (U.S. Army photograph.)

March 26, Friday. It was two o'clock in the afternoon hot as blazes when we arrived at our next hospital area, two miles from Gafsa. The boys were still fighting there. Our trucks were lined up by the side of the road—not too far over, as only a certain number of feet had been cleared of mines. . . .

As the area was cleared, tents were erected. . . . Nearest the entrance was the receiving tent, where all patients were admitted. Homemade tables in the center held our sterile supplies, blood pressure apparatus, and whatever was needed to reinforce dressings on patients who were not to be admitted but were to be sent back to the evacuation hospitals. Directly back of these tents

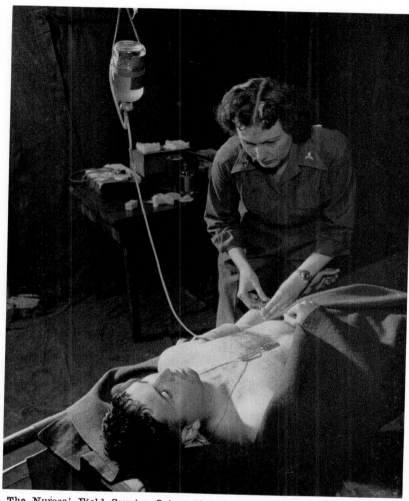

The Nurses' Field Service Orientation Course conducted at the Medical Training School, Degerndorf, Germany, June, 1952. (U.S. Army photograph.)

were the shock wards. . . . These wards were for patients too badly wounded to be operated on at once. The operating tents were over to the side of the resuscitation tents, with preoperative and X-ray and ward tents, holding all the supplies not in use—plasma, saline, extra blankets, enamelware, and surgical instruments. And finally, the kitchen and special-diet tents were set up as near to the wards as possible, but that was an eighth of a mile away.

Within an hour and a half we were ready to operate. Patients were coming in. Badly wounded boys—the worst yet—serious belly wounds from mine explosions, head and chest wounds. The head wounds were really bad, brains

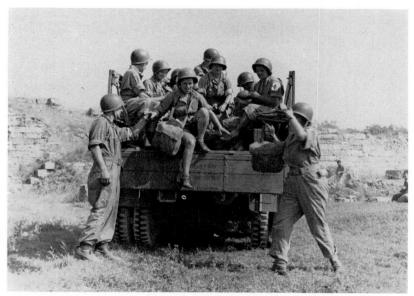

Nurses of an evacuation hospital arriving in Paestum, Italy,
September, 1943. (U.S. Army photograph.)

*oozing from some of them. The sucking chest wounds gave up frothy, bright
red blood with each expiration.*

*This time it was not a question of receiving ten or twenty patients at a time.
Sometimes as many as twenty ambulances pulled up every few hours, which
usually meant eighty patients. . . . The admitting officer decided what was to
be done to each patient. If he needed an operation he went to the preoperative
tent and waited his turn. In the meantime, he was fluoroscoped and the site
of the shell fragment marked, so that no time would be lost in the operating
room.*

*Those operating rooms! Ten tables going night and day, no sleep for the
doctors—they worked the clock around. . .*

*Abdominal cases, bad ones, had to have suction or Wangensteen tubes. . . .
Ours were made of empty saline bottles, and we used the extra tubing from
plasma sets. Dozens of these Wangensteens were going at one time, easing
the pain of abdominal wounds, but we had only eight standards. . . . I had a
corpsman sink four extra tentpoles along the side of the beds toward the
head. To the top of the poles he strung wire, the ends of which were counter-
sunk to afford greater stability. It worked wonderfully. Sometimes as many
as twenty bottles were suspended from that wire.*

*Those tents were something to see—a double row of beds or cots in each tent,
sixteen beds or twenty to twenty-five cots. There were no tables, chairs, or
miscellaneous furniture. A packing case served as cupboard, desk, and catch-
all. Our chlorinated water supply stood there in five gallon cans. One little*

potbellied stove was in the middle of the tent, and on this we heated water for baths and hot water bottles.[8]

Aero-Medical Nursing. In World War II, graduates of a relatively new nursing specialty, aero-medical nursing, also worked close to the front lines. Specially trained flight nurses, the first of any nation to be so prepared, gave immediate care to the sick, injured, and wounded soldiers. These flight nurses traveled to the battle fronts in aircraft which served a dual function: it carried cargo and troops from its base to the front lines and, after unloading, was quickly converted into an ambulance. The cabin of the plane became the nurse's hospital ward. Her patients were arranged on litters in tiers of three to four patients on either side of the center aisle.

Treating patients in the air at an altitude of 10,000 feet was a challenge to the flight nurse all the way. She gave care to patients with head injuries, chest injuries, abdominal wounds, shock, malaria and various anemias. In treating all of these patients, the flight nurse had to understand and be able to apply the principles of aero-medical physiology and therapeutics. As Captain Leora B. Stroup explains, two of these principles related to reduced atmospheric pressure: "the decrease in oxygen pressure with consequent lowering of the oxygen saturation of the blood and the expansion of air or gas trapped in any of the cavities of the body."[9] It was the flight nurse's responsibility to recognize these conditions and to treat them promptly. Records attest the efficiency of the flight nurse in World War II: Of the 173,527 sick, injured, and wounded patients evacuated in 1943, only eleven of the air-borne patients died during flight.

Psychiatry and Psychiatric Nursing. Men were screened for mental illness at induction centers and again in military camps. Those in combat areas who were found to be disturbed were transferred to quieter zones or given a medical discharge. The shell shock of World War I was now known to be fatigue more than shock and a careful therapy of narcosis was instituted. This was a deep, prolonged sleep of fifteen to twenty hours a day for several days. As a man became rested physically his nervous system became tranquil, and he usually recovered completely.

Medical Conditions. Military sanitation was based on sound principles that could be carried out under primitive conditions. The mobile military hospitals followed close behind the battle lines and were staffed by nurses and corpsmen. They were wonders of efficiency which could be set up and ready to receive hundreds of patients within two hours.

The sulfonamides, discovered by Gerhard Domagk, had been refined and doctors and nurses were accustomed to their use in combating infections. However, the sulfa drugs were not enough. It was then that the aspects of a mold, *Penicillium notatum*, discovered by Dr. Alexander Fleming of

---

[8] Theresa Archard, *G. I. Nightingale: The Story of an American Army Nurse* (New York, W. W. Norton & Co., 1945), pp. 96-98.

[9] Leora B. Stroup, "Aero-Medical Nursing and Therapeutics," *The American Journal of Nursing*, Vol. 44 (June, 1944), pp. 575-77.

England in 1929, were further investigated by Dr. Howard Florey of Oxford University. Dr. Fleming had shown that the mold inhibited the growth of staphylococcus, but it was the necessity of war that furnished the impetus to assay the drug and establish the dosage. In 1941 the United States started manufacture of the first antibiotic. The huge distilleries at Peoria, Illinois, were used for emergency production.

Intensive research in blood replacement had been conducted and the use of whole blood was a well-standardized procedure. The storage of whole blood had been instituted in 1930, and seven years later the first American blood bank was established at Cook County Hospital, Chicago, Illinois. Early in

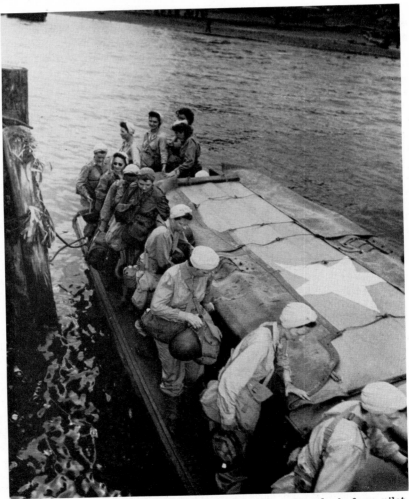

First nurses to arrive in New Britain prepare to disembark from pilot boat to proceed to their station at 251 Station Hospital, Borgen Bay Area, July, 1944. (U.S. Army photograph.)

1941, research was begun on the use of dried plasma, and banks for processing and storing both plasma and whole blood were established.

One of the major activities of the American Red Cross was the Blood Donor Service which collected and shipped enormous quantities of plasma to areas of combat in all parts of the world. Whole blood was processed and flown to Europe and the Orient where it was given to patients directly. These blood-collecting stations were supervised by especially trained Red Cross nurses.

The greatest cause of severe illness and death in the Pacific area was malaria. Unfortunately, our principal source of quinine was from the East Indies, especially Java, and the enemy quickly cut off this supply. As a result, American soldiers who had built up no previous immunity were soon violently ill from all forms of malaria. Biochemists from the United States and England, in their search for another means of combating malaria, investigated quinacrine, and acridine dye, developed in Germany in 1930. Their investigation led to the development and installment of quinacrine as a specific for malaria.

These were the conditions under which American soldiers—men and women —lived and worked during World War II. What were the nursing leaders doing on the home front when the war broke out? How did they participate in the war efforts?

Steps to Avert Crisis. It cannot be said that nursing leaders were asleep at the helm when Gertrude B. Arnest and her nurses suddenly had to cope with a surprise attack by the Japanese at Pearl Harbor. America's nursing leaders had their fingers on the international pulse and when its beat became irregular, they took decisive steps to prepare for any emergency.

Early in 1940, leaders in the American Nurses' Association and Red Cross began to take steps toward preparedness. On May 12, 1940, the American Nurses' Association, the National League for Nursing Education, and the National Organization for Public Health Nursing held a joint convention in Philadelphia. Their main concern was nursing preparedness if the United States should enter the war.

The following month, Julia C. Stimson, president of the American Nurses' Association, called together a group of nurses representing the American Red Cross Nursing Service, the five national nursing organizations, and the Federal agencies concerned with nursing resources—Army Nurse Corps, Navy Nurse Corps, and the United States Public Health Service. This meeting resulted in the establishment of the Nursing Council of National Defense. After war was declared the council was broadened and the name changed to the National Council for War Service. The objectives of the council were to determine the use of nurses if war were declared and to unify all nursing activities related to the war. This involved a study of actual nursing resources without disrupting the schools of nursing or essential public health nursing services. The work in the planning stage was directed by Ida F. Butler.

In October, 1940, Mrs. Elmira Bears Wickenden was appointed executive secretary of the council. Her staff began working on two projects: making a national survey of available nurses, and securing federal funds for nursing education.

The survey of nursing resources was carried out through the American Nurses' Association, with each state nurses' association assuming responsibility through the district associations. Both the Red Cross Nursing Service and the United States Public Health Service aided in this survey. When it was completed it was found that almost 100,000 nurses were eligible (unmarried and under age forty) for military duty, and 25,000 inactive nurses could be available for full-time civilian duty.

The second project—to secure federal funds for nursing education—was as essential as the survey of nursing resources. Schools of nursing had suffered from the depression of 1929, and few had facilities that were adequate. Schools needed funds to increase their instructional staffs and to provide housing for greatly increased student bodies.

This request for assistance to nursing was made through the U. S. Public Health Service. Congresswoman Frances Payne Bolton, that good friend of nursing in World War I, used her influence in convincing Congress that an appropriation was necessary. That Congress did appropriate $1,250,000 in 1941 and $3,500,000 the next year clearly indicated that nurses and lay people should work cooperatively in nursing for the good of both the military service and the community.

U. S. Cadet Nurse Corps. To reopen the Army Nurse School of World War I was not considered in World War II. The National Nursing Council for War Service decided instead to offer nursing education in the existing schools rather than in a new central school. Money had been appropriated to schools for preparation of instructors, classrooms, laboratories, and nurses' residences. To increase greatly the student enrollment Mrs. Bolton successfully sponsored a second bill in Congress that created the U. S. Cadet Nurse Corps. To encourage recruitment in this corps, the council used as its slogan, "Join a Proud Profession."[10]

The Cadet Nurse Corps was placed under the Division of Nurse Education of the U. S. Public Health Service. The government gave scholarships to young women who met the requirements both of the nursing schools to which they applied and of their state boards. Approximately 95 per cent of all nursing students during this period were members of the Cadet Nurse Corps, and they proudly wore the becoming uniforms of gray and scarlet (see page 172 for description of uniform). The total enrollment was 179,000. The first two schools to enroll were the Freedman (Negro) and Providence (Catholic) of the District of Columbia; the University of Minnesota School of Nursing had the largest enrollment. Mrs. Lucile Petry Leone headed the Cadet Nurse Corps with the title of director, Division of Nurse Education, U. S. Public Health Service.

Permanent Rank for Nurses. The struggle for military rank following World War I had ended with the granting of relative rank. Although nurses

---

[10] Editorial: "A Proud Profession," *The American Journal of Nursing*, Vol. 44 (June, 1944), pp. 525-26.

had not been satisfied with this, it was better than nothing, and it did give them the authority to get things done.

When mobilization for World War II began the government recognized the need for trained women who could release more men for combat duty. Women participating in the military services were given an average of four months' training. They were not an integral part of the military services, but they were given the equivalent rank of enlisted personnel, noncommissioned, and commissioned officers. This spurred the American Nurses' Association to introduce legislation to give nurses comparable standing. In December, 1942, both the Army and Navy Nurse Corps were given relative rank with the same pay and allowances as officers of comparable rank in other services. In 1944, both services were given commissioned rank "for the duration and six months." Nurses are a determined and influential group. From 1917 to 1947, a period of thirty years, they had worked for permanent, commissioned rank. On April 16, 1947, an act was signed which provided permanent commissioned rank for both Army and Navy nurses.

Draft for Nurses. Nurses enrolled quickly and generously for war service. When the war was over the American Red Cross had certified 104,500 nurses for military duty and 70,500 had been assigned. This was a proud record since the survey of nurses in 1943 showed the total number of active nurses, exclusive of those in service, was only 171,000.

The Navy had well-trained corpsmen and required only three nurses for each thousand naval and marine personnel, but the needs of the Army were much greater. The War Department rationed nurses in the ratio of six nurses to each 1000 troop strength. The Army's planning figure was 51,000 by June 1944.

By September of that year 30,000 sick and wounded men were being returned from overseas military hospitals each month. Both military and civilian hospitals were seriously understaffed. The Surgeon General of the Army became more insistent that enough nurses be secured to provide adequate care for his men. Although 27,000 more nurses had been classified as I-A by the Procurement and Assignment Service, the War Department had not indicated that these were needed until the Battle of the Bulge, late in 1944. Time was needed to separate these nurses from their present positions, outfit them, and transport them over 3000 to 5000 miles of ocean to the war areas. The Surgeon General, however, believed that recruitment had failed and he appealed to the President of the United States.

President Franklin D. Roosevelt's message to Congress on January 6, 1945 stated in part:

One of the most urgent immediate requirements of the armed forces is more nurses. . . . It has been estimated by the War Manpower Commission that 27,000 additional nurses could be made available without interfering too seriously with the needs of the civilian population for nurses. Since volunteering has not produced the number of nurses required, I urge that the Selective Service Act be amended to provide for the induction of nurses into the Armed Forces. . . .[11]

---

[11] Mary M. Roberts, *American Nursing: History and Interpretation* (New York, The Macmillan Co., 1954), p. 376.

Nursing made the headlines. Public opinion was aroused. Some considered it the only feasible method of securing enough nurses. But nurses regarded this as an affront to their already generous response. But on either side of the argument nurses were essential. The government gave no concern to the fact that the WAAC, WAVES, and SPARS had not reached their quotas.

The American Nurses' Association and the National Nursing Council for War Service immediately called a meeting with thirty-two states represented. This meeting endorsed the principle of a draft for nurses as the first step toward Selective Service in a general mobilization of all women. Two bills were introduced and both passed the House of Representatives by a large majority. The Senate, nevertheless, was reluctant to vote for the conscription of women.

As the hearing on these bills began the Army announced that the nurse enrollment had increased by 20,000 and conscription was not necessary. Many nurses were caught in the conflict between civilian needs and military needs, but the call of the President of the United States influenced the decision, and nurses volunteered by the thousands.

World War II closed without agreement on conscription by the American Nurses' Association. It was the police action in Korea that forced the decision. Nurses realized that only nurses could care for the sick and wounded. During the convention held in 1952 the House of Delegates of the American Nurses' Association authorized its board of directors to approve legislation for Selective Service for nurses if a national emergency made the introduction of such legislation necessary.

Aside from the gallantry and heroism displayed by nurses in World War II, their contribution to patient care had a tremendous influence on the recovery of patients fresh from the front lines, but it also had a marked influence on civilian nursing as it is practiced today. Nursing technics and practices have undergone vast changes since the Pearl Harbor attack. For example, the simple bed bath, which has always been considered to be the epitome of good nursing, has been reluctantly turned over to others. Professional nurses have hesitated to assign this procedure to auxiliary workers, because time spent in giving the patient's bath was used to establish rapport with the patient. In fact, professional nurses have experienced feelings of guilt when turning this procedure over to other personnel, but this had to be done so that the professional nurse could devote her time to more complicated procedures, many of which were previously performed by physicians.

The team concept and patient-centered care are also methods devised since World War II to help patients help themselves. Along with the concepts of psychosomatic medicine came early ambulation. And as the hospitalization period became shorter, doctors and nurses began to see hospitalization as just one phase of patient care.

Perhaps the most important outcome of the nurse's participation in World War II has been the development of the concept of creative nursing, a factor which has necessitated the need for launching definitive studies of all aspects of nursing, thus helping to raise the standards to a professional level.

REFERENCES

World War I:

ASHBURN, P. M.: *A History of the Medical Department of the United States Army.* Boston, Houghton Mifflin Co., 1929.

CLAYTON, S. LILLIAN, and JAMMÉ, ANNA C.: The training schools and the present crisis. *Amer. J. Nurs.* 17:1082 (Aug.) 1917.

DELANO, JANE A.: The need of increased enrollment. *Amer. J. Nurs.* 17:1092 (Aug.) 1917.

DOCK, LAVINIA L., *et al.: History of American Red Cross Nursing.* New York, The Macmillan Co., 1922.

DOLAN, JOSEPHINE A.: *Goodnow's Nursing History,* 10th ed. Philadelphia, W. B. Saunders Co., 1958.

Editorial: The epidemic of influenza. *Amer. J. Nurs.* 19:83 (Nov.) 1918.

FLIKKE, JULIA O.: *Nurses in Action: Story of the American Nurse Corps.* Philadelphia, J. B. Lippincott Co., 1943.

GAGE, NINA D.: Organization of class work and student life at the Vassar training camp. *Amer. J. Nurs.* 19:18 (Oct.) 1918.

GREELEY, HELEN HOY: Rank for nurses. *Amer. J. Nurs.* 19:840 (Aug.) 1919.

HARLOW, RALPH V.: *The United States from Wilderness to World Power.* New York, Henry Holt and Co., 1953, Ch. 37-40.

HOEHLING, A. A.: *A Whisper of Eternity—The Mystery of Edith Cavell.* New York, Thomas Yoseloff, Inc., 1957.

JAMMÉ, ANNA C.: The Army School of Nursing. *Amer. J. Nurs.* 18:179 (Nov.) 1918.

KERNODLE, PORTIA B.: *The Red Cross Nurse in Action.* New York, Harper & Bros., 1949.

"A last message from Edith Cavell." *Amer. J. Nurs.* 17:472 (Mar.) 1917.

ROBERTS, MARY M.: *American Nursing: History and Interpretation.* New York, The Macmillan Co., 1954, Sect. 4.

SCOVIL, ELISABETH ROBINSON: Narratives from the war. *Amer. J. Nurs.* 17:143 (Nov.) 1917.

Letter to Editor: The signing of the Armistice. *Amer. J. Nurs.* 19:339 (Feb.) 1919.

STIMSON, JULIA C.: *Finding Themselves.* New York, The Macmillan Co., 1927.

World War II:

ARCHARD, THERESA: *G. I. Nightingale: The Story of an American Army Nurse.* New York, W. W. Norton and Co., 1945.

BEEBE, GILBERT W., and DEBAKEY, MICHAEL E.: *Battle Casualties, Incidence, Mortality, and Logistical Considerations.* Springfield, Ill., Charles C Thomas, 1952.

BOLTON, FRANCES PAYNE: Home from ETOUSA. *Amer. J. Nurs.* 45:5 (Jan.) 1945.

Editorial: The Army Nurse Corps. *Amer. J. Nurs.* 45:86 (Jan.) 1945.

Editorial: Activities on the home front. *Amer. J. Nurs.* 44:1110 (Dec.) 1944.

Editorial: All the way—as volunteers? *Amer. J. Nurs.* 45:253 (Apr.) 1945.

Editorial: A proud profession. *Amer. J. Nurs.* 44:525 (June) 1944.

EISENHOWER, DWIGHT D.: *Crusade in Europe.* New York, Doubleday and Co., 1948.

JOSE, MARY: Hi, angels. *Amer. J. Nurs.* 45:267 (Apr.) 1945.

Letters from Readers: Men nurses in military service. *Amer. J. Nurs.* 43:1038 (Nov.) 1943.

PYLE, ERNIE: *Here Is Your War.* New York, Henry Holt and Co., 1943.

ROBERTS, MARY M.: *American Nursing: History and Interpretation.* New York, The Macmillan Co., 1954, Ch. 30, 32-37.

RICHARDSON, HENRIETTA: Skyway nursing. *Amer. J. Nurs.* 44:102 (Feb.) 1944.

STROUP, LEORA B.: *Aero-medical nursing and therapeutics. Amer. J. Nurs.* 44:575 (June) 1944.

WECTER, DIXON: The Age of the Great Depression. In *History of American Life,* Vol. XIII. New York, The Macmillan Co., 1948.

CHAPTER 14

Nurses' Uniforms

It is natural that since men and women usually try to present an attractive appearance they will be especially interested in their appearance when caring for the sick. Therefore the history and development of nurses' uniforms has personal appeal to students who will soon be wearing the latest model in a choice of the newest materials.

The history of uniforms is principally the history of dress in general, except in the case of the European religious orders. These habits[1] have been maintained through centuries by tradition, and to change them has been difficult. The late Pope Pius XII, however, advocated changes in the habits for sanitary and safety reasons, and many American and European orders have set about to make the suggested alterations.

UNIFORMS AND EARLY CHRISTIANITY

While there is no record in ancient history that those who cared for the sick wore a particular style of dress, it is reasonable to suppose that the men who assisted the priest-physicians in the Egyptian hospitals and in the Greek sanatoriums wore some sort of garment to distinguish them in their work.

---

[1] It is believed that use of the word "habit" when referring to clothing originated with Shakespeare.

Early Christianity stressed social service and public health as penance for sin and as a means by which heavenly reward was guaranteed. Men known as deacons and women known as deaconesses carried on this work, but did not wear a distinctive dress.

When the Roman Emperor, Constantine the Great, granted religious tolerance to Christians in 313, immediately there was a great outpouring of religious zeal and charitable work among the wealthy and aristocratic. But instead of adopting a special uniform, these men and women wore the rich-flowing robes of the times.

This era was followed by a period of asceticism, or self-denial, which strongly influenced social life and personal hygiene. This attitude continued into the twentieth century. Asceticism lauded neglect of the body and condemned worldly pursuits, enabling a person to devote time to prayer and meditation. Multitudes of men and women secluded themselves in monasteries and convents where they devoted their lives to these pursuits and, frequently, to the care of unfortunates. This self-denial was especially evident in clothing, which usually consisted of a simple, coarse, homespun garment. The women wore caps covering their entire head to hide their hair, thought to be a woman's crowning glory.

Following the fall of Rome in 476 A.D., monastic orders for women grew in number as a place for protection and for the promotion of Christianity. These were difficult times for the many women who had been left homeless and widowed by frequent wars; the monastery offered a home and security. Many women of wealth and influence founded monasteries and became the heads of the institutions. These women were well known abbesses, or mothers, and have been noted for their excellent executive ability. Since they were women of wealth and had known nothing else, they continued to wear the rich ornate dress of the times. Their robes make the uniform or habit of the present-day director of nurses appear ascetic by comparison. Pictures of these regal dignitaries as they attended affairs of state or church functions can be found in histories and art galleries.

These convents were not enclosed, nor was there a compulsory form of dress. It is recorded that in 1140 a Bavarian monk protested to the Pope about the dress of religious women; he suggested that these women wear a distinctive dress by which they could be distinguished from other women of the town.

MILITARY NURSES DURING THE CRUSADES

For six centuries before the Crusades, all good Christian Europeans aspired to make a pilgrimage to the Holy Land, and the Moslems who held this area welcomed the tourist trade. Hostels, or inns, along the route developed into great institutions to welcome the wayfarer and to care for those who were wounded by bandits or who became ill. These institutions were staffed by monks who had had military training. Although the monks fought those who molested the pilgrims, they cared for all who were injured, whether friend or foe.

During the second century of the Crusades, numerous orders of knights were formed to meet the needs for first-aid stations and hospitals. These orders, offering adventure, chivalry, a uniform, and an opportunity for self-sacrifice in a religion that encouraged charity and self-denial, appealed to young Christians.

The best known of these orders were the Knights Hospitallers of St. John of Jerusalem,[2] the Teutonic Knights Hospitallers, the Knights Templars, and the Knights of St. Lazarus.

All the orders active during the Crusades bore the cross of Christ, but in the various orders the color and form of the cross differed as did the robe and cloak. This differentiation is comparable to the distinction made in the uniforms of our present military services.

When in battle the knight wore a coat of mail under his monastic robe. The uniform for those in the order of St. John of Jerusalem was a red robe with a black cloak, on which was sewed an eight-pointed star.[3] The Teutonic Knights Hospitallers wore a black habit covered by a white cloak bearing a black cross on the left shoulder. The Knights Templars, founded in 1118, wore the mantle of Aesculapius over their armor to indicate that they were both warriors and nurses.

NURSING ORDERS OF THE LATE MIDDLE AGES

The late Middle Ages was characterized by great epidemics, and the ever-present leprosy affected people throughout Europe. Infanticide and abandoned children were equally great social evils. Although Christianity was a thousand years old, its members seemed unable to grasp the concept of everyday charity as a means of developing a better social order.

Late in the twelfth century two young, well-to-do men, St. Dominic in Spain and St. Francis in Italy, developed mendicant, or begging orders, to assist in caring for the poor. The men who joined these orders were called Dominicans and Franciscans. The Dominicans wore a black cape and attached hood over a robe of white wool. Because of this cape, they were called the Black Friars. St. Francis, suddenly realizing the useless life he had been living, impulsively donned a peasant's robe of rough woolen cloth and tied a piece of rope around the waist, a costume which later became the habit of the Franciscans.

The Beguines order of Belgium was established in 1180, after the Crusades had been in progress for nearly a century. Many men from France, Belgium, and Holland had joined the Crusades and never returned. Their widows, homeless and destitute, roamed these countries as pathetic vagabonds until the parish priest at St. Christopher's in Liege, Belgium, began caring for them.

In an enclosure near the church, rows of neat little houses were built in which three or four women lived. These women were called Beguines (Beg'ēns) and

---

[2] The great hospital of St. John of Jerusalem at Rhodes was reopened and used during World War II.

[3] This is known as a Maltese cross, a name given to it after the order moved to the Island of Malta in the Mediterranean.

the institution was called a Beguinage. There were no vows of poverty and all were free to marry. The Beguines visited the homes of Liege and combined nursing with housekeeping. Later a hospital was built where the Beguines cared for the patients so satisfactorily that their fame spread and cottage communities were established in many countries.

The Beguines in Liege still live in clean, well-ordered houses, carrying on the same devoted service that has characterized them for eight centuries.

The uniform was a dark gray homespun with the Flemish headdress of white wings (heavenly geese).

The Augustinian Nuns of Hotel Dieu in Paris, established in 1155, was the first purely nursing order. These nuns set a precedent for unremitting toil: they nursed, scrubbed, cooked, sewed, and washed clothes in the River Seine, even in winter. Members of the order did this century after century with no rest or recreation, and their devotion has influenced the public's conception of nursing to the present day. The National Nursing Accrediting Service of the National League for Nursing has found this image of a selfless, night-and-day grind of dedication to the sick to be the greatest hindrance in developing schools of nursing.

There is no record of a uniform in the early days of the order, but for many centuries the habit has been white. This seems strange since black, dark blue, or dark brown was usually worn by all orders.

EARLY MODERN NURSING UNIFORMS

The Sisters of Charity,[4] established by St. Vincent de Paul, was the first nursing order to rise following the Reformation of 1517. At first its members wore the peasant dresses which they had brought with them from home, but they soon adopted a habit of grey-blue homespun woolen cloth, with a blue apron and the spreading headdress which is seen today.

The Deaconess Hospital[5] at Kaiserswerth, Germany, was established in 1836 and is still a thriving institution. Its nurses wear a uniform of plain blue with a bibbed apron of white. The cap is hood-shaped, with a ruffle about the face, and is tied under the chin with a perky, distinctive bow.

Beginning in 1680, nurses at St. Bartholomew's Hospital in London were required to wear a uniform of dark-colored cloth. "In others, for the most part, the dresses were of dark heavy material, as dark cluny, rough dark maroon cloth, black serge, black woolen dresses, black alpaca, and holland brown. These dresses were made with high collars, long sleeves, and a full skirt touching the ground, as it was considered a disgrace for a lady's neck, arms, and ankles to show . . . ."[6]

---

[4] See p. 54, Chapter 6, Leaders for Reform.

[5] See p. 59, Chapter 6, Leaders for Reform.

[6] Julia C. Stimson, "The Nurse's Uniform," *American Journal of Nursing*, Vol. 36 (April, 1936), p. 370.

AMERICAN UNIFORMS[7]

The early uniforms of the American nurses, although strongly influenced by the prevailing fashion of women's dress, were copied from those worn by nurses in English hospitals. These uniforms were designed to be practical, but comfort was not considered and sanitation was unknown. The high collar,

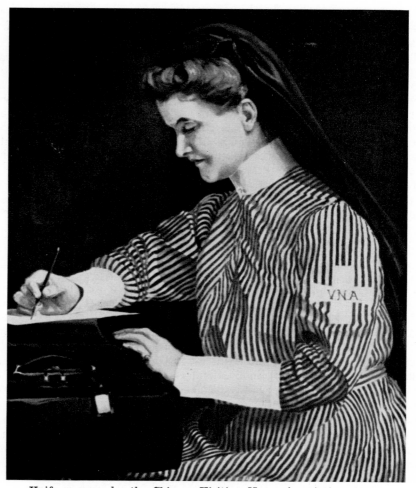

Uniform worn by the Chicago Visiting Nurse Association, 1901.

[7] In 1940 the *American Journal of Nursing* published a study of nurses' uniforms in which 284 directors of nursing schools provided the data. This study included shoes, capes, and sweaters. In the United States the uniform, although ''simple, quiet in color, well made, and spotlessly clean,'' still follows the general fashion trends. The uniform (page 1205 of this article) worn by Alice Bowen, graduate of the Farrand Training School, Detroit, 1889, shows the era of the puffed sleeves. (''The Student Nurse's Uniform,'' *American Journal of Nursing*, Vol. 40:10:1204-1211 [Nov.] 1940.)

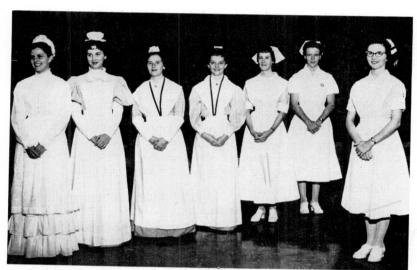

Parade of uniforms of St. Luke's Hospital School of Nursing, Jacksonville, Florida. Left to right: 1886; 1895; 1905; 1907; 1920; 1941; 1950 to the present.

the long stiff cuffs, and the skirt two inches from the floor could not have been comfortable.

Bellevue Hospital, New York City, established in 1873, is believed to have been the first school to adopt a uniform. The students, women of refinement, were reluctant to wear a uniform. The maids and butlers wore uniforms in their homes, as did the servants in the local all-women academies from which the young ladies had graduated. The nursing school committee urged the adoption of a uniform "on the grounds of economy, as well as neatness, and its effect on a group of nurses is the same as on a company of soldiers."[8]

"In the first class of nurses, the tradition runs, there was a beautiful daughter of a prominent Knickerbocker family, Miss Van Rensselaer, who later entered an Episcopal order, and finally became a sister of the Roman Catholic Church, the order of St. Vincent. Having been instructed by the Committee, and also, perhaps by Sister Helen, the probationer was permitted to go home on a two-day leave. At the end of this period she returned to the wards, dressed in a garb of gray-blue striped material with a white apron and cap. It is said that the heterogeneous prints worn by her classmates looked dowdy in comparison and the victory was won."[9]

An apron was part of the original uniform. It began as a length of white muslin gathered into a belt; a square of the muslin was sewed into the belt in front and pinned at the two upper corners as a bib. Much later, two-inch

[8] Julia C. Stimson, "The Nurse's Uniform," *American Journal of Nursing*, Vol. 36 (April, 1936), p. 370.

[9] Lillian Sabine, "The Picturesque Past of the Uniform," *Trained Nurse and Hospital Review (Nursing World)*, Vol. LXXXII (March, 1929), p. 201.

straps were attached to the bib and carried over the shoulders and crossed in the back.

There was wide variation in the materials of the aprons. Some were made of linen, or a soft dimity, with hemstitching at the top of the hem and the top of the bib. The student did this intricate work before she entered the school.

The most conspicuous part of the apron was the utility bag which dangled from its belt. The early bag contained a pencil, scissors, and a tiny case containing matches to light the candles and kerosene lamps. As the clinical thermometer and the hypodermic syringe were invented, these, too, were added to the bag. The thermometer was encased in a tiny metal tube and the syringe in a small flat case. The student was required to purchase both of these instruments.

Some schools issue emblems in the form of a patch worn on the left sleeve or bib strap. On this patch are embroidered the initials of the school, a star, a cross, or some other significant symbol. Some schools add a black band for each year in the school, while in others black bands are worn by seniors only.

The use of bands and chevrons on nurses' uniforms was, and still is, the subject of heated discussions. (These marks are a carry-over from the military influence.) Should there be means of identification for each class? Does it serve a useful function in a school of nursing? What is the effect of class distinction on the patient? Does the patient have as much confidence in the student with one black band as in the student with two black bands? These are some of the questions asked by those debating the merits of bands and chevrons.

An elaborate chevron was worn by students of the Boston City Hospital School of Nursing:

Every nurse who had been a member of the school for six months had one row of white cotton soutache braid sewn on the upper outer side of her left sleeve in the form of an interlaced knot known in heraldry as the "bowen." She added a row of braid every six months by following the outline of the original bow. This she continued until she had six rows to her credit .... These uniforms were very distinctive, and gave their wearers a smart appearance; and who can say they did not give an added sense of well-being, as well as to raise the general tone of the school? Most of the nurses evidently thought they had much to live up to when dressed in full uniform.[10]

The early uniforms for both graduates and students were made from a dark material. Later students adopted an easily washable material of gingham or percale, but the director of nurses continued, as late as the early 1900's, to wear a black alpaca dress with a high white collar and stiff white cuffs. Grace Fay Schryver, in *A History of the Illinois Training School for Nurses, 1880-1929*, includes Helen Scott Hays' account of some of the events of 1906:

Among the less important affairs, there were various questions of tradition and custom, sacred as these were to many of us, where change seemed desirable.

---

[10] Grace Fay Schryver, *A History of the Illinois Training School for Nurses* (Chicago, Board of Directors of the Illinois Training School for Nurses, 1930), p. 86.

For example, with the uniform: the black alpaca dress of the superintendent and her staff was changed to white cotton, which shortly became the uniform of all graduate head nurses as well. . . .[10]

The question of footwear for nurses was also of great concern; the high-buttoned shoes worn by early nurses were not made with the support and comfort seen in the present-day nurse's oxford. Sara E. Parsons, in writing *History of the Massachusetts General Hospital Training School for Nurses*, gives reason for the importance of well-fitting shoes:

Miss Maxwell[11] *concerned herself promptly with the health of her students and sought to free them of some of the heavy domestic labor. Within a few months the nurses were relieved from carrying food and medications to and from the wards, and eventually ward maids and scrubwomen were added to the staff in sufficient numbers to take from the nurses the mopping and some of the dishwashing. Miss Maxwell also recommended proper shoes for the probationers on account of the great trouble many of them had with their feet, some of them being incapacitated with severe pain.*

Modern nurses deplore the great amount of desk work—medical records, forms, and reports—but it does offer an opportunity to rest the feet.

At the Boston City Hospital "a physician was called upon to examine every nurse as to the condition of her feet before she was accepted as a member of the school, and in that way there came about the regulation shoe."[12]

The change from black shoes to white shoes came slowly. The white uniform for graduates had been generally accepted, but both graduates and students continued to wear black shoes. The first white shoes were made of canvas; white leather came much later. A great deal of research was conducted before a white shoe polish was found that would leave the leather white without causing cracks and yellow stains.

A woman's hair has always been one of her pet vanities; it is important today as in the days of the Roman matron. As late as World War I the hair was never cut and it was often a prideful boast that a girl could sit on her hair.[13] Hairwashing was an eventful undertaking and infrequently done. The dust-cap type of head covering served to make hairwashing less necessary and also satisfied the ascetic idea of plainness.

The cap of the early schools was designed to be functional. Although many of the caps did not cover the entire hair, all nurses were required to comb their long hair high upon the head in such a manner as to be completely covered by the cap. Many of these caps were edged with ruching that added

---

[10] Grace Fay Schryver, *A History of the Illinois Training School for Nurses* (Chicago, Board of Directors of the Illinois Training School for Nurses, 1930), p. 86.

[11] Anna C. Maxwell, noted leader in nursing and co-author of the long-popular textbook, *Practical Nursing*.

[12] "Evolution of the Uniform," *American Journal of Nursing*, Vol. 31 (Nov. 1931), p. 1260.

[13] During World War I, Irene Castle, a famous American dancer "bobbed" her hair. The civilized world was scandalized, but in a few months short hair became the rage. The more daring nurses who cut their hair were dismissed from their schools.

greatly to their attractiveness. Also, many caps were tedious to construct and impossible to launder. "The oldtime knife-pleated border which each nurse was forced to construct every 'cap night' was substituted by one of washable muslin."[14]

To the modern nurse with short, clean hair, the cap no longer serves its original purpose of covering the hair; it is now worn for ornamental reasons. Yet every nurse wears her cap with genuine pride because it is the symbol of nursing as truly as the caduceus represents the physician.

The outdoor uniform has never been popular in the United States, but military nurses and those in the Red Cross Nursing Service wear well-designed and attractive outdoor uniforms. The street uniform of the public health nurse has had many changes in the effort to be distinctive enough to give the nurse protection and yet conservative enough to be in good taste.

The cape, whose history began during the Crusades, still has considerable vogue in schools where the nurses' residence is some distance from the hospital. The most important reason for the continued use of the cape is the attractiveness which it gives to the uniform, especially for nurses on review. The linings of red, gold, blue, coral, or other gay tone lend a colorful distinction to the group.

The outdoor uniform of the Cadet Nurse Corps of World War II was a masterpiece of uniform design. The recruitment slogan of the Council for War Service was "Join a Proud Profession," and the uniform was designed to fit the slogan.

Each student was issued one winter and two summer outfits. The winter uniform was a jacket and skirt of light gray flannel with silver buttons and insignia. The sleeve marking was a silver Maltese cross on a scarlet oval. The gray felt beret bore the insignia of the United States Public Health Service. This insignia has as its central figure the staff of Aesculapius, with the wings of Mercury, and an anchor. Around the hook of the anchor is wound an anchor chain. Sailors call this a "fouled anchor," which is symbolic of the sick and injured sailor.

The two summer uniforms were cut from a gray and white striped cotton fabric, and the summer hat was of light gray felt with a scarlet band. The cadet also received a gray flannel reefer coat, a raincoat, a blouse, and a shoulderstrap handbag as part of the complete uniform. When these students were on parade there were no homely nurses. Every face glowed with an inner pride in the awareness of being well-groomed and of wearing a uniform of beauty and significance.[15]

Historically, the indoor uniform has been worn in the hospital only, and this is still true. In its September, 1960 issue, the *American Journal of Nursing* quotes from the *Journal* of September, 1910:

I can't imagine a well-bred as well as a properly trained nurse . . . being willing to "exhibit" herself in uniform either in a hotel diningroom or in any

[14] Grace Fay Schryver, *A History of the Illinois Training School for Nurses* (Chicago, Board of Directors of the Illinois Training School for Nurses, 1930), p. 86.

[15] This complete uniform can be seen on a model in the Smithsonian Institution in Washington, D. C.

other public place. I consider the uniform sacred to the sick room and the hospital ... Let us be known by our deeds and not by our uniforms.

A century of nursing has seen profound changes in uniforms. These changes have been comparable to the changes in women's dress for all occasions. The most radical changes in the uniforms have been made for sanitary reasons: As the germ theory became generally accepted, the sleeves were shortened to permit frequent hand-washing. The floor-sweeping skirts were shortened to the shocking length of twelve inches from the floor, and the high collar with its saw-like edge has been replaced with a low comfortable one. Most duty shoes are wide-toed and perforated. The nurse in uniform is permitted the same comfortable working clothes as women of any other profession.

REFERENCES

"Beguines of Belgium." In *Encyclopaedia Britannica*. Chicago, Encyclopaedia Britannica, Inc., 1957.

DIETZ, LENA DIXON: *Professional Adjustments I*, 4th ed. Philadelphia, F. A. Davis Co., 1957.

DOLAN, JOSEPHINE: *Goodnow's Nursing History*, 10th ed. Philadelphia, W. B. Saunders Co., 1958.

"Evolution of the uniform." *Amer. J. Nurs.* 31:1259 (Nov.) 1931.

"Isabel M. Stewart recalls the early days." *Amer. J. Nurs.* 60:1426 (Oct.) 1960.

JAMIESON, ELIZABETH M., SEWALL, MARY F., and GJERTSON, LUCILLE S.: *Trends in Nursing History*, 5th ed. Philadelphia, W. B. Saunders Co., 1957.

LAMB, HAROLD: *The Crusades—The Flame of Islam*. Garden City, N. Y., International Collectors Library, American Headquarters, 1930.

MERRILL, MARIE G.: *The History of St. Luke's Hospital School of Nursing*. Oak Park, Ill., Hub Printing Service, 1946.

"Nurses through the centuries—Uniforms from 1242-1925." *RN* 19:46 (Feb.) 1956.

NUTTING, M. ADELAIDE, and DOCK, LAVINIA: *A History of Nursing*, Vol. I. New York, G. P. Putnam's Sons, 1935.

PARSONS, SARA E.: *History of the Massachusetts General Hospital School of Nursing*. Boston, Whitcomb and Barrows, 1922.

ROBINSON, VICTOR: White Caps—*The Story of Nursing*. Philadelphia, J. B. Lippincott Co., 1946, Ch. 4.

SABINE, LILLIAN: The picturesque past of the nurse's uniform. *Trained Nurse and Hospital Review (Nursing World)* Part I, 82:197 (Feb.) 1929; Part II, 82:331 (Feb.) 1929.

SCHRYVER, GRACE FAY: *A History of the Illinois Training School for Nurses*. Chicago, Board of Directors, Illinois Training School for Nurses, 1930.

SMITH, CLARE LOUISE: *The Evanston Hospital School of Nursing*. Chicago, Lakeside Press, 1948.

STIMSON, JULIA C.: The nurse's uniform. *Amer. J. Nurs.* 36:367 (Apr.) 1936.

THOMPSON, JAMES W., and JOHNSON, EDGAR N.: *An Introduction to Medieval Europe*. New York, W. W. Norton and Co., 1937, Chap. 21.

Why a cap?—The evolution of the nurses cap in some schools established before 1895. *Amer. J. Nurs.* 40:384 (Apr.) 1940.

CHAPTER 15

The Red Cross

The International Red Cross, with its many national associations, has become an accepted part of our social institutions. Wars have been fought since the beginning of mankind, but the care of the sick and wounded was long left to the army surgeons, with little improvement since Machaon and Podaleirius applied their healing salves on wounded Greeks at the siege of Troy.

The nineteenth century was more humane, particularly after the work of Florence Nightingale at Scutari during the Crimean War. In June, 1859, at the battle of Solferino in northern Italy, the forces of France and Sardinia fought the Austrian army. At the end of sixteen hours of fighting some 40,000 soldiers lay dead or wounded, and the army surgeons were unable to cope with the immense task suddenly thrust upon them. The suffering was grievous and there was much needless loss of life.

On the day of the battle of Solferino, Henri Dunant, a Swiss banker on urgent business to Napoleon III concerning a business venture in North Africa, arrived in Castiglione, Italy. Unable to see the Emperor, M. Dunant became so absorbed in the care of the wounded that he remained for three days to aid the suffering soldiers. He returned to Geneva, once again a banker, but the memory of the terrible slaughter haunted him continually, impelling him to write a book, *A Souvenir de Solferino.*[1]

---

[1] *Souvenir de Solferino* has been translated from the French into English and is published by the American Red Cross, Washington, D. C.

Henri Dunant strongly advocated improvement in the care of the wounded in European armies. The Society of Public Welfare, an influential civic organization, invited M. Dunant to speak at one of its meetings about his experiences in Solferino. In this talk he insisted that the European nations should act to prevent the recurrence of such a catastrophe. Listening to Mr. Dunant that night were three influential men: M. Gustave Moynier, a man of independent fortune who was president of the Society of Public Welfare; Dr. Louis Appia, a physician; and Adolph Ador, an attorney. These men became interested in M. Dunant's views and they in turn secured the cooperation of General William Henri Dufour, Commander-in-Chief of the Swiss Army.

On February 9, 1863, a committee, headed by G. Moynier and with M. Dunant as a member, was appointed by the Society of Public Welfare "to consider a proposition relative to the formation of permanent societies for the relief of wounded soldiers," whether friend or foe. Although Dunant had written and lectured against the existing conditions in the care of the wounded in battle and had inspired thousands with the idea that something should be done, he had no plan for turning this inspiration into a functioning organization. To M. Moynier goes the credit for organizing and systematizing what, from then on, has been known as the *Red Cross*. To him, sympathy without constructive action was maudlin. Gustave Moynier, as President of a Special Commission, had read Florence Nightingale's papers on the sanitary service in the British Army, and he thought he saw the solution to the problem in Dunant's book. General Dufour, another committee member, stressed the importance of obtaining the unanimous agreement of all the princes and nations of Europe, just at Dr. Appia, the fourth member, saw the necessity of obtaining the cooperation of the highest military authorities in the various countries.

After a long discussion the committee of five decided that an international conference was needed as a starting point. However, they had many misgivings about how their idea would be received: Would such a convention think it was only a philanthropic fancy of dreamers and Utopians? The committee knew the necessity of influential publicity, and accordingly brought their plan to the attention of the International Statistical Congress at Berlin in September, 1863. The congress was impressed by the project, and said so.

With the approval of the International Statistical Congress, the committee continued its plans and called a conference for October 26-29, 1863, in the rooms of the Athenaeum at Geneva. This conference of thirty-six members represented fourteen governments. Every member was alert to the responsibilities of an undertaking to lessen the sufferings and privations which are the inevitable consequences of an armed conflict. But more than good will and approval were needed to accomplish the real purpose of this meeting. "Definite, concrete plans must be laid in order . . . to reconcile two opposites— charity and war. Here was the real problem to be solved."[2] This problem was further complicated by the various forms of government in Europe which were either absolute monarchies or limited monarchies.

[2] Clara Barton, *The Red Cross in Peace and War* (Meriden, Conn., Journal Publishing Co.) 1912.

At this Preparatory Conference of October, 1863, the committee passed several resolutions. It called for the establishment in each country of volunteers (committees) which would, in time of war, supplement the army medical corps in caring for the wounded. It also called for formal recognition of these societies by their governments and the adoption of a uniform insignia—a red cross on a white band.

The committee urged that neutral status be given to all volunteers and their equipment used in the care of wounded. It further called upon the societies, when formed in each nation, to communicate with others through the committee in Geneva.

In less than a year Europe was covered by a network of committees for the relief of wounded so'diers. All of the committees were enthusiastic over the resolutions of the Geneva conference and were eager to make it a permanent organization. Consequently, from August 17-22, 1864, the Geneva Treaty was drafted and signed by twelve European nations, ''For the Amelioration of the Conditions of the Wounded in Armies at the Field,'' the subtitle of the International Red Cross Treaty.

The insignia designed for this organization was the same as the flag of Switzerland, but in reverse—a red cross on a white background. The name of the Red Cross is derived from the flag which is its symbol in Christian nations. This symbol has since been modified by other groups: the Red Cross Societies of Moslems use a red crescent, the Iranians have a red lion which is the symbol of Persia, the Zoroastrians a red sun, and the Israelis a red star of David (each of these on a white background).

THE UNITED STATES AS A MEMBER OF THE INTERNATIONAL RED CROSS

The United States did not become a member of the International Red Cross until eighteen years after the organization's ratification at Geneva. At the time of the formation of the International Red Cross, the United States was torn by the Civil War. The Sanitary Commission and many welfare societies in both the north and the south provided relief for wounded soldiers. In the reconstruction that followed the war the invitation from Geneva was neglected. In 1877, M. Moynier, President of the International Committee, appointed Clara Barton as official bearer of an invitation to Pres. Rutherford Hayes, asking that the United States accede to the articles of the convention. Apparently President Hayes did not realize the importance of the invitation, for he declined the offer. When Pres. James A. Garfield was inaugurated in March, 1881, Clara Barton again presented the invitation of the International Committee. The President received the subject cordially and referred it to Secretary of State James Blaine, who assured Miss Barton that the President would recommend the adoption in his message to Congress. Before this was accomplished, however, President Garfield was assassinated. Chester A. Arthur was his successor.

Shortly after his inauguration, however, President Garfield had advised Miss Barton that a Red Cross Organization should be formed in order to aid in the accession to the Geneva Treaty. This was done in Washington, D. C., May 21, 1881, with Clara Barton as president. Accordingly, in November, 1881, Miss Barton placed before President Arthur the matter of the Treaty of Geneva. She assured him that it was the unfulfilled desire of President Garfield that the United States become a member of the international organization.

In his first message to Congress, President Arthur recommended "the adhesion of the United States to that humane and commendable engagement." On March 1, 1882, the President signed the document whereby the United States became a member of the International Red Cross. Clara Barton, after five years of persistent labor with presidents and legislators, could cable the glad tidings of acceptance to President Moynier of the International Committee at Geneva.

ORGANIZATION OF THE AMERICAN RED CROSS

The American Red Cross, created by an act of congress in 1900, is a corporate structure composed of approximately 3700 chapters.

The board of governors of the American Red Cross has fifty members. The President of the United States becomes honorary chairman upon his inauguration as President; he appoints eight members of the board, one of whom becomes president of the board. The other seven appointed members are officials of government departments directly concerned with matters of the Red Cross.[3] Thirty members of the board of governors are elected by chapter representatives at the annual convention. These thirty-eight members elect twelve members-at-large, making a body of fifty members who are elected by the people.

The organization and its chapters are not and never have been financially supported by the government; they are supported by contributions from the public in an annual fund drive. Prior to World War II the roll call of the members of the Red Cross was held each year. The national organization received from the chapters fifty cents for each membership, whether the individual membership was $1 or $25. Since World War II, however, the amount going to the national organization has been established on a quota basis based on (1) the number of people in a community, (2) the income of the community, and (3) its expense in fund-raising. The only other appeals for support are the infrequent disaster relief appeals made when the funds contributed go entirely for relief in a specific disaster area. All accounts of the Red Cross are audited by the Department of Civil Defense and they are filed by the Secretary of Defense with the Congress of the United States.

ACTIVITIES SPONSORED BY THE AMERICAN RED CROSS

The Red Cross sponsors many activities, but not all activities are found in all chapters. Each chapter develops activities best suited to the needs of its community. The major ones are described here.

---

[3] These seven members are Secretary of Labor; Secretary of Health, Education, and Welfare; Deputy Under Secretary of State; Under Secretary of the Treasury; Deputy Secretary; and two Assistant Secretaries of Defense.

Services to the Armed Forces had its incentive in the Original Treaty of Geneva. Aid to men in active service and to their families is given during war or peace. Each country developed these services along lines best suited to its purpose. In the United States these offices are known as Home Service, Service at Military Installations, Service in Veterans Administration Offices, and Service in Veterans Hospitals.

Disaster Relief. This has been the most outstanding activity of the American Red Cross since its beginning. The charter for the American Red Cross granted by Congress in 1905 lists one of the organization's purposes: "To continue and carry on a system of national and international relief in time of peace and to apply the same to mitigating the sufferings caused by pestilence, famine, fire, flood, and other great national calamities and to devise and carry on measures for preventing the same."[4]

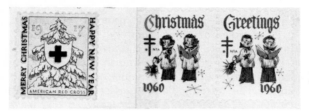

The cross changed from the traditional Red Cross to the double-barred cross of the American Tuberculosis Association.

Christmas Seal Sale. Christmas seals originated in Denmark in 1905,[5] at a time when tuberculosis was the leading cause of death in all countries. At the International Conference held in London in 1907, the Red Cross was urged to assist in the campaign against tuberculosis. The American Red Cross, upon promotion by the Delaware chapter, began the sale of Christmas Seals in 1908. Red Cross nurses not only aided in the promotion and sale of seals but cooperated in a number of antituberculosis projects financed from the sale of seals. The Red Cross withdrew from this field in 1919.

Junior Red Cross Services. Nearly 60,000 of the nation's primary and secondary schools enroll members in the Junior Red Cross. These junior members participate in the popular international communications programs of art, music, and school exhibits. They engage in international study visits, serve as recreational aides on playgrounds, work and play with the home-bound, make toys and games for child disaster victims, write and produce radio programs, and assist with radio and newspaper publicity for Red Cross campaigns. Members of the Junior Red Cross take part in disaster operations, blood programs, and aid to military, veterans, and civilian hospitals.

---

[4] These are natural disasters. The Red Cross does not provide relief for economic disasters, such as the depression of 1930-1940.

[5] Margrethe Kruse, "The Birthday of an Idea," *American Journal of Nursing*, Vol. 54 (Dec. 1954), pp. 1460.

The College Program. The College Program of the Red Cross is a dynamic and challenging program in which college and university students participate. It provides students in the social sciences with a laboratory by using the community itself.

The college program seeks to develop attitudes and values of service that often seem to be overlooked by college students. Through this activity they are making an important contribution to the Red Cross—and equally important, they are learning that service to others is a rewarding educational experience.

Fitness for the Future. This is a course designed to help men and women prepare for the later years through an understanding of processes affecting physical and mental health and the social changes common to the second half of life. Discussion groups have an opportunity to talk about the aging process and how to adjust to the changes that occur as the result of growing old. They also talk about the benefits of medical supervision, good nutrition and safety practices, as well as how to gain an understanding of community resources and create a more satisfying way of life through leisure time activities for physical and mental health.

Volunteer Activities. The volunteer is the basic strength of the Red Cross. Virtually all Red Cross services would be impossible without the work of thousands of volunteers who serve the organization every year.

Certain Red Cross volunteer services, such as Gray Ladies and Canteen were developed to support the American Red Cross in its work with members of the Armed Forces and with disaster victims. Today these services not only help to support all Red Cross programs, but also those of many other community institutions, organizations, and agencies. If a disaster occurs these trained and experienced volunteers are ready to fill emergency roles and give leadership to those who are less experienced. For example, Gray Ladies, famous for their work in military and veterans hospitals, give friendly personal services that contribute to the comfort and recovery of the sick.

Volunteer Nurses Aides assist with nursing care under the supervision of professional nurses in hospitals and clinics, health agencies, emergency medical stations, Red Cross blood centers, and mobile units and disaster shelters. Motor Service drivers are trained to provide safe and efficient transportation on such assignments as taking children and the aging for treatments, collecting and distributing blood, and helping evacuate people from disaster areas. Production volunteers make surgical dressings, knit and sew garments, and make articles for Red Cross activities and for federal and civilian institutions.

THE RED CROSS NURSING SERVICE

The Spanish-American War (1898) called further attention to the need for organized nursing service to care for sick and wounded soldiers. Since schools of nursing were developing rapidly, there were many graduate nurses in 1898, but there was no organization to process the graduates' credentials and to assign these nurses to areas where they were needed.

Dr. Anita Newcomb McGee, with the cooperation of the Surgeon General of the Army, organized the Army Nurse Corps and insisted upon graduate nurses to care for the wounded and ill.

Origin of the Red Cross Nursing Service. In 1905, Surgeon General W. C. Braisted of the United States Army was sent by the government to observe medical and sanitary conditions in the Russo-Japanese War. The nursing service of the Japanese Red Cross was considered the best in any country; Dr. Braisted admired the excellent work and efficient system that he saw in the Japanese hospital wards. He learned that the Japanese nurse, after completing her course in the Red Cross hospital, was free to leave and marry, and have a home and children; but she was required to keep in touch with the Red Cross organization so that in time of need she could be called into service. Although Dr. Braisted realized that to organize 20,000 to 30,000 reserve nurses would be an enormous undertaking, he suggested in his report "that the effort might be worth making."

When the American National Red Cross was reorganized in 1905, its charter was granted by Congress, which specifically stated that the purpose of this organization was

. . . to furnish volunteer aid to the sick and wounded in time of war, in accordance with the spirit and conditions of the Geneva Convention . . .

Such an aim would make necessary a constant reserve force of nurses, since medical treatment and nursing care were rapidly becoming more complex.

The manner in which this could best be done was widely discussed by nurses and physicians who still remembered the chaos of the Spanish-American War. The chief obstacle to be overcome was the objection by influential persons to the enrollment of nurses by the thousand. These objectors declared such action unnecessary because they believed the United States would never go to war again. A second difficulty arose over the variation in standards of nursing in different schools and hospitals. In 1909 the Red Cross asked the American Nurses' Association to cooperate in working out a uniform basis for nursing service. The result of this affiliation was the formation and development of the Red Cross Nursing Service composed of registered nurses and having its own officers and national committee. Jane Armindo Delano was the first chairman of this branch of the Red Cross, a position which she held until her death at Base Hospital, No. 69, Savenay, France, in March, 1919.

In April, 1947, the government created a permanent nurse corps in the Army and Navy with provision for a reserve force. This made it unnecessary for the Red Cross in its nursing service division to maintain a national roster of nurses for military purposes. But community needs continued, such as disasters, epidemics, and need for instruction in home nursing, and instruction for Volunteer Nurses Aides. In May, 1947, therefore, the American National Red Cross reorganized the Nursing Service to meet community needs rather than military needs. It decided that enrollment would be granted on the basis of actual community service through the Red Cross rather than on the basis of availability for military or disaster service. The enrollment roster would be maintained in the local chapters rather than at national headquarters.

However, acceptance for enrollment and award of the badge continued on the basis of national uniform requirements.

Training Program Qualifications.   Professional nurses who have not enrolled previously may qualify for enrollment in any of the following ways:

1. By serving in any of the several nursing programs of the American Red Cross, such as instruction in Home Nursing and in a training course for nurses aides, assistance in the blood program, and service in disaster, epidemic, or other special projects.

2. By committee membership or other activity which serves to promote or interpret the basic philosophy of the Red Cross to nursing students, nursing organizations, or community groups.

3. By serving in related Red Cross activities, such as instruction in first aid and accident prevention, motor service, or public information.[6]

Organization of the Red Cross Nursing Service.   The Nursing Service, since its organization in 1909, has functioned under the guidance of a national professional advisory committee, composed of leading nurses who represent different fields of nursing as well as different parts of the country. It helped to keep the Red Cross Nursing Service in line with the trends and service needs in the country as a whole. The members of the committee are selected on the basis of their experience in nursing and their interest in Red Cross Nursing Service. They are appointed by the President of the Red Cross.

The professional nursing staff at National Headquarters in Washington, D. C., consists of the national director, the assistant national director, director of Home Nursing and Volunteer Nurses Aide Instruction, and director of Disaster Nursing and Nurse Enrollment.

The Red Cross is divided geographically into four sections, or areas. These are the Eastern Area, the Southeastern Area, the Midwestern Area, and the Pacific Area.[7]

At each of the four area offices there is a director of nursing services, one or more assistant directors, and a professional field staff, all of whom assist the chapters in developing their nursing programs. These programs are designed to meet needs for nursing service not completely taken care of by other agencies and to supplement or extend the nursing service offered by hospitals and public health organizations in time of disaster or epidemics.

[6] Ruth B. Freeman, ''Nursing Plus,'' *American Journal of Nursing* Vol. 48 (Jan., 1948), pp. 12.

[7] These are the states included in each area:

EASTERN: Connecticut, Delaware, District of Columbia, Indiana, Kentucky, Maryland, Massachusetts, New Hampshire, New Jersey, New York, Ohio, Pennsylvania, Rhode Island, Vermont, Virginia, West Virginia.

SOUTHEASTERN AREA: Alabama, Florida, Georgia, Louisiana, Mississippi, North Carolina, Tennessee.

MIDWESTERN AREA: Arkansas, Colorado, Illinois, Iowa, Kansas, Michigan, Minnesota, Missouri, Nebraska, New Mexico, North Dakota, Oklahoma, South Dakota, Texas, Wisconsin, Wyoming.

PACIFIC AREA: Alaska, Arizona, California, Idaho, Montana, Nevada, Oregon, Utah, Washington, and Hawaii.

Major Programs of the Red Cross Nursing Services.   The major programs of this service concern the areas of disaster and home nursing, and volunteer nurses aides.

Disaster Nursing.   The Disaster Nursing Program has three aims: to devise a nursing plan for disaster emergencies, to train nurses to serve under this plan, and to provide supplementary nursing care for disaster or epidemic victims.

At the time of disaster, nurses are assigned from their local chapters to

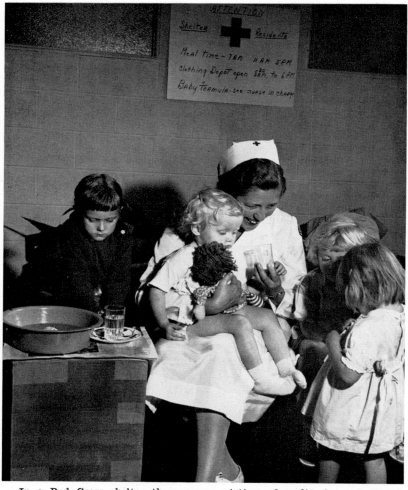

In a Red Cross shelter these young victims of a disaster get expert attention from a volunteer Red Cross nurse. Whenever and wherever people are displaced by flood, tornado, or natural catastrophe, the Red Cross will be on the job, when it counts most. (Courtesy of Public Information Department, Chicago Chapter, American Red Cross.)

serve in emergency medical stations, supplement the general nursing staff in hospitals, serve as special duty nurses to the critically ill, and provide nursing care and health supervision to the less seriously ill or injured in the home. They also provide health supervision in shelters and assist the health department in carrying responsibilities that have increased as a result of the disaster, such as communicable disease control through immunization programs. In addition, these nurses help families to identify their dead and provide supervision and nursing staff in emergency hospitals.

Since the victims undergo a grueling emotional experience during the chaos of disaster, nurses are prepared to watch for signs of emotional disturbance also.

Home Nursing. The Red Cross Nursing Service has three home nursing courses: "Fitness for the Future," "Mother and Baby Care," and "Care of the Sick and Injured." The two latter courses provide instruction in the nursing care of mothers, infants, aged and infirm, as well as general home care. This instruction is given free to community groups and to schools and colleges. The course is conducted by qualified authorized instructors, who usually serve on a volunteer basis.

The training courses for instructors consist of thirty hours of instruction and supervisory assistance in practice teaching to insure that the home nursing courses will have uniform content and a high quality of instruction. Only nurses may be authorized to teach "Mother and Baby Care," which requires an additional fifteen hours of training, but nonnurses with teaching experience may teach "Care of the Sick and Injured."

With the great increase in nursing homes, the American Nursing Home Association is aware of the need for well-prepared nursing aides to care for patients in nursing homes. To meet this need the United States Public Health Service and the American Nursing Home Association have requested the American Red Cross to offer the course, "Care of the Sick and Injured," to paid nursing aides employed in nursing homes. This course is taught by a registered nurse who has completed the "Care of the Sick and Injured" thirty-hour instructor training course, and who is authorized by the Red Cross Nursing Service to teach the course.

Volunteer Nurses Aide Service. This service was developed during World War II and in many instances meant the difference between closing hospitals and keeping them open. The influence of these dedicated aides continued after the war because of their understanding of nursing and hospital routine.

New treatments and new drugs have developed greatly during the past two decades. Also, the hospital census has changed from a two-week stay for the average patient to a stay of one week, which has increased the number of acutely ill hospital patients requiring intensive nursing care. Doctors have delegated many technical procedures to registered nurses, and they in turn have come to depend upon licensed practical nurses and nurses aides.

The Red Cross, through its Volunteer Nurses Aide Service, prepares women and men to give volunteer assistance to professional nurses in hospitals, public

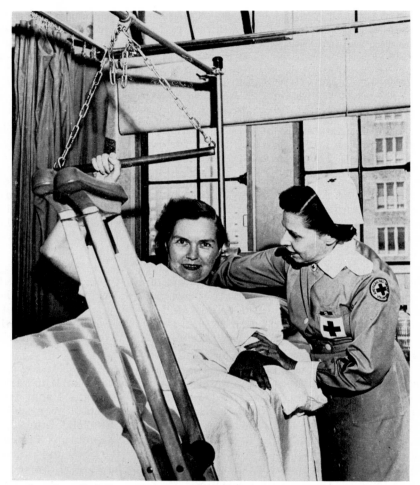

American Red Cross Volunteer Nurse Aide program came into use during World War II and has remained as a most helpful part of the hospital personnel. (Public Information Department, Chicago Chapter, American Red Cross.)

health organizations, and the Blood Program. They are given a forty-hour course by qualified professional nurses.

Enrollment in Nursing Service. To be eligible for enrollment in the Nursing Service, a nurse must be graduated from a state-accredited school of nursing and registered following graduation. This includes both men and women nurses in hospitals, clinics, public health, schools, Armed Forces, and private duty. Nurses may be married, retired, or homemakers. Nurses interested in the Nursing Service qualify for enrollment at the local Red Cross chapter.

Senior student nurses may earn enrollment privileges by giving service in the senior year. They will receive the emblem upon state registration.

Employment in Nursing Service. At each area office there is a director of nursing services, with one or more assistant directors, and a professional field staff who assist in the development of the nursing programs of the chapters in that area.

A highly responsible position in the field staff is the Nursing Representative, who is assigned to a specific territory which may cover from one-half to one or two states. This representative is responsible for the professional aspect of all Red Cross Nursing Services in her territory except the Blood Program. She trains and supervises Home Nursing and Volunteer Nurses Aide instructors, trains nurses in adapting skills to disaster conditions, and gives on-the-job training to nurses assigned to disaster areas. She maintains a reserve of volunteer nurses who are qualified and willing to serve in disaster. A bachelor's degree is the academic requirement for this position.

The chapter Director of Nursing Service is responsible for the administration, teaching, and supervisory responsibilities within a single chapter. This director must understand the fields of nursing and nursing education, the professional organizations of that community, and to develop good working relations with the health agencies of that city.

A nurse interested in a position with the Red Cross Nursing Service may apply directly to the chapter of her choice or to the area office covering the state in which she lives. Salaries and personnel benefits in general are comparable to those of similar organizations of that city.

Nursing in the Blood Program. Registered nurses serve in the Blood Program; they are an important part of the professional team in this service which is vital to the community and to national preparedness.

Nurses on the Blood Program staff care for donors, perform technical procedures of blood collection, and participate in the training and supervision of Red Cross volunteers. A typical regional center employs a chief nurse, an assistant chief nurse, and six to ten staff nurses to collect 40,000 to 60,000 units of blood a year. These nurses form teams that travel with the bloodmobile to communities participating in the regional Blood Program.

Each blood collection operation has, in addition to the fifteen to twenty lay volunteers from the community who assist the operation, four or more volunteer registered nurses recruited by the local chapter. These nurses (some 70,000 have served since the beginning of the program) are trained in blood collection technics and make a valuable contribution to the operations and to the disaster reserves of our country.

The chief nurse is required to have a bachelor's degree with courses in public health nursing, and at least two years in an administrative position. A bachelor's degree is desirable for the assistant chief nurse, but at least two years of college is a requirement with one year of experience in an administrative capacity. The Blood Program staff nurse is required to have at least one year of nursing experience following graduation.

LEAGUE OF RED CROSS SOCIETIES (LORCS)

Following World War I the American Red Cross and the Red Cross and Red Crescent Societies of Europe and the Near East were acutely aware of the necessity for continuation and coordination of peacetime activities for the war-torn countries. In 1919, delegates from these countries met in Cannes, France. From this Cannes Conference developed the greatest international agreement so far in history: *The League of Red Cross Societies.*

The American Red Cross contributed generously in providing leadership and training for personnel in public health and hospitals. Nurses in Europe and the Near East were granted scholarships for study in the United States, then returned to their countries to teach in schools of nursing and public health organizations, established by the American Red Cross.

The Nursing Advisory Committee of the League of Red Cross Societies. This committee advises, through the Executive Committee, the Board of Governors of the LORCS about all nursing matters it thinks appropriate for consideration by the Board.

Membership on the committee consists of no fewer than ten nor more than sixteen persons, representatives of the nursing services of their society. The committee members are selected every four years for a four-year term and meet biennially, preferably in conjunction with and in the same location as the executive committee.

In this way there is a world sharing of knowledge and professional resources with all countries, and a close relationship is maintained with the nursing departments of the League of Red Cross Societies and the International Committee of the Red Cross.

REFERENCES

ADKERSON, JEANIE: When disaster strikes. *Amer. J. Nurs.* 46:310 (May) 1946.

AIRD, ELLEN L.: The new look in Red Cross home nursing. *Amer. J. Nurs.* 57:1568 (Dec.) 1957.

BARTON, CLARA: *The Story of the Red Cross.* New York, Appleton-Century-Crofts, 1904.

BARTON, CLARA: *The Red Cross in Peace and War.* Meriden, Conn., Journal Publishing Co., 1912.

BOARDMAN, MABEL T.: *Under the Red Cross Flag at Home and Abroad.* Boston, Houghton, Mifflin Co., 1922.

BRADSHAW, VINAN OLSON, and TAYLOR, EARL S.: The nurse and the blood donor service. *Amer. J. Nurs.* 44:555 (June) 1944.

DAVIDSON, HENRY POMEROY: *The American Red Cross in the Great War.* New York, The Macmillan Co., 1920.

DOCK, LAVINIA L., et al.: *History of American Red Cross Nursing.* New York, The Macmillan Co., 1922.

DOWNEY, FAIRFAX: *Disaster Fighters.* New York, G. P. Putnam's Sons, 1938.

DULLES, RHEA FOSTER: *The American Red Cross: A History.* New York, Harper and Brothers, 1950.

EDERSTROM, MARY ELLEN: In the wake of the flood. *Amer. J. Nurs.* 51:662 (Nov.) 1951.

Editorial: We all share the burden. *Nurs. Outlook* 4:75 (Feb.) 1956.

ELLIMAN, VIRGINIA B.: Disaster Nursing. *Amer. J. Nurs.* 53:1356 (Nov.) 1953.

FERBER, ELLEN THEROUX: I like volunteer teaching. *Amer. J. Nurs.* 52:202 (Feb.) 1952.

FREEMAN, RUTH B.: Nursing plus. *Amer. J. Nurs.* 48:12 (Jan.) 1948.

FREEMAN, RUTH B.: Extending instruction in home nursing. *Amer. J. Nurs.* 49:170 (Mar.) 1949.

GLADWIN, MARY E.: The Red Cross and Jane Arminda Delano. Philadelphia, W. B. Saunders Co., 1931.

GOODMAN, LOIS: Preparing public health nurses to teach home nurses. *Amer. J. Nurs.* 49:498 (Aug.) 1949.

GUMPERT, MARTIN DUNANT: *The Story of the International Red Cross.* New York, Oxford University Press, 1938.

HENTSCH, YOUVNE: The Treaty of Geneva. *Amer. J. Nurs.* 44:34 (Jan.) 1944.

''Introduction to the Red Cross.'' Washington, D. C., American Red Cross, 1950, Publication No. 543.

KERNODLE, PORTIA B.: *The Red Cross Nurse in Action—1882-1948.* New York, Harper and Brothers, 1949.

MAGNUSSEN, ANN: Delano Day—A time for reflection. *Amer. J. Nurs.* 51:164 (Mar.) 1951.

MAGNUSSEN, ANN: Nursing in disaster. *Amer. J. Nurs.* 56:1290 (Oct.) 1956.

MAGNUSSEN, ANN: Nursing under the Red Cross today. *Nurs. Outlook* 9:158 (Mar.) 1961.

NELSON, RUTH E.: Never too old to learn. *Amer. J. Nurs.* 51:572 (Sept.) 1951.

ODIER, LUCIE: The Geneva conventions. *Amer. J. Nurs.* 51:21 (Jan.) 1951.

''Red Cross nursing—1950.'' *Amer. J. Nurs.* 51:442 (Aug.) 1951.

SCHER, BETTY.: Alice and her wonderland. (Alice Fitzgerald) *Amer. J. Nurs.* 61:74 (June) 1961.

THOMPSON, HAZEL: We learn to teach Red Cross classes in home nursing. *Amer. J. Nurs.* 51:209 (Mar.) 1951. p. 209.

WILLIAMS, BLANCHE COLTON: Clara Barton—Daughter of Destiny. Philadelphia, J. B. Lippincott Co., 1941.

CHAPTER 16

Ethical Codes for Nurses

Modern medicine properly begins in the age of Pericles, in which scientific medicine had its origin. During this period, organizations, composed of physicians only, were formed as distinct from the priest-physicians with their superstitious cults. These scientific groups were bound by solemn oath or promise, made in the presence of the group, to uphold the ethical standards which were considered proper for the practice of medicine. It is rather surprising that the ethical standards which doctors and nurses follow today were established in 500 B.C.

Hippocrates, the best known of these physicians, required his students to take an oath which is universally known as the *Hippocratic Oath*. This oath perhaps constitutes the most ancient historic document that codifies the ethics of a professional body.

The text of the Hippocratic Oath is as follows:

I swear by Apollo the physician, and Aesculapius, and Hygeia, and Panacea, and all the gods and goddesses, that according to my ability and judgment, I will keep this oath and its stipulation—to reckon him who taught me this art equally dear to me as my parents, to share my substance with him, and to relieve his necessities if required; to look upon his offspring in the same footing as my own brothers, and to teach them this art if they shall wish to learn it, without fee or stipulation, and that by precept, lecture, and every other mode of instruction, I will impart a knowledge of the art to my own sons, and those of my teachers, and to disciples bound by a stipulation and oath according to the law of medicine, but to none other.

I will follow that system of regimen which, according to my ability and judgment, I consider for the benefit of my patients, and abstain from whatever is deleterious and mischievous. I will give no deadly medicine to anyone if asked, nor suggest any such counsel; and in like manner I will not give to a woman a pessary to produce abortion. With purity and with holiness I will pass my life and practice my art. I will not cut persons laboring under the stone, but will leave this to be done by men who are practitioners of this work. Into whatever houses I enter, I will go into them for the benefit of the sick, and I will abstain from every voluntary act of mischief and corruption; and, further, from the seduction of females or males, of freemen and slaves. Whatever, in connection with my professional practice, or not in connection with it, I see or hear, in the life of men, which ought not to be spoken of abroad, I will not divulge, as reckoning that all such should be kept secret.

While I continue to keep this Oath unviolated, may it be granted to me to enjoy life and the practice of this art, respected by all men, in all times. But should I trespass and violate this Oath, may the reverse be my lot.

This promise was required of medical students in the Greek schools and later in the Roman schools. After the fall of Rome in 476 A.D., scientific medicine disappeared from Europe.

During the twelfth century Europe began the renaissance of science, especially medicine and mathematics. This new interest was awakened by the translations of the whole body of Greek medicine and the works of Hippocrates which had been preserved by the Moslem universities. The Europeans, in their appreciation of the early Greek culture, adopted the Hippocratic Oath for use in the European medical schools.

As medicine developed in America, the schools were aware of the need for an ethical code. Again, the Hippocratic Oath contained all the requirements for ethical practice and the Oath became the standard in the United States.

THE NIGHTINGALE PLEDGE

During the decades between 1880 and 1900, schools of nursing developed rapidly. The founders of these schools were keenly aware of the "dark period" of nursing which had persisted for three centuries. They knew that the public's attitude toward nursing could be changed only by attracting and admitting women of education and refinement to schools of nursing. Many of the early classes were made up of schoolteachers. In their desire to achieve professional status, they wanted a guide for the ethical practice of nursing. Many of the early schools developed oaths, pledges, and prayers. Some were fashioned after the Hippocratic Oath, or the Prayer of Maimonides. Some, still preserved in the early schools, seem to be original. At graduation the pledge was read by the director of nurses, one line at a time, and the students repeated it after her.

These pledges or promises have passed into nursing history. They have been replaced by the now universally accepted *Nightingale Pledge*. This beautiful pledge was formulated by a committee of the Farrand School of Nursing, Harper Hospital, Detroit. Mrs. Lystra Gretter, director of the school, was chairman and the guiding spirit of the committee; her name is signed to the original pledge. One of the members of the committee was Dr. C. A. Devendorf, a member of the Harper Hospital staff, who was deeply interested in the Hippocratic Oath and its traditions.[1] His interest may have influenced the committee to use the second paragraph of the Hippocratic Oath as a guide. Also, Mrs. Gretter's father was a physician, who served as a surgeon in the Union Army during the Civil War.[2]

At the time this pledge was made into a formal statement, Florence Nightingale had been the leader in nursing for thirty years. She was still the ideal of nurses and her standards for schools of nursing were accepted without question. It seemed quite natural, therefore, that this pledge should be dedicated to Miss Nightingale. However, she was in no way concerned with the formulation of the pledge and only knew of it when a copy was sent to her.

The original pledge follows:

I solemnly pledge myself before God and in the presence of this assembly to pass my life in purity and to practice my profession faithfully.

I will abstain from whatever is deleterious and mischievous, and will not take or knowingly administer any harmful drug. I will do all in my power to maintain and elevate the standard of my profession, and will hold in confidence all personal matters committed to my keeping and all family affairs coming to my knowledge in the practice of my calling.

With loyalty will I endeavor to aid the physician in his work, and devote myself to the welfare of those committed to my care.

THE CODE OF THE AMERICAN NURSES' ASSOCIATION

The American Society of Superintendents, now the National League for Nursing, was organized in 1893. One of the early concerns of the Society was the formation of a code of ethics for nurses. A committee consulted Dr. John

---

[1] The other three members of this committee were two nurses, Miss N. E. Haight and Miss Louise F. Ford, and Rev. William Davis, D.D.

[2] Mrs. Lystra E. Gretter graduated from the Buffalo Hospital School of Nursing in 1899. Upon graduation she became Director of Nurses of the Farrand Training School for Nurses, a position for which she had been recommended three months before graduation. She remained as Director of the Farrand School for eighteen years. During this time, without fanfare, she instituted reforms that spread to other schools. She began the eight-hour day for students in 1891. This was the first in the country and such time-consideration did not become general until thirty years later. She was a charter member of the National League for Nurses, and President of that organization in 1902. It was through her vision and effort that a department of public health was established in the University of Michigan.

Shaw Billings, the noted medical bibliographer, who said, "You don't need a code of ethics—just be good women."

As hospitals increased and nurses assumed more responsibility, to "just be good women" was not enough. Specific situations arose between nurses and doctors, between nurses and patients, between nurses and administrators, and between nurses and visitors. As a clearing house for specific situations the *Committee on Ethical Standards* became a standing committee of the American Nurses' Association in 1924.

This committee began to assemble material for a code and, at the biennial convention in Atlantic City in May, 1926, presented the first code to the House of Delegates. The title of this code, "A Suggested Code: A code of ethics presented for the consideration of the American Nurses' Association," was in no sense final, and suggestions and criticisms were invited from individual members, nursing organizations, and allied groups.

The committee continued to work toward an acceptable code. The indexes of the *American Journal of Nursing,* between 1926 and 1940, list numerous articles on the subject. One of these, "Developing a Code of Ethics for the Nursing Profession,"[3] shows insight into the difficulties incurred in preparing a code that would be acceptable to nurses: "They confuse professional ethics with personal morality ... they are too general in statements, failing to come to grips with specific areas of conflict; they rely too much on mere pronouncement for enforcement. In short, makers of ethical codes usually have not been realistic enough."

Another code was prepared by the Committee on Ethical Standards and presented to the American Nurses' Association in 1940. This, too, was not accepted.[4]

The 1950 Code. In 1949 the Advisory Council of the American Nurses' Association encouraged the Committee on Ethical Standards to again formulate a set of guiding principles for the practice of nursing. In the development of this code, the committee invited suggestions from all sections of nursing: the chairmen of all American Nurses' Association sections, and standing and special committees, the Director of the Professional Counseling and Placement Service, the executive secretaries of the, then, five national associations of registered nurses, and the Executive Secretary of the National Association of Practical Nurse Education.

These suggestions and comments were tabulated and arranged in the form of a check list. These were submitted to the presidents of all the state and district associations, to all national nursing organizations, to sixty-nine schools of nursing, to forty employers of nurses, and to the executive secretaries of the American Hospital Association and the American Medical Association.

---

[3] Limbert, Paul M.: "Developing a Code of Ethics for the Nursing Profession," *Amer. J. Nurs.* Vol. 32 (Dec., 1932), p. 1257.

[4] During 1931, 1932, 1933, and occasionally in 1934, the *American Journal of Nursing* published specific situations which had been presented to the Committee on Ethical Standards. These discussions and findings did much to clarify the nurse's position in difficult situations and these served as examples for the final draft of the code.

Returns of this check list were then studied by the Committee on Ethical Standards and used as the basis for the code which was presented to the biennial convention in San Francisco, May, 1950. This code was adopted; this completed twenty-five years of work by the Committee on Ethical Standards. During 1952 and 1953 the *American Journal of Nursing* published seven articles entitled ''What's in Our Code.'' These articles, prepared by the Committee on Ethical Standards, made specific interpretations of the code.[5]

The 1960 Code. During the decade from 1949 to 1959 social changes had developed especially along the lines of economic security for nurses, and advertising and the nurse. A revision of the 1950 Code was drafted by the Board of Directors of the American Nurses' Association. This revision was presented at the biennial convention in Miami, 1960, and ratified.

The individual nurse's responsibility toward this code is stated by the *American Journal of Nursing*, September, 1960:

''Professional status in nursing is maintained and enriched by the willingness of the individual practitioner to accept and fulfill obligations to society, co-workers, and the profession of nursing.''

The seventeen points of the 1960 Code are:

1. The fundamental responsibility of the nurse is to conserve life, to alleviate suffering, and to promote health.

2. The nurse provides services based on human need, with respect for human dignity, unrestricted by considerations of nationality, race, creed, color or status.

3. The nurse does not use professional knowledge and skill in any enterprise detrimental to the public good.

4. The nurse respects and holds in confidence all information of a confidential nature obtained in the course of nursing work unless required by law to divulge it.

5. The nurse as a citizen understands and upholds the laws and performs the duties of citizenship; as a professional person the nurse has particular responsibility to work with other citizens and health professions in promoting efforts to meet health needs of the public.

6. The nurse has responsibility for membership and participation in the nurses' professional organization.

7. The nurse participates responsibly in defining and upholding standards of professional practice and education.

8. The nurse maintains professional competence and demonstrates concern for the competence of other members of the nursing profession.

9. The nurse assumes responsibility for individual professional actions and judgement, both in dependent and independent nursing functions, and knows and upholds the laws which affect the practice of nursing.

---

[5] These articles are listed in the references at the end of this chapter.

10. The nurse, acting through the professional organization, participates responsibly in establishing terms and conditions of employment.

11. The nurse has the responsibility to participate in study of and action on matters of legislation affecting nurses and nursing service to the public.

12. The nurse adheres to standards of personal ethics which reflect credit upon the profession.

13. The nurse may contribute to research in relation to a commercial product or service, but does not lend professional status to advertising, promotion, or sales.

14. Nurses, or groups of nurses, who advertise professional services, do so in conformity with the dignity of the nursing profession.

15. The nurse has an obligation to protect the public by not delegating to a person less qualified any service which requires the professional competence of a nurse.

16. The nurse works harmoniously with, and sustains confidence in nursing associations, the physician, and other members of the health team.

17. The nurse refuses to participate in unethical procedures and assumes the responsibility to expose incompetence or unethical conduct in others to the appropriate authority.

Codes of all professions require changes to conform to social changes in general. This is to be expected and accepted, especially in a profession as dynamic as that which characterizes nursing in the United States.

REFERENCES

''A suggested code of ethics.'' *Amer. J. Nurs.* 26:599 (Aug.) 1926.

BECK, SR. M. BERNICE: What's in our code? *Amer J. Nurs.* 56:1406 (Nov.) 1956.

BURGESS, MAY AYRES: What makes a good nurse? *Amer. J. Nurs.* 32:1238 (Dec.) 1932.

CASTIGLIONE, ARTURO: *A History of Medicine.* Alfred A. Knopf Co., New York, 1941.

DEANS, AGNES, and AUSTIN, ANNE L.: History of the Farrand Training School for Nurses. Alumnae Association, Harper Hospital, Detroit, 1936.

FINK, ELIZABETH E.: How our code of ethics was formed. *Nurs. World* 75:348 (Aug.) 1951.

GARRISON, FIELDING H.: *An Introduction to the History of Medicine.* W. B. Saunders Company, Philadelphia, 1929.

LIMBERT, PAUL M.: Developing a code of ethics for the nursing profession. *Amer. J. Nurs.* 32:1257 (Dec.) 1932.

MUNSON, HELEN W.: Lystra Gretter (History of the Nightingale Pledge). *Amer. J. Nurs.* 49:345 (June) 1949.

' Revision proposed in code for professional nurses.'' *Amer. J. Nurs.* 60:77 (Jan.) 1960.

''The code for professional nurses.'' *Amer. J. Nurs.* 60:1287 (Sept.) 1960.

''What's in our code?'' *Amer. J. Nurs.* 52:1246 (Oct.) 1952; 53:299 (Mar.) 1953; 53:456 (Apr.) 1953; 53:843 (July) 1953; 53:965 (Aug.) 1953; 53:1099 (Sept.) 1953; 53:1217 (Oct.) 1953.

UNIT II

Orientation of the Graduate Nurse

CHAPTER 17

Professional Nursing

The earliest definition of nursing was "care of the sick without remedial measures." But as scientific discoveries were made the practice of medicine became more complex; the need for nurses to assume more responsibility became necessary. To carry out this responsibility, educational requirements for nurses were increased; nursing education was broadened to give the student an intelligent background for the added skills which modern medicine demanded. The education of the student was given consideration as well as the demands of nursing service. The physician became aware that the nurse was not the handmaiden of the physician, but together they made up a team for the treatment and care of the sick which is largely responsible for the increased life expectancy of the American people.

Out of this change in the concept of the care of the sick has emerged the professional nurse with the rights and privileges accorded persons in other professions. In 1955 the Board of Directors of the American Nurses' Association (the national organization for professional nurses) formulated a definition of professional nursing:

The practice of professional nursing means the performance for compensation of any act in the observance, care, and counsel of the ill, injured, or infirm, or in the maintenance of health or prevention of illness of others, or in the

supervision and teaching of other personnel, or the administration of medica-
tions and treatments as prescribed by a physician or dentist; requiring
substantial specialized judgment and skill based on knowledge and application
of the principles of biological, physical, and social science. The foregoing
shall not be deemed to include acts of diagnosis or prescription of therapeutic
or corrective measures.[1]

This defines nursing in the United States. It is not an international definition of nursing. After graduation from schools in the United States American nurses may visit other countries under the ANA International Unit's Exchange Service. They will often find nurses carrying out functions that would be considered medical practice in the United States.[2] Also, the head nurse or sister is given more freedom in the use of her judgment and experience than is her counterpart in this country.

TYPES OF NURSING

Nursing is a popular field of employment for women, second only to teaching. This care of the sick is broadly divided into professional nursing and practical nursing.

There are three types of professional nursing schools. These are the junior or community college, usually of two calendar years; the college or university of four academic or four calendar years (a few college schools offer a five-year program) ; and the hospital school of three calendar years.

SELECTION OF A SCHOOL

When is a school of nursing a good school? It is the responsibility of the state to safeguard its citizens by investigating and accrediting the schools of nursing that operate in that state. This is a legal procedure and minimum requirements differ from state to state. Schools of nursing also are accredited by the Accreditation Service of the National League for Nursing. This is a voluntary program which aids the school of nursing in eliminating the weak points and raising standards cn a national level. Two authentic sources of information on this subject are:

"Nursing—Profession for You?" published by the Committee on Careers, National League for Nursing, 10 Columbus Circle, New York 19, N. Y.

The list of schools that are fully accredited by the National League for Nursing is published annually in the February issue of Nursing Outlook.

---

[1] "ANA Board Approves a Definition of Nursing Practice," *Amer. J. Nurs.* Vol. 55 (Dec. 1955), p. 1474.

[2] Read *The Burma Surgeon* by Gordon S. Seagrave, M.D. (New York, W. W. Norton Company.)

FUNCTIONS OF PROFESSIONAL NURSES

Nurses as other professional groups have distinctive functions to perform. To outline nursing functions seemed an overwhelming undertaking, but in 1953 the American Nurses' Association began a study of functions, standards, and qualifications of nursing (this is known as the F S & Q Study). Some 20,000 nurses participated in this study and the report *Twenty Thousand Nurses Tell Their Story*, published in 1958, makes fascinating reading.

The significance of this colossal study in its everyday use is of importance to all nurses. These standards serve as the guide for nursing practice and job specifications. In nursing education they are helpful in planning curriculums. These clearly defined functions have legal significance; there was a need for identification of standards and functions in malpractice suits. These statements now make it possible to separate medical practice and practical nursing from professional nursing.

These statements will need revision to meet changes and advances in nursing. The nurse will keep on her professional toes by reading these revisions as they appear in the official magazines. FS&Q is important for all types of nursing and the nurse should be alert to changes.

MAINTAINING PROFESSIONAL STATUS

Every thoughtful person is aware of the prestige given to education. Time was when wealth was the compelling drive for recognition. Now, in a country of unrivaled prosperity, education has become a social yardstick. Each occupation is striving for professional status although it means restraints, sacrifices, and controls. People are willing to subject themselves to this discipline in order to be given professional recognition. Why? Because professions require advanced education and education always assumes a commanding position in men's minds. Another reason is the autonomy or self-government accorded professions:

Society gives the professions a mandate to do certain jobs and grants them autonomy in order to do these jobs. This autonomy can be thought of as a socially distributed reward for the discipline of professional life and for what that discipline makes it possible to achieve. To a great extent, the professions themselves decide what they are to do, how they are to do it, and who is to do it. In short, they are granted the privilege of defining their functions, their standards, and their qualifications.[3]

There are three convenient and available methods by which nurses may continue to increase their professional stature: *Formal education* in a college or university is within the reach of many nurses. With a working day of eight hours and two free days each week, the duty schedule can be planned so that the nurse is able to carry one subject. It is not necessary that the subject pertain to nursing. One of the characteristics of a professional person is his

---

[3] Robert K. Merton, ''The Search for Professional Status.'' *Amer. J. Nurs.* Vol. 60 (May, 1960), p. 662.

broad background of information. Nursing education necessarily includes a great deal of science. It will be an intellectual treat for the nurse to enroll in a class of philosophy, geography, or a foreign language. Classes in advanced English offer courses in public speaking.

All professions have well-defined organizations. This is especially true of nursing. The *district organization* is within reach of all nurses, and it has a tremendous potential for increasing the nurse's interest. True, it is much easier to invite a doctor who is a good speaker to talk at the district meeting, but the members themselves have a rich source of experience and knowledge which can be developed to provide a beneficial program. Classify the practicing interests of the membership and plan a year's program along these lines:

The Nursing Care of the Craniotomy Patient

The Training and Rehabilitation of the Cerebral Vascular Accident Patient

The Care and Rehabilitation of the Patient with Both Eyes Patched

The Terminal Care of Cancer Patients

Civil Defense and the Hospital

Since these are broad subjects the presentation can be divided among several members. Each can enrich her material by information from current magazines, medical, and hospital magazines. Such programs will increase interest and attendance. Nurses want to learn about nursing.

The *professional magazines* offer the most convenient way of keeping abreast of the fast-moving developments in nursing. The official magazines—"The American Journal of Nursing" and "Nursing Outlook"—give information on a wide range of subjects. There are several good commercial magazines, as well as magazines devoted to specialties, with which the nurse can keep informed along the lines of her chief interest.

It is not enough to graduate from a professional school of nursing. The nurse owes it to herself to keep her interests, attitudes, and activities alive as a professional person.

PHILOSOPHY

As the early Greeks coined the word "philosophy" it meant to satisfy curiosity or the pursuit of mental excellence; a literal translation would mean "to love learning." But "philosophy," like the English word "wisdom," implies not only broad knowledge, but also sound judgment of the values of different things in life, i. e., what is most worth striving for in life. The present-day use of the word has come to mean a guide for human conduct based on experience, reasoning, and established personal beliefs.

Each student, as an upper classman, should formulate a plan for the future. Now the fundamental background of nursing has been acquired; experience has made a deep impression; the student has learned to reason as never before. In the light of all these a philosophy should be thought through, and concrete plans should be made. Circumstances may change this goal, but it will not be aimless drifting through the course of events.

Every one has a philosophy of life, a philosophy of nursing in terms of work satisfaction, and a philosophy of education, either formal or in-service. This belief in life should be sound and constructive, directed by an earnest attempt to live it with professional satisfaction but never contentment.

CLASS EXERCISE

Each member of the class will contribute one pertinent fact on the present nursing situation. These should come from reliable sources, such as editorials from official magazines, both nursing and medical, and from radio releases. In selecting these points keep in mind that nurses are interested in professional advancement, professional satisfaction, continued employment, and salaries comparable to those of other professions.

REFERENCES

BENNE, KENNETH D., and BENNIS, WARREN: Role confusion and conflict in nursing: What is real nursing? *Amer. J. Nurs.* 59:380 (Mar.) 1959.

BOYLE, RENA E.: Critical issues in collegiate education in nursing. *Nurs. Outlook* 10:165 (Mar.) 1962.

BRIDGES, DAISY C.: The nurse in space. *Nurs. Mirror* 112:529 (May 12) 1961.

BROTHERSON, J. H. F.: Nursing responsibilities to meet changing health needs. *Nursing Mirror* (London) 103:2670:1009 (July 6) 1956.

Editorial: Toward perfecting our practice. *Amer. J. Nurs.* 59:1397 (Oct.) 1959.

Editorial: Well now. *Amer. J. Nurs.* 60:189 (Feb.) 1960.

"Education or Training." *Nurs. Outlook* 1:437 (Aug.) 1953.

GOLDBERG, EMANUEL: Men in nursing. *RN* 22:40 (May) 1959.

HALE, THOMAS: The five sides of the nursing problem. *Mod. Hosp.* 89:74 (Dec.) 1957.

HAYS, DORTHEA E.: An untapped source of potential nurses. *Nurs. Outlook* 8:596 (Nov.) 1960.

HILLWAY, TYRUS: *The American Two-year College.* Harper & Brothers, New York, 1958.

HUGHES, EVERETT C., HUGHES, HELEN M., and DEUTCHER, IRWIN: *20,000 Nurses Tell Their Story.* J. B. Lippincott Company, Philadelphia, 1958.

INNOCENT, BROTHER: One hundred forty-three men nurses. *Amer. J. Nurs.* 55:76 (Jan.) 1955.

JAHODA, MARIE: Nursing as a profession. Opening address of the First Plenary Session, 12th Quadrennial International Congress of Nursing. *Nurs. Mirror* 112:237 (Apr. 21) 1961 (Part I); Apr. 28, 1961 (Part II).

JAHODA, MARIE: A social psychologist views nursing as a profession. *Amer. J. Nurs.* 61:52 (July) 1961.

JOHNSON, DOROTHY E.: A philosophy of nursing. *Nurs. Outlook* 7:198 (Apr.) 1959.

MARYO, JOAN S., and LASKY, JULIAN J.: A work satisfaction survey among nurses. *Amer. J. Nurs.* 59:501 (Apr.) 1959.

''Nurses for a growing nation.'' *Amer. J. Nurs.* 57:721 (June) 1957.

''Nursing education for whom, where, and when.'' *Amer. J. Nurs.* 62:50 (Apr.) 1962.

PORTER, ELIZABETH K.: What it means to be a professional nurse. *Amer. J. Nurs.* 53:948 (Aug.) 1953.

''Principles governing professional nursing education. *Amer. J. Nurs.* 62:56 (Apr.) 1962.

RAISIG, L. MILES: Keeping up with professional literature. *Amer. J. Nurs.* 59:544 (Apr.) 1950.

SPALDING, EUGENIA K.: *Professional Nursing: Trends, Responsibilities, and Relationships.* J. B. Lippincott Company, Philadelphia, 1959.

SYMONDS, PERCIVAL M.: Evaluation in professional education. *Nurs. Outlook* 5:166 (Mar.) 1957.

WILLIAMS, MARYJO: When to advise a girl against nursing. *R.N.* 23:35 (Mar.) 1960.

WOLFF, ILSE S.: As others see us. *Nurs. Outlook* 2:408 (Aug.) 1954.

UNIT III

Opportunities and Preparation

CHAPTER 18

Opportunities

The public, the doctors, even the nurses themselves, bewail the shortage of nurses. They appear incredulous when told that there are more actively practicing nurses now than ever before. Where are they? Thirty thousand nurses took the written licensing examination in 1960.[1] Where did they go? The country does not have a shortage of nurses; it does have a vast increase in nursing opportunities—opportunities to suit the interests of every registered nurse.

It is interesting to note that nurses do not abandon nursing. To paraphrase William Shepeard's ninth criterion of a profession,[2] nursing does have sufficient self-impelling power and interest to retain nurses through their working years. It is not a mere stepping stone to other occupations.

Nurses, at the age of graduation and registration, are naturally concerned with marriage, home, and family rearing. Yet state inventories show that more than half of the nurses working are married "with husbands present."[3]

---

[1] See *Facts About Nursing.* (New York, American Nurses' Association, 1960), Section B, under "Professional Nurse Education."

[2] William P. Shepeard, "Professionalization of Public Health," *American Journal of Public Health*, Vol. 30 (Jan., part 2, 1948), p. 145.

[3] Thirty-four states require annual registration. In this way the state has current information concerning its nurses.

Many of these have small children. It is interesting to watch this social revolution: ''The mother's place is in the home.'' ''Working mothers are the greatest cause of juvenile delinquency.'' Yet, nurses' children seem to grow up as normal children in families where home duties are shared by all, and assuming responsibility is taken for granted.

CAUSES OF OPPORTUNITY INCREASE

The American public has come to depend upon nurses as part of a way of life; nurses have become indispensable and at the same time nursing opportunities continue to increase. The causes of this increase are many:

Prosperity. The world never has known the amazing prosperity that characterizes America, the richest country on earth. People can pay for nursing service, and since this service usually is given in hospitals approximately half of the nurses are employed in hospitals. People no longer remain at home when ill, even for minor illnesses; therefore more hospitals are needed. New hospitals are under construction and additions are made to existing ones in every city and town.

The Hill-Burton Act. This is a hospital expansion law, passed in 1946, by which federal money was appropriated to aid communities in building hospitals. This act has increased the number of hospital beds by 100,000 and it has provided 300 health clinics. Many of these new hospitals and clinics are in outlying towns of less than 10,000 population, but distant from any hospital facilities.

Because of the relative isolation of many of these hospitals, securing an adequate nursing staff has been difficult; but through marriage or home ties, nurses have been secured and a stable auxiliary staff has been trained. Generally, the nursing care is of excellent quality.

Hospital Insurance. Hospital insurance caught on rather slowly. It is unpleasant to contemplate illness. However, as new diagnostic tests were discovered and new medicines and treatments came into use, the cost of hospitalization increased. To meet these costs a prepaid plan was devised whereby the person could pay for hospital care while well, as he paid for life insurance while living.

There are numerous plans for health and hospital insurance; most of these operate with the approval of organized medicine. All plans provide for a free choice of physicians which in no way interferes with individual medical practice.

Prepaid hospital care has increased immensely the need for hospitals and nurses. In 1946 the number of hospital admissions was 15,500,000. By 1957 the annual admissions totaled 23,000,000, due largely to the increase in hospital insurance.[4]

---

[4] *Annual Guide Issue of Hospitals*, August 1, 1959 (Part 2).

Increased Birth Rate. Babies! Babies! Babies! They are well fed, well clothed, and loved. This population increase has opened nursing opportunities in more and larger pediatric hospitals, camp nursing, health supervision in homes for dependent children. It has greatly increased the need for school nurses, and for nurse teachers in pediatric hospitals affiliated with schools of nursing.

Industry. Occupational health has replaced the early term "industrial nursing." The United States is an industrial nation with increasing industrial needs due to demands made by an expanding population. World War II taught industry the advantages of the occupational health nurse. War materials were urgently needed and keeping workers on the job was important. Industries first employed one or two nurses and quickly increased the number to ten or more. The nurse found the reason for absenteeism, especially among women workers, and she maintained a smooth running health service for the employees. The nurse has proved her worth as a part of the plant personnel. By the time the war was over, the field of industrial nursing was established. Occupational health now ranks fourth in the employment of nurses.

Office Nursing. Each year many new graduates become office nurses. This is now the third largest field of nursing. Modern medicine has become too complex for the routine work to be turned over to the "office girl." The physician requires intelligent, well-qualified assistance upon which he can depend as a part of the health team, which is as necessary in the office as in the hospital.

A doctor with an extensive practice may employ from one to four nurses. Several physicians may form a group-practice clinic and several nurses are employed. Although there is little opportunity for advancement in office nursing, the nurse derives professional satisfaction and stimulation in keeping abreast with medical advances as does her employer.

Rehabilitation. This is a new and exciting opportunity in a field of work of which the medical profession is scarcely aware.[5] This is not occupational therapy or physical therapy, but a challenging type of nursing in which nurses and doctors are equally important in restoring the patient to usefulness.

Dr. Howard A. Rusk, Professor of the Department of Physical Medicine and Rehabilitation, New York University Medical Center, has said " . . . disabled people—the people who represent the greatest minority group in the world today. Justice, to them, means the right to compete with their so-called normal brothers; the opportunity to be treated and trained to live the best lives they can with the abilities they have. They ask to be judged on their abilities, not on their disabilities."

Courses in rehabilitation designed for nurses are offered in rehabilitation centers; courses are also given on the master's degree level with the idea of teaching rehabilitation in medical centers.

[5] Lena Dixon Dietz, "Rehabilitation and the Nurse," *The Davis Nursing Survey*, Vol. 24 (Oct. 1960), p. 150.

Mental Health. The mental hospitals of the United States contain more than 700,000 patients. Most of these patients are in state-supported institutions. The whole pattern of mental treatment has changed. Custodial care is being replaced by scientific methods in which nurses have an important part. Advances in psychiatry are becoming too complex for the politically appointed ward attendant. Psychiatric nurses need good understanding of the social sciences in addition to the basic nursing course. Because of the pressing need for nurses in mental hospitals, a number of states make educational grants to nurse students, who, after completion of the basic nursing course, return to work in a mental hospital in that state.

Research. Clinical research attracts many nurses as a new and exacting field of nursing. The United States government, through the Department of Health, Education, and Welfare, makes large annual appropriations for medical research. A part of the annual appropriation is assigned to medical centers for a specific research project. The government is concerned with improving the nation's health. In 1900 the average newborn child could be expected to live only 47 years. Today the average life span is 70 years.[6]

An interesting field of clinical research is the National Institutes of Health of the Public Health Services, Bethesda, Maryland. There are seven of these institutes:

National Institute of Neurological Diseases and Blindness
National Institute of Mental Health
National Cancer Institute
National Institute of Arthritis and Metabolic Diseases
National Institute of Allergy and Infectious Diseases
National Heart Institute
National Institute of Dental Research

Patients to be studied in these institutions are admitted to the Clinical Center. This hospital has a capacity of 500 beds with 1100 laboratory units. In the Clinical Center each institute has patient rooms and research laboratories in close proximity. The facilities for diagnosis, medical and nursing care, social service, rehabilitation, and recreation are comparable to those in any good hospital. But the emphasis is placed on research, so that nursing care is exacting and scientific. Observations and reports assume a new significance.

SALARIES

The nurse has a right to be interested in the salary in the field of nursing which she selects. The American Nurses' Association, through its Economic Security Program, has assumed great responsibility in helping nurses secure salaries that will assure them living conditions comparable to that of other professions.

---

[6] *Holy Bible*, Psalm 90: "The years of our age is three score years and ten."

The salary range in various parts of the country is shown in Chapter IV in *Facts About Nursing*, 1961. The United States Department of Labor, in cooperation with the Women's Bureau, furnishes the Research and Statistical Unit of the American Nurses' Association with this information. An estimate of salaries in all fields of nursing can be obtained annually from *Facts About Nursing* under the heading: "The Economic Status of the Nursing Profession." Also, information can be secured from the Economic Security Unit of the ANA.

OCCUPATIONAL TRENDS

Work trends in nursing are changing. This is the age of specialization in nursing as well as in medicine, engineering, and law. There is specialization within the various divisions of nursing as there is in medicine: a surgeon may do only chest surgery; private duty nurses, if they desire, may now limit their patients only to those having had open-heart surgery.

The upper classman in a school of nursing with a well-rounded program has had ample opportunity to be aware of nursing in the various departments (psychiatry, public health, rehabilitation, and the like), but there are fields of nursing outside the school experience that may offer interest.

Books cannot be written fast enough to keep up with these changes. To keep informed, however, is a professional duty. The following sources are listed as references by which the nurse can follow the direction of nursing interests:

1. Dorothy Deming, long a leader in nursing, prepared *Careers for Nurses*.[7] This book gives job descriptions of seventeen fields of nursing which are described in an accurate and readable style. The book is available in all nursing school libraries. Chapter 1, "Choosing a Career," will assist the student in evaluating her potential in a field of nursing that may appear interesting. This chapter includes the subjects of educational qualifications, necessary experience, responsibilities, and functions of the type of nursing under consideration.

2. *Facts About Nursing* is an annual statistical publication (paper bound) of the American Nurses' Association. The National League for Nursing and the United States Public Health Service assist in supplying information for this publication. Statistics are of genuine interest when they are translated into current information, i. e.: How many employed professional nurses are there in the United States? How do the salaries of general duty nurses in New England compare with salaries on the Pacific coast? How many nurses in this state are enrolled in a master's degree program? How many men nurses graduated from professional schools last year? What is the proportion of practical nurses to professional nurses?

3. Annual Guide Issue of *Hospitals*, the journal of the American Hospital Association, is a central reference source for information on

---

[7] Dorothy Deming, *Careers for Nurses*, 2nd. ed. (New York, McGraw-Hill Book Company, Inc., 1952).

hospitals, the American Hospital Association, and allied organizations and agencies. This issue is divided into four sections: Listing of Hospitals, Directory for the Hospital Field, Guide to the American Hospital Association, and Hospital Statistics. The last section includes statistics on professional nurses.

4. United States Department of Labor issues an annual publication, *Women's Handbook on Women Workers*. This handbook lists the activities of women workers in all types of work and it makes an excellent statistical reference for comparison of nurses and nursing with women workers in other fields.

NURSES FOR A GROWING NATION: A REPORT

This report is the result of a study carried out by the National League for Nursing's research and statistics department under the auspices of the Committee on the Future.

This study was made in order "To forecast changing needs in nursing service and nursing education based upon examination of social and health trends in the forseeable future."[8] This report and its goal is concerned with the supply and demand of nurses based upon three factors:

1. The expected population growth

2. The desirability of more nursing service through an increase in the ratio of nurses to population

3. Personnel lost through marriage, family responsibilities, retirement, and death

---

CLASS EXERCISE

The number of licensed practical nurses, nurse aides, and attendants now exceeds the number of professional nurses. List five reasons why this is not a threat to the future employment of professional nurses.

REFERENCES

BRIDGMAN, MARGARET: Collegiate Education for Nursing. Russell Sage Foundation, New York, 1953.

COOPER, SIGNE S.: Are nurses interested in nursing? *Nurs. World* 131:9 (June) 1957.

Editorial: Nurses for a growing nation. *Amer. J. Nurs.* 57:721 (June) 1957.

---

[8] *Nurses for a Growing Nation* (New York, National League for Nursing, 1957).

Guide Issue of *Hospitals*, Journal of the American Hospital Association, published annually in August.

HERWITZ, ADELE: An international look at employment problems. *Amer. J. Nurs.* 59:355 (Mar.) 1959.

HORGAN, PATRICIA D.: They work in a hospital for medical research. *RN* 23:42 and 23:62 (July) 1960.

JOHNSON, EVERETT: There's no short cut to nursing leadership. *Mod. Hosp.* 79:68 (Oct.) 1952.

LAMBERTSON, ELEANOR: The education and role of tomorrow's nurse. Hospitals 34:39 (Jan. 1) 1960.

LEONE, LUCILE PETRY: Wanted: Good nursing. *Nurs. Outlook* 5:576 (Oct.) 1957.

LOIJA, ELEANOR A.: The director of nursing service and her choice of positions. *Amer. J. Nurs.* 61:96 (Sept.) 1961.

McIVER, PEARL: Nursing moves forward. *Amer. J. Nurs.* 52:821 (July) 1952.

MOSES, EVELYN B.: The profile of a professional nurse. *Amer. J. Nurs.* 60:368 (Mar.) 1960.

National Institutes of Health: Bulletin No. 1215-2, Dept. of Health, Education and Welfare, U. S. Public Health Service, Washington, D. C.

POHLEN, KURT: Measuring the need for hospital beds. *Hosp. Progr.* 29:47 (Feb.) 1948.

PRICE, JULIAN P.: The health of the nation. *Hospitals* 32:48 (Jan.) 1958.

RAMOS, LUIS F.: A man nurse in public health nursing. *Amer. J. Nurs.* 58:1254 (Sept.) 1954.

SCHLOTFELD, ROZELLA M.: Reflections on nursing research. *Amer. J. Nurs.* 60:492 (Apr.) 1960.

SLEEPER, RUTH: What kind of a nurse? *Amer. J. Nurs.* 52:828 (July) 1952.

"Three ways to enter professional nursing." *RN* 23:45 (Sept.) 1960.

U. S. Dept. of Labor: Employment Outlook in Health Occupations. Bulletin No. 1215-2.

"We need more teachers." *Amer. J. Nurs.* 51:487 (Aug.) 1951.

WITNEY, FRED: Is nursing meeting its obligations to society? *Amer. J. Nurs.* 56:1127 (Sept.) 1956.

CHAPTER 19

Registration and Interstate Licensure

"The primary purpose of licensing legislation for professional nurses is to protect the public by establishing certain requirements which must be complied with by individuals seeking to engage in nursing practice."[1]

DEPARTMENT OF STATE REGISTRATION

Beginning in 1901, with North Carolina first, state nurses' associations were organized rapidly. The first objective of these organizations was to work for laws to regulate the practice of nursing. Twenty years later all states had passed such laws; this was a great achievement for nursing because women could not vote. Many hospitals were privately owned by men who could vote. These hospitals were operated as commercial enterprises and nurse registration was a serious threat to the profits of these institutions.[2]

When a bill to regulate the practice of nursing has been signed into law it becomes the function of the state government to carry out its provisions. The

---

[1] *Facts About Nursing,* Section G, 1960.

[2] Adelaide Nutting and Lavinia Dock, *A History of Nursing* (New York, G. P. Putnam's Sons, 1935), Vol. III, pp. 142-187.

law provides for an administrative agency—usually known as "state board" or "board of nurse examiners." This board has two areas of responsibility: education for nursing and licensing of those who would practice nursing.

Functions of the State Board of Examiners. In 1957 the American Nurses' Association appointed a subcommittee to prepare a statement of the functions and standards for members and for professional employees of state boards of nursing.[3] These functions fall into four areas:

1. General administration, such as developing a philosophy for board action, collection and distribution of funds, maintaining legal records, and selection of personnel.

2. The board surveys schools of nursing for approval or accreditation of the nursing program. Criteria for approved schools are set up by the individual state. These standards specify the number and qualifications of the faculty, classrooms, laboratories, library, clinical practice, housing of students, and state board examination performance.

3. The board conducts examinations and issues licenses to those who have achieved the grade required by *that* state. To issue such a license is a legal function of the state as a protection of its citizens; therefore, those who apply for examination must have graduated from a school of nursing which has been accredited by the state.

4. The board of nurse examiners is not an isolated unit of the state government. In the interest of the citizens' welfare and in good nursing practice, the board interprets nursing and nursing education for schools and agencies who wish to establish schools. The board assists in strengthening schools by interpreting trends in nursing and nursing education to groups and individuals interested in the education of nurses.

Qualifications. The board of nurse examiners, which administers the nurse practice law, may function within one of several departments, such as the medical board, department of registration and education, public health, or public welfare. The examiners may be appointed by the governor of the state or by the board under which the practice law functions, although this is hardly in keeping with democratic ideals. The majority of the states make recommendations from among the members of the state nurses' association.

General and personal qualifications for members of the board differed widely in different states. In 1957 the American Nurses' Association appointed a subcommittee to prepare a statement of qualifications for members and professional employees of the state board of nurse examiners in order to make qualifications more uniform. As a general statement: "Eligibility for appointment to the board of nursing should be based on personal fitness, educational preparation, and breadth of experience, rather than on representation from a clinical field or geographical area."[4]

---

[3] "ANA Statements of Functions and Standards for Members and Professional Employees of State Boards of Nursing, *American Journal of Nursing*, Vol. 57 (Dec. 1957), p. 1586.

[4] "ANA Statements of Qualifications for Members and Professional Employees of State Boards of Nursing," *American Journal of Nursing*, Vol. 57 (Nov. 1957), p. 1446.

These qualifications were carefully detailed by the committee; the personal and professional requirements are listed with an explanation for each. This official statement now serves as a criterion for the appointment of board members and makes for uniformity in the Bureau of State Board of Examiners.

Support. The state department of nurse registration is entirely self-supporting; it is not financed by taxation. The fees paid by each candidate for examination provide sufficient funds to maintain the department.

STATE EXAMINATIONS

State rights are of practical importance in the licensing of nurses. At the time the original thirteen colonies declared themselves independent, each colony had developed a self-sufficiency peculiar to its own needs. Education ranged all the way from good to none. In order to hold the colonies together politically, the founding fathers conceded education developments and requirements as the right of each state. Nursing education followed the same pattern. As nursing legislation was enacted in each state, the standards and qualifications were planned independently of any other state.

This independence, granted under state rights, made interstate licensure extremely difficult, and often unfair to the nurse who wished to practice nursing in another state. This difficulty involved length of course, subject content, clinical experience offered, and performance at state board examinations. Some of these difficulties still exist. Not all states require clinical experience in psychiatry. Therefore, if the nurse who has not had this experience applies to a state which requires this experience of its practitioners, the nurse cannot be granted a license in that state until this deficiency has been made up.

Licensure between states is based generally on the presumption that the license will be granted provided that the nurse who applies for a license *has graduated from a school meeting all the requirements of the state to which she applies* for registration.

STATE BOARD TEST POOL

The traditional examination was prepared and administered by the members of the state board. These papers, usually the essay type, were corrected and scored by the examiners—a time-consuming process. With the beginning of World War II, when time was precious and enrollment increasing, an effort was made to find a method by which questions could be prepared by a well-qualified group and the answers graded by machine.

In December, 1942, the National League of Nursing Education Committee on Nursing Tests consented to operate a pool licensing tests. Less than ten states used the first pool in 1943. Now the State Board Test Pool is used by all the states and by seven provinces of Canada.

Although this examination has a national distribution it is *not* a national examination. Each state and province assists in developing the tests, and determines where and when the tests will be given and what the passing score shall be.

The responsibility for establishing the passing grade for licensure rests with the state board of examiners as a state right. One powerful medium by which standards of nursing are being improved is through the gradual raising of the passing scores which have been comparatively low in some states.

R. N.

The term *registered nurse* with the initials *R. N.* is not a title in any sense of the word and it should not be so used. It indicates to the public that the nurse has met certain requirements which have been prescribed by a particular state, and that, having done so, she is entitled to the legal and social privileges and responsibilities accorded registrants of that profession.

The initials *R. N.* cannot be used by the nurse in states in which she is not registered. She may be a registered nurse in Oregon, and as such she is entitled to use the initials *R. N.* in Oregon when indicated. She does not have this privilege in Washington unless she is registered in Washington.

RENEWAL OF CERTIFICATE

Forty-four states now require annual renewal of license. This is considered good practice for the following reasons:

1. It keeps a current list of all nurses in the state.

2. It provides a check on lost certificates.

3. It furnishes a current identification card for the nurse.

4. Information requested at the time of renewal provides the department of nurse registration with a list of active and inactive nurses and the field of nursing in which they are engaged.

The expiration date for license renewal differs in different states. Each state, with its license expiration date, is listed in the annual issue of *Facts About Nursing*, Chapter I, "Distribution of Nurses."

The renewal certificate by the state department of nurse registration is issued as a billfold-size card which carries the original registration number as well as the current number. The nurse should carry this card at all times for a ready means of identification.

Renewal of the certificate is necessary in order to practice nursing, but renewal is not enough. As a professional person the nurse is expected to keep informed. The nurse who graduated in 1955 cannot be considered a safe practitioner in 1965 merely because her state registration has been kept current. Both nursing service and doctors are requiring inactive nurses to have a refresher course before again caring for patients.

REVOCATION

All states make some provision for revocation of the license or certification of registration. This is for the protection of the public and for the profession. Many states have laws which provide disciplinary measures as a reprimand or probation for less serious offenses. Drug addiction and mental incompetency are the usual causes for the revocation or suspension of a license.

Nurse practice laws have a section on violations. This is applied usually to nurses who pose as registered nurses with all the employment benefits of the registered nurse. Reports of these imposters occur at times; they usually are apprehended and sentenced in a court of law. In some instances such persons produce considerable evidence, such as a diploma or pin. This should warn all registered nurses to take special care of these credentials, lest they fall into unscrupulous hands and be used illegally.

INTERSTATE LICENSURE

Registration without examination or interstate licensure means that the nurse has the privilege of registration in another state without taking the written examination. True, all nurses in all states take the same examination but state rights permit each state to decide on the course content, clinical experience, and passing grade in the state examination.

Application. A registered nurse who wishes to practice nursing in another state should write to the board of nurse examiners in the other state and find if she is eligible to practice there. The nurse should give the name and address of the school from which she graduated, the date of registration, and the registration number.

The request for this information should be addressed to the secretary of the board of nurse examiners, sometimes called the "board of nursing." The name and address of this official is given in the Official Directory of the *American Journal of Nursing*. This directory is published each January and July.

The nurse should not confuse the *secretray of the board of nurse examiners* with the *secretary of the state nurses' association*.

The nurse who wishes to secure registration in another state should make plans several months in advance. First, information will need to be secured from the home school and from the department of nurse registration in the home state. Second, applications are processed at the meetings of the board; these meetings are held each month or each second month. Third, additional information may be required. The time required for the entire procedure is frequently three months.

Permit to Practice. Some states do not permit the nurse to work as a registered nurse until formal registration is complete. Some states issue permits until the next examination; some issue courtesy permits until the formal registration is complete; others issue permits to nurses who are only temporarily in that state. All nurse practice acts make some provision for exemptions from the rule of registration such as caring for members of the family, gratuitous nursing, and professional nurses from other states who are doing graduate work.

STATE ACCREDITATION AND LEAGUE ACCREDITATION

State accreditation means that the school of nursing has been inspected and approved and the school is accredited by the state licensing board. It is the duty of the state examining board to see that all schools meet the minimum standards set by that state. Students who take the written examination and are registered by the state then have a legal right to practice nursing in that state.

Beginning in 1940, the National League for Nursing began a program for national accreditation. This program is voluntary and does not carry legal status. National accreditation has greatly improved schools of nursing in every state,[5] but it does not alter state rights. To graduate from a school which has "full accreditation" from the League Accrediting Service does not guarantee the nurse the right to register in any state. The nurse may graduate from a school which has full accreditation from the National League for Nursing, yet that school may be located in a state in which the passing score is 350 points. As a student, she drifted along without effort, secure in the belief that the full accreditation of the school would permit her to register in any state. Her state board score was 362. She wishes to return to her home state which requires a passing grade of 400. It is then that the nurse learns that she cannot register in her home state—a bitter disappointment and a severe handicap. Every student should strive for grades that will permit interstate licensure with any state, other requirements being equal.

NURSES FROM OTHER COUNTRIES

Every large medical center has a great many foreign nurses, both men and women. To license these nurses is a complex problem since the primary function of the state licensing board is to insure safe nursing care for its citizens.

Many states require a declaration of intention to become a citizen or a certificate of citizenship. Second, the professional status of the applicant must be established; third, credentials related to professional education are studied and evaluated. Credentials must be translated into English by a translating agency approved by the examining board in the state in which the nurse wishes to practice.

The International Refugee Organization, working in displaced persons camps, has a considerable fund of information, gathered by careful investi-

---

[5] *Nursing Outlook*, February issue each year, for a complete list of schools fully accredited by the National League for Nursing.

gation by nurses who had a wide knowledge of schools of nursing in countries from which the displaced persons came. Some documents and information from this committee can be used to validate credentials from nurses whose schools no longer exist and in whose country there have been changes in government.

The International Council of Nurses, London, through a half century of records, has been able to help in securing credentials of schools of nursing in both Europe and Asia.

Nurses with relatives and friends in other countries who wish to come to this country ask how to go about establishing professional status in order to practice nursing in the United States. A letter should be written in English to the American Nurses' Association, 10 Columbus Circle, New York 19, N. Y., to ask for information and instructions about the procurement of a professional nurse license.

The time required for investigation of the academic background, professional school, course content, clinical experience, and professional examination depends upon many factors. Often this information must be returned to the home school for revision and completion. There must be an unbroken thread of valid information before a license can be granted, either with or without examination.[6]

SUMMARY

This chapter, "Registration and Interstate Licensure," is perhaps the chapter of greatest practical importance for the nurse. Every field of nursing requires state registration. The most valuable source of current information on nursing and registration is to be found in the annual publication, *Facts About Nursing,* published by the American Nurses' Association. The nurse can keep her information current by consulting this publication from year to year.

CLASS EXERCISE

1. When did the nurse practice act in your state become a law?

2. Is the nurse practice act administered by the board of education? By the medical board? By the state welfare board? Does it function as an independent department of the state?

3. How many members are there on the state board of examiners?

4. Are these members elected or appointed? How long is their term?

5. How could certificate renewal be of importance in Civil Defense?

---

[6] For a valuable article which treats this subject in detail, see R. E. Feider and M. E. Manley, Licensure of Nurses from Other Countries. *American Journal of Nursing,* 54:1228 (Oct.) 1954.

6. What is the state passing score?

7. What is the passing score in adjoining states?

8. When and where are registered nurse examinations held?

9. Does the state have permanent state registration or is there an annual certificate renewal?

10. For what reasons may a registered nurse's license be revoked?

REFERENCES

"Accreditation Q & A. *Nurs. Outlook* 8:44 (Jan); 8:639 (Nov.) 1960.

"ANA statements of qualifications for members and professional employees of state boards of nursing," *Amer. J. Nurs.* 57:1446 (Nov.) 1957.

"ANA statements of functions and standards for members and professional employees of state boards of nursing," *Amer. J. Nurs.* 57:1586 (Dec.) 1957.

ANDERSON, BERNICE E.: *Facilitation of Interstate Movement of Registered Nurses.* J. B. Lippincott Co., Philadelphia, 1950.

ANDERSON, BERNICE E.: The problem of interstate licensure. *Amer. J. Nurs.* 52:586 (May) 1952.

BARNES, MARCIA LOU: What does mandatory license mean? *Amer. J. Nurs.* 59:546 (Apr.) 1959.

"Development of state board test pool examinations for professional and practical nurses," *Amer. J. Nurs.* 54:1484 (Dec.) 1954.

Editorial: Mandatory license. *Amer. J. Nurs.* 57:299 (Mar.) 1957.

FEIDER, R. E., and MANLEY, M. E.: Licensure of nurses from other countries. *Amer. J. Nurs.* 54:1228 (Oct.) 1954.

"Qualifications for state board members." *Amer. J. Nurs.* 56:293 (Mar.) 1956.

STAHL, ADELE G.: Prelude to licensure. *Amer. J. Nurs.* 59:1259 (Sept.) 1959.

"State boards of nursing." *Amer. J. Nurs.* 59:1137 (Aug.) 1959. Annual report of the American Nurses' Association of the Special Committee of State Boards of Nursing. The 1959 report is especially concerned with licensure of nurses from other countries.

LESNIK, M. J.: The board of nurse examiners and the nursing practice act. 54:1484 (Dec.) 1954.

CHAPTER 20

Applying for a Position

The newly graduated nurse has spent three to five years in a school of nursing in which she has learned the many procedures used in the care of the sick; she may have triumphantly passed the state board examinations. She now has come from the protecting walls of the school into a new world of opportunities and responsibilities. What will be the first step toward success? Will she take it blindly, or with a carefully thought-out plan? How may she secure her first position?

It may be that the nurse is not a recent graduate but one who has had ten or twelve years of active experience. During those years, positions may have been plentiful and employment may have been easy to secure, but now she finds herself listed among others as a job-hunter.

There is still a third group, which is made up of employed nurses who are not happy in their present position but remain there, always a little disgruntled and hoping that something will happen to cause a change. Because they fear unemployment, they never take the initiative to change positions.

In any case the process of securing a position is the same: *the nurse must sell herself*. She must take stock of herself as an individual, her abilities, and her capabilities, for these are what she has to offer in exchange for a position. She must sell herself whether to a director of nurses as a head nurse, to a

220

school board personnel director as a school nurse, to the public as a community nurse, or to the mother of an invalid child.

Before seeking a position the nurse should do the following: 1. Make a careful study of the field; choose the work that has genuine appeal and then plan an approach to it. 2. Investigate the various avenues of approach to the selected field through vocational agencies, friends, professional magazines, classified lists, government notices, and newspapers. 3. Realize the importance of first impressions created by letters of application and personal interviews.

CHANNELS OF EMPLOYMENT[1]

The position should depend upon the nurse's interest. Fields of nursing and opportunities in them are unlimited. There is no valid reason to continue in a field in which the nurse has no interest and which offers no opportunity for advancement, provided, of course, that the nurse has initiative to overcome the inertia required to make the change.

There are numerous channels through which positions can be investigated:

1. The *American Journal of Nursing,* each month, carries a long, classified list of positions available. This list includes all types of positions in every part of the world.

2. For public health nursing, the nurse should write to the public health service agencies in the city, county, or state.

3. Information on job openings in school nursing may be secured from the local board of education.

4. Employment opportunities in occupational health nursing may be ascertained by writing to the personnel directors of companies engaged in the industry in which the nurse may be interested.

5. For a commission in the Army, Air Force, or Navy, the nurse should write directly to the branch of service in which she is interested.[2]

6. There is an increasing need for nurses in the Veterans Administration (see p. 249).

7. Announcements of examinations for U. S. Civil Service positions are posted in all first- and second-class post offices.

PROFESSIONAL COUNSELING AND PLACEMENT SERVICE (PC & PS)

This service was established in 1945 by the American Nurses' Association to provide a repository for the professional records of nurses, and to provide a counseling service for nurses. This service is well known, and it is widely used by employers of nurses in any capacity.

A detailed record of each nurse is prepared and kept on file. This record is confidential and will not be released except upon written request from the

---

[1] See also Chapter 21.

[2] For addresses of these services, see Chapter 22, *Government Nursing.*

nurse-applicant. The portion of the record released upon written request is called the ''professional biography.'' This is then sent to prospective employers who have indicated an interest in the nurse's application for employment.

The title of this agency, Professional Counseling and Placement Service, describes the actual functions for which the agency is designed. ''Professional Counseling'' was placed first in the title because wise counseling is important to satisfactory placement for both the nurse and the employer.

All directors of these offices are experienced counselors. They have current information on opportunities for professional advancement. They can help the nurse plan for degree-completion and evaluation of her educational credits. They can help in long-range planning for goals that may seem unattainable. The nurse has the privilege of discussing aspirations and present problems with the counselor even if no change in employment is contemplated.

This service is provided, without charge, only to nurses who are members of the district association and therefore are members of the ANA. A nurse who requests this service must show proof of ANA membership; this can be done best by enclosing her membership card or a photostatic copy of the card in her first letter requesting counseling or placement service. This will save time and correspondence; the membership card will be returned.

State nurses' associations are assuming responsibility for state offices of counseling and placement in cooperation with the national office of the American Nurses' Association at 10 Columbus Circle, New York 19, N. Y. Names and addresses of the state professional counseling and placement offices are listed in the Official Directory which is published in every January and July issue of *The American Journal of Nursing*. If a state office has not yet been established, the nurse may write to the national office.

LETTER OF APPLICATION

A letter of application is the most important piece of writing that most nurses undertake. It is unbelievable that nurses would permit themselves to be represented by some of the poorly written letters of application received by executives who employ nurses. The form may be incorrect, the grammar may be poor, and the spelling may appear to be that of a fifth grade pupil. *A letter of application is the nurse's personal representative.* As the prospective employer reads it, she visualizes the applicant; colored stationery, improper salutation, no margins, poor spelling, limited information make a poor impression.

Letters of application have an established form. The following points are given as a guide:

1. State the purpose of the letter in the first paragraph (please consider my application for . . . . . .).

2. State the source of information concerning the opening or the reason that led the nurse to apply for the position.

3. Give concise statement of qualifications: nursing education and experience.

4. References should include the names and addresses of at least three persons.

5. Request a personal interview if practical.

Appearance of Letter of Application. An application is a business letter and it should have the appearance of one. Use regular business stationery—plain, white, and unruled. Do not use an employer's stationery.

The letter should be typewritten and suitable margins should be maintained; a copy should be kept by the applicant. Some employers prefer to see the applicant's handwriting. A postscript may be added: "So that you may judge the appearance and legibility of my reports, I am submitting this postscript as a sample of my handwriting."

Previous Experience. Experience is important and it should be described in considerable detail. The more responsible the position, the greater the stress laid upon previous experience. If the applicant's experience has been long and varied, mention only that which has a direct bearing upon the position in view.

References. The applicant should give the name and address of three or four persons who are familiar with her work. She should make sure that she has permission to use the names of these persons as references. The name of the most recent employer is the most important reference that the applicant can furnish. If the nurse refuses permission to request a reference from her former employers but prefers to give the name of a colleague, she should explain this variation in detail.

The nurse, whose record is on file with the Professional Counseling and Placement Service, should request this agency to obtain a reference from her employer as a part of her permanent record. This reference should be obtained as soon as possible so that the evaluation can be done by the person familiar with the nurse's performance.

If the position is secured the nurse should write a note of appreciation to those whose references aided her in securing the position. This is not only common courtesy, but also a builder of good will.

Photographs. Photographs may be requested by the prospective employer. The photograph should be of passport or billfold size and, preferably, should show the nurse in uniform. The photographer should be told that this picture will be used in securing a position; he can re-touch the negative a bit, making a more pleasing picture and, at the same time, a more natural one. The picture always should be a recent one.

PERSONAL INTERVIEWS

A personal interview is an advantage to both the applicant and the prospective employers. The nurse should learn all she can about the position in order to ask intelligent questions. She should prepare a list of questions in order that there will be no omissions or regrets after the interview is closed.

Learn the correct pronunciation of the employer's name. It is annoying to have a name repeatedly mispronounced. Some names, although not differing in spelling, may have a wide variation in pronunciation. If the nurse only has seen the name written, the pronunciation may be uncertain. The interview may be opened by a frank exchange of names and the preferred way of saying them.

The nurse should prepare carefully for this interview. One may not always be well dressed, but one always can be well groomed. This should include a clean business suit and fresh blouse or a simple street dress, polished shoes, clean nails, a fresh handkerchief; the nurse should avoid absorption of the odor of tobacco by her clothes or person.

The nurse should be moderate in the use of cosmetics and, above all, should not chew gum. The nurse should keep in mind that this is a business interview and that she is a professional person.

The state registration card and the district membership cards of the American Nurses' Association and the National League for Nursing should be available as evidence of the nurse's professional status if it is requested.

The nurse should not expect a final answer at the end of the interview. The employer may have several applicants for the position; the final decision may involve a number of points unknown to the applicant. It is quite proper, however, for the nurse to ask if she may have a definite decision at an early date.

SALARY

There are several sources from which the nurse can secure information on salaries in any given region. She may write or call the office of the Economic Security Program of a particular state nurses' association. It can supply information on the prevailing salary scales for all types of nursing in that state.

Every issue of *Facts About Nursing* contains a chapter, "The Economic Status of the Nursing Profession." This chapter lists salaries for hospital nurses, public health nurses, faculty members in schools of nursing, industrial nurses, and office nurses, and federal government salary schedules. With this knowledge, the nurse is in a position to make intelligent replies should the employer ask, "What salary do you expect?" or "This is the salary that we pay for this position."

RESIGNING

When planning to leave a position, regardless of the reason, the nurse should make a special effort to sever relations with a good feeling toward all concerned. Later she will be able to recall that institution or that city with pleasure rather than bitterness.

The nurse's employer should be given ample time to fill the vacancy. A notice of one month is usually sufficient. The importance and responsibility of the position should be considered. No faculty appointment should be terminated during a specified instructional period except for cause.

A Letter of Resignation. A letter of resignation should state the date at which the nurse wishes to leave and her reasons for doing so. The letter should express the nurse's regret at leaving. If the separation is because of differences and incompatibility, state so in a dignified and courteous manner. If the relationships have been pleasant, the employer will appreciate your mentioning this.

A letter of resignation should never express bitterness or resentment. One cannot reform another, and once the emotional storm has subsided, any expression of ill feeling will be regretted. The relationship with an employer and the length of time employed should determine the method of resignation. In any case, a written notice should be tendered as a part of the nurse's record.

There are no extenuating circumstances that warrant any nurse in taking "French leave," regardless of the nature of the position. The reason for leaving in an ethical manner is understood when the nurse applies for a new position. To be able to give the name of her last employer as reference will go far toward securing a new position.

CLASS EXERCISE

Writing an application for a position is the most important piece of writing that the student undertakes. The application presents the image that the employer sees as she reads the application. In order that the student may have practice in application writing while she still has a kindly critic, it is suggested that a letter of application for a position as staff nurse in the hospital or agency of her choice be written.

REFERENCES

"A service for nurses." *Amer. J. Nurs.* 55:557 (May) 1955.

"ANA PC and PS restricted to ANA membership." *Amer. J. Nurs.* 59:214 (Feb.) 1959.

BEATRICE, SR. MARY: Transfers, discharges, and methods of resigning. *Canad. Nurse* 43:783 (Oct.) 1947.

DUDLEY, MARTHA: How to quit your job. *RN* 22:47 (Sept.) 1959.

"Getting the nurse and the job together." *Amer. J. Nurs.* 46:443 (July) 1946.

GINSBURG, RALPH: The job of getting a job. *Esquire, Feb.,* 1957. Condensed in *Reader's Digest* (Mar.), 1958.

"It's there when you want it." (Professional Counseling and Placement Service of the ANA.) *Amer. J. Nurs.* 61:56 (Apr.) 1961.

LETHBRIDGE, LOIS: Personal interview. *Canad. Nurse* 43:293 (Apr.) 1947.

"Looking for a job." *Amer. J. Nurs.* 52:413 (Apr.) 1952.

MATTHEWS, RODERIC D.: Counseling and placement—a profession's function. *Amer. J. Nurs.* 56:734 (June) 1956.

McALISTER, EDITH: Interviews can be pleasant. *Nursing World* 129:13 (Jan.) 1955.

McKENNA, FRANCES: The nurse in professional employment. *Nursing World* 129:22 (Sept.) 1955.

"PC and PS; how it works." *Amer J. Nurs.* 57:1032 (Aug.) 1957.

ROGERS, C. R.: A counseling approach to human problems. *Amer. J. Nurs.* 56:994 (Aug.) 1956.

"Some hints on writing references." *Amer. J. Nurs.* 51:306 (May) 1951.

"The value of references." *Amer. J. Nurs.* 60:365 (Mar.) 1960.

WATKINS, MARY R.: Two sides of the coin. *Nursing Outlook* 3:651 (Dec.) 1955.

WHITE, RUTH M.: The art of application and interview. *Nurs. Mirror* 101:2625 (Aug. 19) 1955.

CHAPTER 21

General Fields of Nursing

In this chapter the general fields of nursing are listed in the order of the number of nurses employed in these groups. Further information concerning these types of nursing may be obtained from *Functions, Standards, and Qualifications* prepared by the American Nurses' Association, and *Facts About Nursing* prepared by the Research and Statistical Units of the ANA and the Economic Unit of the ANA. *Careers for Nurses*[1] gives detailed job descriptions of seventeen fields of nursing, and the book is available in all schools of nursing. Therefore, with current information available, only special points of information will be included in the areas of nursing given in this chapter.

NURSES IN HOSPITALS AND RELATED INSTITUTIONS

Hospitals are accredited, as are schools of nursing. This accreditation requirement helps to insure good medical practice, better laboratory and x-ray facilities, and an environment that is conducive to good patient care.

The Joint Commission on Accreditation of Hospitals is supported by the American Hospital Association, the American College of Surgeons, and the

---

[1] Dorothy Deming, *Careers for Nurses,* 2nd ed. (New York, McGraw-Hill Book Co., 1952).

American College of Physicians. Hospitals are carefully inspected for accreditation. After the hospital has been approved, all members of the hospital staff cherish this credential and make an effort to continue to meet these requirements specified by the Joint Commission.

Hospital assets rank fifth among principal manufacturing industries. There are about 7000 hospitals with more than one and one-half million beds, and a daily census of more than one and one-third million patients. This patient load is cared for by nearly 200,000 nurses.[2] The total expense of this philanthropic industry is 8.3 billion dollars of which 65 per cent is paid to employees.

The number of nursing homes is presently estimated at 26,000 with a continuous annual increase due to the growth of the number of persons with chronic diseases. These nursing homes have a capacity of half a million beds, all of which usually are occupied. Many nursing homes are staffed with licensed practical nurses. Some states, however, now require nursing homes to have at least one registered nurse on duty at all times.

Progressive Patient Care.   This type of nursing care began in 1956 and has produced interesting results. A hospital that offers progressive nursing care may have from one to five units, as recommended by the United States Public Health Service:

Intensive care is for the seriously ill patient; the patient is given constant care by professional nurses.

Intermediate care is for the moderately ill patients who usually constitute about half of the patient census. These patients can care for minimal personal needs and, therefore, require a lower ratio of registered nurses and licensed practical nurses.

Self-care is for ambulatory convalescents and ambulatory patients who require extensive tests. They attend to their personal needs and eat at the cafeteria. In this manner a group of ten or twelve patients can be cared for by one professional nurse.

Long-term care is for those patients who need rehabilitation and physical therapy. These facilities are seldom available in the nursing home; therefore, the patient must be hospitalized.

Home care provides the transition from self-care to the home. It is not visiting nursing or public health; it is an extension of the hospital team—nurses and doctors—into the home and it eliminates the need for prolonged hospitalization.

This program of care is becoming popular and new hospitals are being planned with this trend in view. The plan divides hospital nursing into a new type of specialization. The intensive care and the intermediate care program offers a type of nursing that more nearly represents the image that the nurse had of herself when she chose nursing as a career. Home care offers an interest-

---

[2] Guide Issue of *Hospitals*, the official journal of the American Hospital Association, published annually in August.

ing combination of private duty and public health, with the hospital as home base.

Qualifications. Functions, standards and qualifications by the American Nurses' Association in their study (see p. 198) have been compiled in considerable detail for each type of hospital nurse: the staff or general duty nurse, the head nurse, supervisor, and director of nurses.

The ANA functions, standards, and qualifications for educators, administrators, consultants, and teachers have been approved as have those for instructors in a school of nursing which may be connected with a hospital or medical center.

Salaries. Salaries for nurses differ considerably in different parts of the country. Information concerning current salaries of nurses in all categories by states or regions may be obtained from the latest issue of *Facts About Nursing* under the chapter, "The Economic Status of the Nursing Profession."

PRIVATE DUTY NURSING

Historically, private duty was the first major field of nursing outside the hospital. All nursing was done by the students. When the nurse completed her nursing course there was no employment for her outside the hospital. A chain of events changed this early picture: Beginning in 1900, state nurses' associations were organized; these associations worked for legislation to regulate nursing by required state examinations. These state boards of examiners increased formal class requirements and examinations to the point where students could no longer carry the patient load and meet state board demands. Graduate nurses were employed to stabilize nursing service and to permit students to attend scheduled classes. General duty or staff nursing offered more employment security and benefits than did private duty. Today general duty ranks first and private duty second in the number of nurses employed in hospitals and related services.

As new hospitals are built and old ones remodeled, recovery rooms are provided for newly operated patients. Intensive care units are staffed to care for the seriously ill patients. These services are eliminating the need for private nurses during an acute illness of a hospitalized patient.

Private duty, once considered a field of general nursing care, is developing its own special fields: obstetrical nursing, cardiac nursing, rehabilitation, and cancer nursing.

Registries. The private duty nurse has long been considered an independent contractor and, legally, continues to be. Present-day nurses, however, are facing some requirements hitherto unknown. It was generally accepted that any nurse who possessed a diploma from an accredited school of nursing and a certificate of registration could be eligible for private duty. As a result private duty was open to many nurses who had no qualifications for other fields of nursing.

Now, most nurses are employed through a registry. The registry maintains a committee on qualifications; the applicant's personal fitness, work performance, and confidential references are carefully reviewed. In case of doubt, a period of probation is imposed. The registry assumes responsibility for its registrants as a public service; therefore, if the registry receives reports of unsatisfactory nursing, the registrant's name is removed from the list.

The recommendations of the ANA Committee on *Functions, Standards and Qualifications for Practice* have provided the registries with a guide to indicate the performance expected of the private duty nurse.

The Inactive Nurse.   The nurse who has been inactive in nursing for as long as five years is not a safe nurse in any capacity. The private duty nurse is expected to take complete care of one patient. It is unjust to ask the staff nurse to do a procedure "because we weren't taught that when I was a student." The inactive nurse who considers private duty should spend three months on the various divisions of a medical center as a refresher course. It is not fair to the patient or doctor to use a seriously ill patient as a practice field.

Professional Malpractice Insurance.   "Courts are increasingly holding nurses responsible for their professional acts, and it is especially important for private duty nurses, who are independent contractors, to carry insurance that will protect them against the costs of litigation should they become involved in a suit for negligence.

"In a few instances hospitals require that private duty nurses carry professional liability insurance in order to practice in these institutions."[3]

Malpractice insurance policies are available under the American Nurses' Association plan of group insurance. Because this is offered as a group plan, the annual cost of such a policy is about $10. This gives the nurse peace of mind if she never has occasion to need the insurance and great financial help if she does need it. This insurance is one of the benefits offered to nurses through the Economic Security Unit of the ANA.

Financial Aspect of Private Duty Nursing.   The private duty nurse should be equipped with statement blanks which can be obtained from a stationer or the registry. Statements should be presented each week or sooner if the nurse is employed only for a short time. Statements should be presented to the person responsible for the nurse's employment, never to the hospital.

Provision is made for the private duty nurse to have social security coverage by classifying her as a self-employed person. She keeps a record of all patients and pays her social security tax as she does her income tax.

Fees for private duty services are regulated by the private duty section of the local district association. In some states all the districts within a state agree on a standard fee. Private duty fees are listed by states in *Facts About Nursing* under the chapter, "Economic Status of Professional Nursing."

---

[3] *ANA in Review*, Winter, 1960.

OFFICE NURSING

World War II produced sweeping changes in the work of the office nurse. A more descriptive term would be "physician's assistant." Many overworked physicians found that they could see more patients by delegating many procedures to a professional nurse. This gave the doctor more time for reading and research.

Office nursing ranks third in the number of nurses employed. There are several reasons for the popularity of this type of nursing. First, the nurse has considerable freedom in the organization of her work. Second, her on-duty time can be more easily arranged to meet the needs of her family. Third, the nurse has a sense of essentiality in devoting her entire time to the individual patients.

The Office Nurses' Branch of the General Duty Section of the American Nurses' Association has prepared its statement of functions, standards and qualifications for office nurses. This provides a detailed guide for nurses who wish to investigate this field of nursing.

Legal Hazards. The nurse should be aware of the legal hazards connected with office nursing. The public is strongly inclined to press a law suit and the courts tend to hold the doctor *and the nurse* responsible for their professional acts.

Accuracy in keeping records is important. Hospital medical records are significant, too, but then responsibility is shared by others, but in office nursing the entire responsibility is shared only by two professional persons. Accuracy can protect the nurse as well as her employer. Record of the time, the treatment, and the patient's reaction may be requested by a court years later for insurance claims, malpractice suits, or for other court testimony. Even a record to show that a patient *did not* keep an appointment may have legal significance.

An office nurse learns many personal facts about the patient that she would not learn in other types of nursing. This information should be regarded as "classified material" and held in strict confidence. The nurse should train herself not to use a patient's name in an office telephone conversation, lest someone overhear and bring suit by declaring that his right of privacy had been invaded.

The books, *The Medical Assistant*[4] and *The Medical Secretary*,[5] should be standard equipment for the office nurse. Also, *Medicolegal Forms,* prepared by the American Medical Association, will explain the use of notes, letters, and forms in legally dangerous situations.

Salaries. Salaries of office nurses are generally comparable to those of general duty nurses in the same locality. *Facts About Nursing* for 1960 reports "Salaries varied directly with the size of the city in which the nurses

---

[4] Miriam Bredow, *The Medical Assistant* (New York, McGraw-Hill Book Co., 1958).

[5] Kenneth B. Coffin and R. Forrest Colwell, *The Medical Secretary* (New York, The Macmillan Co., 1959).

were employed. The median salary for "nonsupervisory" nurses in cities of over 500,000 was $340; the one for those in cities of less than 10,000 was $285."

Qualifications. Most office nurses have entered this type of nursing from the general duty field. They have added to their knowledge and skill by inservice training in the special field of their employer.

The current medical magazines and the new books, plus the official nursing magazines, should be required reading for the office nurse in order to keep well informed of the type of work done by the physician and to maintain a broad outlook on current nursing trends.

The office nurse must be tactful always, be able to meet the public with a gracious dignity, and she must possess such self-assurance that the patient in the office will feel that the nurse, as well as the physician, is doing everything for his welfare.

The personal appearance of the office nurse is important. Careful grooming of her hair and hands is imperative. Her uniform should be of good quality and well laundered, and the feet well shod. It is through the office nurse that the patient gains his first impression, and her personal neatness and professional attitude will increase the confidence of the patient in the ability of the physician.

PUBLIC HEALTH NURSING

Official and Nonofficial Agencies. Nurses are employed by two types of agencies: official and nonofficial. Official agencies are supported by taxes levied by the city, state, or federal government. The nonofficial agencies are private agencies, such as visiting nurse associations. These groups depend for support upon campaign funds, banquets, contracts with companies, and small fees paid by patients.

The number of nurses employed by official agencies is increasing steadily. City, county, and state governments are assuming more responsibility for the care of their citizens; this increases the number of nurses required in the tax-supported or official agencies. There has been an increase in the number of nurses employed by boards of education and in the number of public health nurses employed as instructors in schools of nursing.

Functions of the Public Health Nurse. The functions, standards, and qualifications of the public health nurse were defined by a committee of the Public Health Section of the ANA. These give an excellent idea of the many activities of the public health nurse.[6]

Because of the changes and developments in public health, the functions of the nurse have been greatly expanded. It is her responsibility to assist families and individuals in analyzing their health needs and related social problems, to help them understand and use their community resources, and to help them formulate and carry out plans for the protection and promotion

---

[6] A detailed description of public health nursing is given in *Careers for Nurses*, 2nd ed., by Dorothy Deming (New York, McGraw-Hill Book Co., 1952).

of their health. All these functions together form a well-rounded public health nursing program. In order to give the best possible service to the family and in the interest of efficiency and economy, there is an increasing trend toward generalized service; that is, to have one nurse give all types of service to the family in a limited area. If one service, such as school nursing, is carried on as a separate activity, it is done in close cooperation with other phases of public health nursing. With this coordination the school nurse will refer students or families to the visiting nurse or the health department as the need arises.

Educational Requirements. High qualifications for nurses appointed to first-level positions have been set up. Public health is the latest of the organized fields of nursing; its members have not had the long struggle to establish academic standards that the older groups had but they have formally stated that advanced education is necessary for public health nursing.

If, in her basic nursing education, the nurse has not had preparation for a first-level position in public health nursing, she is required to have advanced professional study in public health. For the staff nurse, one year in an approved course in public health is required. This course should lead to a certificate of public health. A degree in public health is required for the supervisory nurse.

Salaries. Information on the current salaries of public health nurses can be obtained from the annual issue of *Facts About Nursing*. This statistical publication gives median salaries in considerable detail under the chapter heading, ''Economic Status of Professional Nursing.'' The salaries are given under type of service, position, and regions. These regions are divided into North Atlantic, Midwestern, Southern, and Western. Salaries are listed for official health units, nonofficial, and for boards of education. Tables of salaries also are given by population groups. This information on salaries is obtained from the National League for Nursing *Yearly Reviews* and from the Research and Statistical Unit of the ANA.

Nurses who may be considering public health nursing as a career will be interested in some of the ''fringe benefits'' granted by many of the official and nonofficial agencies, such as sick time, overtime, and vacations. These tables are listed in *Facts About Nursing*.

OCCUPATIONAL HEALTH NURSING

Occupational health nursing, formerly called ''industrial nursing,'' first appeared as emergency nursing in industry, but it has since become an established and effective means of promoting, conserving, and restoring health to employees in industry. The nurse is the key member of the health team. ''The occupational health nurse herself is the most frequently found representative of the health profession in the plant health service. She is the daily tangible and visible image of ''nursing'' to the labor force, on whom depends the well-being of all members of the community. In all nursing practice, occupational health is an inextricable component."[7]

The highly industrialized states are California, Illinois, Michigan, New York, Ohio, and Pennsylvania. These six states employ 55 per cent of the total number of nurses engaged in occupational health.

This type of nursing is done directly in the industrial plant as part of the health program or as home or visiting nursing. Approximately 96 per cent of the work is carried on in the plant. In some of the large aircraft plants nurses are employed in the plant and as nurses who visit sick employees in their homes.

Duties of the Occupational Health Nurse. The functions of the nurse differ widely according to the size of the plant and the type of industry.

The American Association of Industrial Nurses,[8] which is a national specialization organization, has prepared a considerably detailed statement:

Duties and Responsibilities of the Professional Nurse in an Industrial Service. The Occupational Health Nurses Section of the American Nurses' Association has prepared, for their section, *Functions, Standards, and Qualifications of a One Nurse Service in Industry or Commerce.*

The American Association of Industrial Nurses has prepared several publications, listed below, which may be used as a guide for the inservice education of the nurse who may wish to consider industrial nursing or for the new nurse in occupational health:

Duties and Responsibilities of the Professional Nurse in an Industrial Medical Service (June, 1955)

Principles of Physician-Nurse Relationships in Industry (1957)

Recommendations for a Professional Nurse Working without Nursing Supervision in an Industrial Medical Service (1955)

Recommended Qualifications: For a Professional Nurse Working with Nursing Supervision in an Industrial Medical Service (1955)

A careful study of this literature will indicate that the duties of the nurse in occupational health generally fall into four classes: emergency duties, maintenance of good plant sanitation, maintenance of good health among employees, and investigation of causes for absenteeism.

Requirements. Most nurses in occupational health have entered this field with only the basic nursing course. Since occupational health is closely related to public health, courses and experience in public health are valuable. Some nurses have used their experience in the emergency room as a steppingstone to occupational health.

---

[7] Heide L. Hendricksen, A Memorandum: To Professional Nursing Organizations from Plant Nurses. Subject: Services to Constituents. *Nursing Outlook*, November, 1960.

[8] For address of this group, see the Official Directory in any January or July issue of *Amer. J. Nurs.*

Salaries. The Bureau of Labor Statistics of the U. S. Department of Labor regularly surveys occupational earnings in selected industries and certain cross-industry occupations in various major communities. Field representatives of the Bureau of Labor Statistics collect data through samples of individual industries in nineteen cities. These samplings provide the basis for determining the average weekly earnings from Atlanta to Seattle. The present cross-country range of the average salary is from $76.50 to $93.50 per week. A study of this annual report will show the comparison between the nurse's salary and that of the skilled industrial worker.[9]

This list of ''The Average Weekly Earnings of Industrial Nurses in 19 Cities'' is published annually in *Facts About Nurses,* in the chapter ''The Economic Status of the Nursing Profession.''

NURSE EDUCATORS

There was a shortage of qualified nurse educators during the depression years of 1930-1940. Now, with the greatest prosperity that the world has ever known, there still is a deficiency in the number of teachers needed for an adequate faculty in schools of nursing.

This lack of teachers is cause for genuine concern. All nursing schools need to expand educational facilities for young women and men seeking education in the associate degree program, the diploma schools, and the baccalaureate degree program.

Enrollment in diploma schools is decreasing while at the same time enrollment in the associate degree program has increased by 20 per cent. The need for teachers in grade schools and colleges, so that a good educational level can be maintained, is serious. Of equal concern should be the need for teachers to protect the health of the country. Leaders in both groups know that this condition will become more acute in the immediate future.

Teaching as a Career. Teaching is listed as first in the number of women employed in professions. Teaching is *teaching* in any type of education. The student who has potentialities for teaching should be encouraged to enter a school of nursing where these qualifications can be guided into participation in higher education. Nursing schools would do well to subsidize well-qualified graduates to continue their education for the purpose of teaching in schools of nursing.

The American Nurses' Association, because of its concern for the need of well-prepared teachers, initiated federal legislation to provide trainee-ships for supervisory, teaching, and administrative positions. This program began experimentally on a year-to-year basis, and has proved the necessity for such educational assistance. All fellowships available in this program were used and more are requested. The Federal government has now extended the program for the next five years.[10]

---

[9] This annual report may be obtained from the Bureau of Labor Statistics, Department of Labor, Washington, D. C.

[10] See Federal Traineeships: Where to Apply. *American Journal of Nursing,* December, 1959.

Clinical Instructors. This is a term commonly applied to instructors who correlate and apply formal classroom teaching to clinical situations. The instructor, therefore, should have an extensive background in her subject and be able to help the student at the patient's bedside to understand the reasons for procedures, expected results, patient-teaching and over-all nursing care. Such instructors derive great personal satisfaction from clinical teaching. It is a nice combination of teaching and nurse-patient relationships.

With the continued lack of an adequate faculty many diploma schools have arranged, with a local college, for formal classes in chemistry, anatomy and physiology, psychology, and sociology. This arrangement greatly increases the need for nurse instructors to carry over these scientific principles to clinical situations.

State Board Requirements for Schools of Nursing. The state examining board is responsible for the state accreditation of schools of nursing. One of the requirements for accreditation is a well-qualified faculty. The yardstick for measuring this demand is a degree, preferably in nursing education.

In order to meet this requirement educational administrators have frequently induced young nurses with a degree to qualify as instructors. Frequently they have had no teacher training or experience; this is difficult for the school and unfair to the teacher.

Future of Nurse Teachers. Nursing education will be an open field for teachers for all time to come. Nurses everywhere are aware that an education comparable to that of other professions is necessary for a nurse to qualify as a truly professional person. To achieve this objective there must be qualified teachers in all types of nursing schools, even in the practical-nurse schools. High schools require all teachers to have a baccalaureate degree; those with master's degrees are preferred. The nurse student has a right to expect that a school of nursing has a higher educational level than high school and that her teachers will be as well prepared academically.

For this reason schools of nursing will continue to need teachers with higher degrees in order to prepare truly professional nurses.

Teaching Load. An instructor should be expected to carry a teaching load of not more than sixteen hours per week based on the following: one hour of classroom instruction per week equals one hour of teaching load; two hours of clinical supervision or laboratory equals one hour of teaching load. Instructors who teach more than one course during a term should not be expected to carry sixteen hours. The teaching load should be adjusted to take into consideration additional responsibilities other than instruction and the total should not exceed forty hours each week.

Salaries. The Research and Statistical Unit of the ANA conducts a survey of salaries for nurse faculty members every two years. The report of this survey is made in *Facts About Nursing*. The report gives salaries according to type of position, academic preparation, salary range, type of school, type of control, and geographical area. The 1961 report states: ''Academic preparation had a direct relationship to salaries. The median annual salary of teachers and administrators in hospital professional nursing educational programs was $4,910, while in collegiate professional nursing schools the median was $6,000. However, while the median of all the educators in collegiate schools was 22 per cent higher than that of educators in hospital schools, a nurse with a baccalaureate degree in the collegiate school averaged about three per cent more than a nurse in a hospital school. If she had a master's degree, she averaged about four per cent more than the nurse in the hospital school with the same degree.''

The state office of Professional Counseling and Placement Service is an excellent source of information on salaries of nurse educators in that state.

Salaries of nurse educators are being studied by the Research and Statistical Unit of the ANA. The results of this study will be used to provide comparative data for evaluating the economic factor affecting nurse educators.

Need for this information stems from the existing critical shortage of professional nurses in nursing education. At present the difference in salary between that of the staff nurse and that of the nurse teacher is not sufficient to act as an incentive for further education from the standpoint of economic improvement. Salaries and conditions of employment for this group of nurses must be improved if well-qualified nurses are to be attracted and retained in careers of nursing education.

PSYCHIATRIC NURSING

Mental illness is more prevalent in the United States than in any other country in the world. It is the pride of every American to say, ''We rank first,'' but to rank first in mental instability and to realize that such a condition is increasing should cause every responsible person to obligate himself to learn the significant facts of this problem.

All sorts of explanations have been offered to account for the increase in the incidence of mental illness: life is more complex than formerly; the strain of living is greater; the urban population has increased, causing more restraint than before; the speed of travel has increased; there is a notable lack of discipline in the formative years; increased emphasis on recreation has increased personal demands. Whatever the cause or combination of causes, one person in ten is now receiving treatment for mental illness in a private or state institution or clinic or from private psychiatrists.

Cost of Mental Illness. The taxpayer is becoming aware of the colossal sums paid annually to maintain our state hospitals with their present daily census of more than 750,000 patients. More than 300,000 *new* patients are admitted each year. Over one billion dollars in tax funds is spent annually to provide hospital care for these patients. The public is asking for something to be done to remedy this terrible social and economic loss and to prevent future losses.

Restorative Measures. Many of these patients, through intelligent and scientific care, can be restored to their usual position in their homes and communities. This is made possible through chemotherapy and other thera-peutic technics which require special training for both the nurse and the physician. Executives and psychiatrists associated with progressive institu-tions have discarded the notion that *anyone,* even though she may be a regis-tered nurse, is capable of caring for the mental patient. It is recognized that the best care can be given only by professional nurses with psychiatric training.

Qualifications. The psychiatric nurse must know not only the principles of nursing procedures but how to adapt them to the needs of psychiatric patients. In addition, the nurse must have managerial ability, such as organizing, plan-ning, and executive procedures with whatever adaptations are required for the improvement of each patient. She must be a person to whom socialization comes naturally: easy conversation, a genuine interest in social games, interest in clothes, or whatever the patient may need to acquire social skills.

The nurse is essential in the treatment of the patient. This includes intelli-gent listening and marginal counseling, of which the patient is unaware. She must be qualified to respond constructively to patient-situations of panic, fear, loneliness, isolation, or withdrawal.

The psychiatric nurse is qualified to teach the patient, students, and auxil-iary personnel. Teaching ability is as essential for the staff nurse as for the full-time instructor. Teaching is carried on by the staff nurse in the form of group therapy for patients, ward conferences for students, and team nursing conferences in which nurse aides and attendants are included.

The successful psychiatric nurse must be able to do all of these and to move swiftly from one to the other as the situation arises. These are natural characteristics which have become intensified through instruction and disci-pline to make the nurse a well-integrated person.

Need for Psychiatric Nurses. The need for nurses with psychiatric training and interest is opening up one of the greatest fields of nursing. Mental hospitals accomplish very little without well-prepared nurses, "therapists of a special sort, and not merely bedmakers and keepers of the keys." When only 3 to 5 per cent of the professional nurses are concerned with more than 50 per cent of the hospital patients, one must conclude that there exists a widespread and deplorable condition which challenges both medicine and nursing.

One of the duties of a professional group is to provide for the needs within that profession. Psychiatric nurses are the ones most needed. Fifty one per cent of all hospital beds are occupied by psychiatric patients. Modern treat-ment is interesting and rewarding to both nurses and doctors. Senior students with an interest and inclination toward psychiatric nursing should be coun-seled to enter this field of nursing.

Nurses Take the Initiative. Professional nursing is taking the initiative in an effort to remedy the lack of nursing care for the mentally ill. Most state boards of nursing now require that applicants who take the state examination must have had actual experience in the care of mentally ill patients in a qualified institution. Graduates who have not had this experience are denied interstate licensure. Such a handicap is an incentive to make such experience a requirement for all states.

The National League for Nursing has concerned itself with this problem through its Mental Health and Psychiatric Advisory Service. This program is largely financed by the National Institute of Mental Health.

CLASS EXERCISE

List the types of nursing service generally found in the community, and list the positions in each type of nursing. Assuming that educational requirements will continue to increase at the present rate for the next five years, what plans should the nurse now make for advanced education?

REFERENCES

Nurses in Hospitals and Related Institutions:

ABDELLAH, FAYE G., and LEVINE, EUGENE: *Patients and Personnel Speak.* Public Health Service Bull. 527, Government Printing Office, Washington, D. C., 1957.

BEAL, JOHN M.: Intensive nursing care. *Amer. J. Surg.* 100:1 (July) 1960. (Abstracted and published in *The Davis Nursing Survey*, 24:133 (Oct.) 1960.)

BETTERMAN, C. S.: The evening supervisor. 2. In a medium-sized hospital. *Amer. J. Nurs.* 57:447 (Apr.) 1957.

BLANCHER, GERTRUDE C.: Some satisfactions in geriatric nursing. *Amer. J. Nurs.* 60:1635 (Nov.) 1960.

BRACKETT, MARY E.: Where and how should head nurses be prepared? *Nurs. Outlook* 5:644 (Nov.) 1957.

BULLOCK, ROBERT P.: Position, function, and job satisfaction of nurses in the social system of a modern hospital. *Nurs. Res.* 2:4 (June) 1953.

DEMING, DOROTHY: *Careers in Nursing.* 2nd ed. McGraw-Hill Book Co., Inc., New York, 1952.

DUDLEY, MARTHA: Here they let nurses be nurses. *RN* 24:53 (Sept.) 1961.

Editorial: An open letter to head nurses. *Amer. J. Nurs.* 56:438 (Apr.) 1955.

Editorial: If a hospital strike occurs. *Amer. J. Nurs.* 60:344 (Mar.) 1960.

ELDER, FRANCES: R.N.'s to the astronauts: Pioneers of space nursing. *RN* 24:37 (Sept.) 1961.

"Facts About Nursing." Annual statistical publication of the American Nurses' Association.

FINER, HERMAN: Preparation for administration of nursing service. *Amer. J. Nurs.* 51:701 (Dec.) 1951.

GIFFIN, MARGARET: Nursing service. *Hospitals* 32:70 (Apr. 16) 1958.

GRAVES, HELEN G.: Head nurses are key people. *Amer. J. Nurs.* 54:572 (May) 1954.

GRIFFIN, WINIFRED H.: Mastering those machines. *Amer. J. Nurs.* 62:81 (Feb.) 1962.

HERWITZ, ADELE: The director of nursing wears two hats. *Amer. J. Nurs.* 60:1423 (Oct.) 1960.

LOGSDON, AUDREY: The head nurse. *Amer. J. Nurs.* 59:825 (June) 1959.

McQUILLEN, MARY: How do graduates of collegiate programs rate? *Nurs. Outlook* 9:100 (Feb.) 1961.

"Men nurses have their say." *RN* 24:50 (Apr.) 1961. (Part I); 24:37 (May) 1961 (Part II).

PEARSALL, MARION: Supervision—a nursing dilemma. *Nurs. Outlook* 9:91 (Feb.) 1961.

PETERSON, FREDA A.: Eleven to seven. *Amer. J. Nurs.* 51:127 (Feb.) 1951.

POWERS, RUTH A.: A refresher course in a community program. *Amer. J. Nurs.* 60:821 (June) 1960.

REDDY, ANN KATHLEEN: Who will make the best head nurse? *Nurs. Outlook* 9:38 (Jan.) 1961.

SEVISON, K. D.: The evening supervisor. 3. In a small hospital. 57:449 (Apr.) 1957.

SILVERMAN, MILTON: An outsider's inside look at hospitals. *Hospitals* 28:86 (Nov.) 1954.

SLATTERY, LUCILE C., and GODDARD, MARY A.: On the edge of space. *Amer. J. Nurs.* 61:42 (June) 1961.

SMITH, VIRGINIA E.: An open letter to general duty nurses. *Amer. J. Nurs.* 51:373 (June) 1951.

STERNS, LINA: Changing concepts in nursing supervision. *Amer. J. Nurs.* 59:63 (Jan.) 1959.

TOBIN, R. P.: The evening supervisor. 1. In a large hospital. *Amer. J. Nurs.* 57:446 (Apr.) 1957.

YANKAUER, RUTH G.: The position of the head nurse. *Amer. J. Nurs.* 55:957 (Aug.) 1955.

Private Duty Nursing:

American Nurses' Association, Private Duty Nursing Section: Functions, Standards, and Qualifications for the Practice of Private Duty Nursing. American Nurses' Association, New York, 1956.

COUEY, ELIZABETH D., and STEPHENSON, DIANE D.: The field of private duty nursing. Georgia State Nurses' Association, Atlanta, 1955.

DUDLEY, MARTHA: Is private duty on the way out? *RN* 22:46 and 86 (June) 1959.

FINER, HERMAN: Evaluating the private duty nurse's performance. *Amer. J. Nurs.* 56:1564 (Dec.) 1956.

JANNEY, MARIE: Back to class—then back to work. *Amer. J. Nurs.* 58:1695 (Dec.) 1958.

KASUN, MARJORIE: Registries and intergroup relations. *Amer. J. Nurs.* 59:234 (Feb.) 1959.

MATZ, ANNA V.: A tribute to private duty nursing. *Amer. J. Nurs.* 59:375 (Mar.) 1959.

MOSES, EVELYN B.: The case in private duty. *Amer. J. Nurs.* 60:1784 (Dec.) 1960.

PATTERSON, LILLIAN B.: The private duty nurse and the ANA social security program. *Nurs. World* 126:69 (Feb.) 1952.

PORTER, ELIZABETH K.: The prospect before you. *Amer. J. Nurs.* 59:56 (Jan.) 1959.

REGAN, WILLIAM A.: Legal pointers: Private duty relief. *RN* 23:53 (June) 1960.

REGAN, WILLIAM A.: When is the private duty nurse legally liable? *RN* 24:62 (July) 1961.

SPALDING, EUGENIA K.: *Professional Nursing: Trends, Responsibilities, and Relationships.* *6th ed.* J. B. Lippincott Co., Philadelphia, 1959, Chapter 5.

VIENO, JOHNSON: Let's redefine special nursing. *RN* 20:73 (Sept.) 1957.

''Will tomorrow's private duty nurses be college educated?'' *RN* 24:45 (May) 1961.

Office Nursing:

American Nurses' Association, Special Groups Section: Functions, Standards, and Qualifications for the Practice of Office Nursing; Past, Present, and Future of FS and Q. American Nurses' Association, New York, 1957.

BREDOW, M.: *The Medical Assistant.* McGraw-Hill Book Co., Inc., New York, 1958.

BRUEHL, FRANCES S., and LISH, RUTH E.: The nurse in a gynecologist's office. *Amer. J. Nurs.* 55:187 (Feb.) 1955.

COFFIN, KENNETH B., and COLWELL, FORREST: *The Medical Secretary.* The Macmillan Company, New York, 1959.

''*Facts About Nursing.*'' Annual statistical publication of the American Nurses' Association.

HALL, GEORGE E.: The office nurse and the law. *RN* 23:36 (Mar.) 1960.

MacDONALD, A. R.: Office nurse on a hospital payroll. *RN* 20:48 (Aug.) 1957.

McDOWELL, MARION: Office nurses in Ohio. *Amer. J. Nurs.* 58:840 (June) 1958.

SCHICK, JOHNNYE C.: Office nurses are on their way. *Amer. J. Nurs.* 56:429 (Apr.) 1956.

Public Health Nursing:

American Nurses' Association, Public Health Nurses Section: Functions, Standards, and Qualifications. *Amer. J. Nurs.* 56:1305 (Oct.) 1956.

CONKLIN, M. VIRGINIA: Public health nursing in nursery schools. *Nurs. Outlook* 2:126 (Mar.) 1954.

Editorial: The department of public health nursing: a year of decision. *Nurs. Outlook* 8:127 (Mar.) 1960.

FREEMAN, RUTH B.: *Public Health Nursing Practice.* 2nd ed. W. B. Saunders Company, Philadelphia, 1957.

FREEMAN, RUTH B., and McLAUGHLIN, MARGARET: Leadership components in public health nursing. *Amer. J. Nurs.* 58:552 (Apr.) 1958.

Editorial: Guide on certification of school nurses. *Amer. J. Nurs.* 59:866 (June) 1959.

HUBBARD, RUTH W.: Public health nursing, 1900-1950. *Amer. J. Nurs.* 50:608 (Oct.) 1950.

JOHNSON, WALTER L.: Public health nursing turnover. *Amer. J. Nurs.* 57:464 (Apr.) 1957.

McLANAHAN, WINIFRED, and FLEMING, RICHARD: How the visiting nurse works with emotionally ill patients. *Nurs. Outlook* 6:648 (Nov.) 1958.

PRESTON, DORIS: Dollars for miles. *Amer. J. Nurs.* 56:1263 (Oct.) 1956.

PROCK, VALENCIA N.: Analysis of the health services given by a voluntary and official agency. *Nurs. Res.* 4:23 (June) 1955.

Editorial: Public health nursing for the future. *Nurs. Outlook* 5:399 (July) 1957.

SHEPARD, W. P., and WHEATLY, G. M.: Visiting nurse service. *J.A.M.A.* 149:554 (June) 1952.

SULLIVAN, MARY M.: Nursing in a Blue Cross—Blue Shield program. *Nurs. Outlook* 3:644 (Dec.) 1955.

Occupational Health Nursing:

BARNARD, ANN: A student experience in industry. *J. Amer. Assoc. Industrial Nurses* 4:5 (June) 1956.

BRAND, MORRIS: What labor expects from the public health nurse. *Nurs. Outlook* 6:226 (Apr.) 1958.

DUGGAN, MARY G.: The industrial nurse teaches health. *Amer. J. Nurs.* 58:537 (Apr.) 1958.

"Facts About Nursing." Annual statistical publication of the American Nurses' Association.

FELTON, JEAN S.: Educational trends in industrial nursing. *Nurs. Outlook* 5:655 (Nov.) 1957.

FERGUSON, LEONA E., and MASTERS, RAYMOND E.: The occupational health nurse and atomic energy. *Amer. J. Nurs.* 58:1533 (Nov.) 1958.

"Guiding principles and procedures for industrial nurses." *J.A.M.A.* 159:1028 (Nov. 5) 1955. (Reprinted in *Amer. J. Nurs.* 56:192, Feb., 1956.)

HENDRICKSEN, HEIDI L.: A memorandum to professional nursing organizations from plant nurses; subject: services to constituents. *Nurs. Outlook* 8:612 (Nov.) 1960.

HOEPER, BEATRICE E.: A lesson in positive health: A "close-to-home" subject—cancer—provided the state of readiness necessary for an outstanding educational program in industry. *Nurs. Outlook* 8:614 (Nov.) 1960.

"Legal scope of industrial nursing practice." *J.A.M.A.* 169:1072 (Mar. 7) 1959. (Reprinted in *Amer. J. Nurs.* 59:996, July, 1959.)

LEMBRIGHT, KATHERINE A.: The nurse in small industry. *Amer. J. Nurs.* 59:829 (June) 1959.

STEELE, MARGARET L.: The Industrial Nurse. *Tomorrow's Nurse* 1:8 (Dec.-Jan.) 1960-61.

YANTA, GERALDINE M.: Stewardess-nurse. *Amer. J. Nurs.* 58:1699 (Dec.) 1958.

Nurse Educators:

BOYLE, RENA: A study of programs of professional education for teachers of nursing in 19 selected universities. *Nurs. Outlook* 3:635 (Dec.) 1954.

Editorial: The economic position of the nurse educator. *Amer. J. Nurs.* 56:1566 (Dec.) 1956.

"Facts About Nursing." Annual statistical publication of the American Nurses' Association. Chapter II, Professional Nurse Education.

GRATZ, PAULINE: Good teachers are made—not born. *Nurs. World* 131:7 (Jan.) 1957.

HEIDGERKEN, LORETTA E.: Preparing teachers of nursing. *Nurs. Outlook* 3:635 (Dec.) 1955.

HOLMES, SARA V., and OTTO, EVELYN L.: What the evening instructor does. *Amer. J. Nurs.* 51:340 (May) 1951.

PETRY, LUCILE: The preparation of teachers for nursing schools to meet new demands and responsibilities. Forty-eighth annual report of National League of Nursing Education, National League for Nursing, New York, 1942, pp. 190-195.

PRICE, ALICE W.: The nurse as a teacher. *Nurs. Outlook* 7:98 (Feb.) 1959.

REITTER, FRANCES: The preparation of clinical instructors. *Amer. J. Nurs.* 44:1066 (Nov.) 1944.

SPALDING, EUGENIA K.: Current problems of nurse educators. *Teachers College Record* 57:38 (Oct.) 1955.

Psychiatric Nursing:

"Facts About Nurses." Annual statistical publication of the American Nurses' Association.

Guide issue (Annual) of Hospitals, the *Journal of the American Hospital Association*, Chicago, Illinois.

"Important role of the psychiatric nurse." *Nurs. Mirror*, London, No. 2647, (Jan.) 1956.

KALKMAN, MARION E.: Interpreting psychiatric nursing to the public. *Amer. J. Nurs.* 55:1359 (Nov.) 1955.

KALKMAN, MARION E.: *Introduction to Psychiatric Nursing.* 2nd ed. McGraw-Hill Book Co., Inc., New York, 1950.

LePAGE, ANITA M.: A new role for the psychiatric nurse. *Nurs. Outlook* 7:709 (Dec.) 1959.

MALONEY, ELIZABETH M.: Why not psychiatric nursing? *Amer. J. Nurs.* 54:1248 (Oct.) 1954.

ORPHAN, DENNIS: A word is spoken. *Today's Health* 39:22 (Jan.) 1961.
    [1] Accredited by the National League for Nursing.

"Patients and nurses in psychiatric hospitals." *Amer. J. Nurs.* 51:700 (Nov.) 1951.

ROBINSON, ALICE M.: Changing of the guard. *Amer. J. Nurs.* 50:152 (Mar.) 1950.

Staff of Moorhaven Hospital, Ivybridge, Devon, England: Nursing after-care for psychiatric patients. *Nurs. Mirror* 112:ii (June 30) 1961.

STEELE, KATHERINE M., and MANFREDA, MARGUERITE L.: *Psychiatric Nursing.* 6th ed. F. A. Davis Company, Philadelphia, 1959.

TUTEUR, WERNER: As you enter psychiatric nursing. *Amer. J. Nurs.* 56:72 (Jan.) 1956.

CHAPTER 22

Government Nursing

Government nursing provides an interesting field with great possibilities for advancement. The salaries are adequate and the daily period of duty does not exceed eight hours, except in emergencies. Government services employing the largest number of nurses are: Army Nurse Corps, Air Force Nurse Corps, Navy Nurse Corps, United States Public Health Service, and Veterans Administration.

ARMY NURSE CORPS

Army nursing service includes the care of members of the army and their families and, in some instances, civilian employees. Much of the care is given by enlisted personnel who have had training in bedside care and first aid. The nurse cares for acutely ill patients, obstetrical patients, and supervises the general care of all patients.

Nurses are assigned to army hospitals in the United States and to base and station hospitals overseas. An eight-week orientation course is conducted at the Medical Field Service School, Brooke Army Medical Center, Fort Sam Houston, Texas, for newly appointed officers.

Eligibility. A nurse must be a graduate of a hospital-affiliated school of nursing acceptable to the Army Nurse Corps; show current registration in at least one state; be a citizen of the United States, and she or he must be between twenty-one and thirty-five years of age. She may be married or unmarried but with no dependents under eighteen years of age.

Rank and Rates of Pay. The young nurse with little or no experience as a graduate or no college background enters the corps with the commissioned rank of second lieutenant. Otherwise, the Department of the Army determines the grade according to graduate experience or professional background. After completion of eighteen months of constructive service, the second lieutenant is eligible for promotion to first lieutenant. Pay is increased with each promotion in rank.

Salary for a second lieutenant is $222.30 a month plus allowance for subsistence and quarters. Full maintenance in the army amounts to considerable more than in the usual civilian hospital. Life insurance is available for policies ranging from $1000 to $10,000 at low rates. The nurse also has sick leave with pay, as well as retirement, dependent, and educational benefits.

Inquires should be addressed to any regional office of Army Nurse Procurement or to the Office of the Adjutant General, Washington, D. C.

AIR FORCE NURSE CORPS

The Air Force Nurse Corps was established July 1, 1949 as a part of the Air Force Medical Service.

The flight nurse may be assigned as (1) a staff nurse with duty on medical or surgical services; in pediatric, obstetric or out-patient departments; or in communicable disease wards; (2) a member of the air evacuation squadron or teaching staff; (3) an administrative nurse; (4) operating room nurse; (5) psychiatric nurse; or (6) nurse anesthetist.

Eligibility. The qualifications of the flight nurse are rigid. An alert intelligence is essential, but emotional stability in any situation is of primary importance. She cannot be accepted until she has demonstrated ease and self-confidence in all the tasks assigned to her while the plane is in flight.

The nurse must be a graduate of a school acceptable to the Surgeon General of the USAF, currently registered in at least one state, a citizen of the United States, and between twenty-one and thirty-five years of age without dependents under eighteen years of age.

Rank and Rates of Pay. The nurse with less than three years of experience enters the Air Force as a second lieutenant with a base pay of $222.30, plus allowances for quarters and subsistence. Nurses are considered for promotion to the grade of first lieutenant after eighteen months of service, with corresponding increases in pay. Excellent opportunities for advanced education are offered. The nurse draws full pay and allowances while in attendance for specialty courses or for completion of a degree.

Information may be secured by writing the Surgeon General, U.S. Air Force, Washington 25, D. C., Attention: Nursing Division.

NAVY NURSE CORPS

In 1947 the Nurse Corps was established as a permanent staff corps of the United States Navy. The Nurse Corps Reserve was established as an organized and trained group of nurses ready for service in times of emergency or for voluntary active duty when their services are needed. However, all appointments—for active or inactive duty—in the U.S. Navy Nurse Corps are made in the Nurse Corps, U.S. Naval Reserve (also called Nurse Corps Reserve). Transfer to the Regular Navy (Nurse Corps, USN) is possible for those Nurse Corps Reserve officers who are interested in this branch of service as a career.

Eligibility. For appointment as ensign, the applicant (female only) must be twenty to twenty-eight years of age at time of appointment, a citizen of the United States, a registered nurse in good standing, a graduate of a school of nursing acceptable to the Surgeon General of the U.S. Navy, single or married but with no dependents under eighteen years of age, and must meet moral and physical requirements.

Appointment as lieutenant (junior grade) (twenty-one to thirty-two years of age) or lieutenant (twenty-five to thirty-four years of age) depends upon educational and professional experience qualifications.

Other Programs. Instruction in nursing education, nursing service, nursing specialties (including flight nursing) and anesthesia is available for Nurse Corps officers. Baccalaureate and master's degree programs are available to Regular Nurse Corps officers. The nurse draws full pay and allowance while attending full-time duty under instruction with tuition paid by the Navy. A nursing education program for enlisted women (WAVES) leading to appointment as Ensign in this corps has been established also.

The Navy Nurse Candidate Program offers financial assistance to qualified senior students who are enrolled in a collegiate nursing education course.[1] This is a scholarship-type program which provides for commission as Ensign after successful completion of the course.

Rank and Rates of Pay. Most initial commissions are in the grade of ensign. An ensign is eligible for promotion to lieutenant (junior grade) after eighteen months of active duty, or after twelve months if she has a B.S. degree. Subsequent selection for promotion is based on length and excellence of service, education, experience, professional qualifications, and aptitude and fitness for military nursing.

The pay of the ensign is $222.30 per month plus full maintenance. Maintenance includes an allowance of $300.00 for the initial cost of uniforms, and complete medical and dental care, with no loss of pay during illness.

Inquiries for detailed information should be addressed to the Director, Navy Nurse Corps, Bureau of Medicine and Surgery, Navy Department, Washington 25, D. C.

---

[1] Accredited by the National League for Nursing.

UNITED STATES PUBLIC HEALTH SERVICE (USPHS)

This service is responsible for safeguarding the United States from communicable disease from a foreign source and prevention of the spread of communicable disease from one state to another; conducts research programs; assists the individual states and foreign nations in improving health services or in instituting health service programs; and operates hospitals and outpatient clinics.

Although nurses participate in nearly all aspects of the activities of this service, it is in the hospital division that most of the nurses are employed.

Hospital Division. This division offers professional services for patients in the general medical and surgical hospitals; neuropsychiatric hospitals affiliated with the farms for narcotic addicts at Lexington, Kentucky, and Fort Worth, Texas; the tuberculosis hospital at Manhattan Beach, Brooklyn, New York; the Clinical Center of the National Institutes of Health, Bethesda, Maryland (this is a research hospital); outpatient clinics; and Indian hospitals.

The only leprosarium in the continental United States is at Carville, Louisiana. This hospital is operated by the Public Health Service but the nursing care is under the direction of the Daughters of Charity of St. Vincent de Paul.

In 1955 the hospitals of the Office of Indian Affairs were transferred to the charge of the Public Health Service. The Division of Indian Health operates fifty-six hospitals (these include four tuberculosis sanatoriums and many health centers, health stations, and boarding school infirmaries), ranging in size from 20 to 425 beds.

General Information. Appointment to the Public Health Service is made through the U.S. Civil Service Commission or through the Commissioned Corps. Salaries, grade, and rank for both types of appointment are determined by educational and professional experience qualifications. Nurse-applicants may indicate their preference for assignment in a particular field of activity of this service. The Public Health Service also maintains the Commissioned Reserve—nursing personnel who are trained and in readiness to assist in any major disaster or national emergency.

Information on qualifications, salaries, and the like, may be obtained by writing to: Chief, Division of Personnel, Public Health Service, U.S. Department of Health, Education, and Welfare, Washington 25, D. C.

VETERANS ADMINISTRATION

The Veterans Administration system has a hospital in every state and in Puerto Rico. This gives the nurse a wide choice of locations of hospitals for reasons of climate preference, home ties, or "seeing the country." The nurses may transfer to any other Veterans Administration facility without loss of professional status.

Veterans Administration hospitals are of three types: general medical and surgical care, neuropsychiatric, and tuberculosis. Under wartime conditions some of these hospitals have a mixed service, since all are planned to admit emergency patients of all types. The hospitals provide for the care and treatment of all honorably discharged men and women of all wars in which the United States has been engaged.

Basic Requirements. For positions in nursing in this agency, the nurse must be a citizen of the United States and a graduate of an accredited school of nursing, preferably from a school with full accreditation by the National League for Nursing; she must have current registration in at least one state and a successful professional record. References should be obtained from those individuals under whose supervision the applicant has had professional nursing experience or study; references that cover the more recent experience are desirable, and one covering the current or last employment is essential.

Promotion to higher grades, with corresponding increase in salary, is based upon professional experience and education preparation, rather than the position to which the nurse may be assigned.

Salaries. The authorized pay scale, as of July, 1960, shows the minimum salary for junior grade as $4,760 per year to the maximum of $5,790 with the following benefits: Thirty days' vacation, free laundry or cash allowance for uniforms, low-cost life insurance, retirement plans at low cost, and maintenance available at the hospital.

Application for appointment to the Veterans Administration Nursing Service may be made to the nearest VA hospital or regional office, or Nursing Service, Veterans Administration, Washington 25, D. C.

OTHER INFORMATION SOURCES FOR NURSES IN PUBLIC SERVICES

Both upper-class students and registered nurses should be aware of ready sources of information, such as the following, on the activities and requirements for nurses in government services:

Announcements of examinations of the United States Civil Service Commission are posted in first- and second-class post offices.

The Official Directory, which appears in every January and July issue of *The American Journal of Nursing,* lists the names and addresses of all government services.

Articles and announcements on government nursing appear in *The American Journal of Nursing, Nursing Outlook, Military Medicine, The Armed Forces Medical Journal.*

CLASS EXERCISE

Carefully collect and classify information on nursing opportunities in private fields of nursing and in public service nursing. Divide the class into two groups and arrange for a formal debate:

Resolved, that nursing in public service offers more advantages in advancement, security, travel, and graduate study than does civilian nursing.

REFERENCES

Army Nurse Corps:

ALLEN, GERTRUDE F.: Five hours to zero. *Nurs. Outlook* 5:417 (July) 1957.

ARCHARD, THERESA: *G. I. Nightingale: The Story of an American Army Nurse.* W. W. Norton & Co., New York, 1945.

AYNES, EDITH A.: Military nursing—1951. *Amer. J. Nurs.* 51:232 (Apr.) 1951.

AYNES, EDITH A.: The army area chief nurse. *Nurs. Outlook* 2:136 (Mar.) 1954.

CLAUSSEN, MARCIA: Hospitals follow the battle line in Korea. *Nurs. World* 126:16 (Oct.) 1952.

Editorial: They directed the Army Nurse Corps. *Amer. J. Nurs.* 55:1350 (Nov.) 1955.

FLIKKE, JULIA O.: *Nurses in Action.* J. B. Lippincott Co., Phila., 1943.

GATES, KERMIT H., and WEINER, LEONA: Health nursing service at an army hospital. *U.S. Armed Forces Med. J.* 6:1773 (Dec.) 1955.

HAYNES, INEZ: Commissions and men nurses. *Amer. J. Nurs.* 56:775 (June) 1956.

"Hospital Train." *Amer. J. Nurs.* 61:92 (Feb.) 1961.

WERLEY, HARRIET H.: The nurse's role in nuclear disaster. *Amer. J. Nurs.* 56:1580 (Dec.) 1956.

ZECK, MARTHA J.: Army nurses in San Antonio. *Amer. J. Nurs.* 51:70 (Feb.) 1951.

Air Force Nurse Corps:

"Air Force nurses share their know how." *Amer. J. Nurs.* 55:812 (July) 1955.

ALBERT, JANICE: What's different about flight nursing. *Amer. J. Nurs.* 56:873 (July) 1956.

GERSEMA, VIVIAN M.: When you choose Air Force nursing. *Nurs. Outlook* 3:380 (July) 1955.

LAY, FRANCES I.: Next step outer space. *Amer. J. Nurs.* 59:971 (July) 1959.

MARTIN, ANITA M.: We earn our wings. *Amer. J. Nurs.* 57:894 (July) 1957.

SMITH, ELINOR V.: Career opportunities for the Air Force nurse. *Nurs. World* 126:18 (Aug.) 1952.

"When you join the Air Force Nurse Corps." *Amer. J. Nurs.* 53:861 (July) 1953.

"Your Chance of a Life Time." Air Force Nurse Corps, Washington, D. C., 1960, booklet.

Navy Nurse Corps:

CASAREGOLA, MARY: The nurse in navy blues. *Amer. J. Nurs.* 54:594 (May) 1954.

"*Facts About Nursing.*" Annual statistical summary, American Nurses' Association, New York. Section on "Distribution of Professional Nurses."

HARRINGTON, ELEANOR: Aboard a hospital ship. *Amer. J. Nurs.* 53:583 (May) 1953.

JACKSON, W. LEONA: We've reached the golden year. *Amer. J. Nurs.* 58:671 (May) 1958.

"Senior students may join Navy in new program." *Amer. J. Nurs.* 57:1539 (Dec.) 1957.

U. S. Navy Nurse Corps (booklets): *White Task Force* (published in 1952) and *Navy Nurse Corps* (published in 1959). Department of the Navy, Bureau of Medicine and Surgery, Washington, D. C.

United States Public Health Service:

ABDELLAH, FAYE G., and LEVINE, EUGENE: *Patients and Personnel Speak.* U. S. Public Health Service, Washington, D. C., 1957, Publication No. 527.

BAHL, IDA E.: I couldn't have gotten along without Sam. (The success of the public health program among the Navajos.) *Nurs. Outlook* 9:352 (June) 1961.

HADLEY, J. NIXON: Health conditions among Navajo Indians. *Public Health Reports* 70:831 (Sept.) 1955.

LEWIS, FRANCES: Narcotic nightmares. *R. N.* 14:48 (Dec.) 1950.

McBRIDE, MARGUERITE: Nursing on an Indian reservation. *Amer. J. Nurs.* 57:1168 (Sept.) 1957.

MARSH, LUCILLE J.: Health services for Indian mothers and children. *Children* 4:203 (Nov.-Dec.) 1957.

SELLON, JACQUELYN: North Woods Hospital: a small rural hospital which serves an Indian population. *Amer. J. Nurs.* 59:676 (May) 1959.

TAYLOR, L. B.: Missile nurses. *R.N.* 23:64 (Oct.) 1960.

''The Nation's Health.'' President's Commission on the Health of the Nation, Washington, D. C., 1952.

''*Nurses in the United States Public Health Service.*'' U. S. Public Health Service, Washington, D. C., 1961, Publication No. 361.

''*The Public Health Nurse Today.*'' Federal Security Agency, U. S. Public Health Service, Washington, D. C.

WIENS, AGNES A.: Nursing service on a Chippewa reservation. *Amer. J. Nurs.* 61:92 (Apr.) 1961.

Veterans Administration Nursing Service:

ADDAMS, RUTH: Nursing care in VA out-patient clinics. *Nurs. World* 124:504 (Nov.) 1950.

ADDAMS, RUTH, and TORRENS, IVA F.: Home nursing care for veterans. *Nurs. Outlook* 4:497 (Sept.) 1956.

ARMY, MADELINE J.: Staff nurses are more than bedside nurses. *Milit. Med.* 119:296 (Nov.) 1956.

''*Opportunity for you in VA.*'' Veterans Administration, Washington, D. C., 1956, Pamphlet 10-30.

CHAPTER 23

Graduate Study

The senior nurse should realize that a diploma from a school of nursing and a state board certificate are no longer sufficient for more than first-level positions.

At the biennial convention of the ANA in Miami, 1960, the Committee on Current and Long-Term Goals presented a report to the House of Delegates on nursing education for the future:

Only with a truly professional education can nurses meet society's needs and the nursing profession maintain its strength at a time when the general educational level of the population is rising constantly.

To insure that within the next 20-30 years, the education basic to the professional practice of nursing, for those who then enter the profession, shall be secured in a program that provides the intellectual, technical and cultural components of both a professional and liberal education. Toward this end, the ANA shall promote the baccalaureate program so that in due course it becomes the basic educational foundation for professional nursing.

After considerable discussion it was voted "to accept the report of the Committee on Current and Long-Term Goals with appreciation and to use it as a basis for discussion in the states." [1]

[1] *American Journal of Nursing,* June, 1960.

254

This report is a warning that nurses graduating now should make definite plans for degree completion.

For many newly graduated nurses, formal education has been a continuing process for fifteen years. They still enjoy learning, but they have a well-earned sense of freedom and they treat themselves to the luxury of ''just studying what I want to.'' This wish can be achieved but it should be done in an organized manner. Without some plan or orderly direction the nurse becomes a ''course-taker'' and perhaps long after finds herself with considerable advanced education but no college credit.

The nurse can begin her plan by writing for the catalogue of colleges or universities in which she is interested. The course outline will list the Humanities, Social Sciences and Electives. Within these three fields courses will be offered that will be new and broadening; helping her to develop creative self-expression and an appreciation of the beautiful, to provide an understanding of man's natural and social environment, and to provide an introduction to other people and their cultures.

The nurse should discuss her plans with the dean of the college or the extension representative. Extension courses, not correspondence courses, are now offered in most towns with a population of 10,000 or more.

As credits for these semester hours accumulate they act as an incentive for degree completion and the goal is then within sight.

How Many Courses? If the nurse is working full time one course is considered a student load. All courses require reference reading, book reports, tests, and perhaps laboratory work. The student should undertake only one course for the first semester as an experiment.

Information on Courses. The National League for Nursing, 10 Columbus Circle, New York 19, N. Y., offers a list of college programs for professional nurses which have been accredited by the NLN. This list gives schools offering a baccalaureate degree, and those offering a master's or doctor's degree in nursing. From this list select the schools that are near or within easy traveling distance. Write for the school catalogue and study the list of courses offered.

Credit Evaluation. The nurse will wish to know the credit value of her nursing education. Most universities determine this on an individual basis by using the Graduate Nurse Qualifying Examination. The student should beware of the school that offers a large amount of blanket credit. The better schools make a careful investigation of the courses and qualifications of the instructors of the school from which the applicant graduated before deciding upon the amount of credit to be given.

Financing Graduate Study. There are numerous scholarships, fellowships, grants, and loan funds available for graduate study. Alumnae associations frequently offer scholarships ranging in value from $300 to $500 for graduates of their school. Grants are available through state nurses associations, lodges, churches, industries, and through the state and federal government.

The *American Journal of Nursing,* August, 1956, published a list, prepared by the Committee on Careers of the NLN, of organizations interested in providing funds to nurses for graduate study.

The Professional Counseling and Placement Service of the ANA is an authentic source of information on scholarships, fellowships, and other educational grants.

These educational aids go a long way toward making graduate study possible. The registered nurse has a distinct advantage in being able to use her basic nursing to good economic advantage. By week-end staff nursing or private duty, she earns as much as many students do in a week of waiting tables or stenographic work.

Federal Traineeships.   There long has been a serious shortage of public health personnel and nurse educators. The need for public health nurses increased and schools closed for lack of nurse teachers. Finally, in 1956, through the combined efforts of nursing and medical leaders, the federal government began the Professional Nurse Traineeship Program. This program was authorized for three years. By 1959 the demand had become so great that it was extended for five years.

These traineeships are awarded through grants to approved institutions to which the graduate nurse applies for admission. This fellowship covers tuition, fees, and a liberal stipend for living expenses.

Candidates for traineeships are selected by the university in accordance with its own admission program and policies with consideration for the potential of the applicant. The nurse must use this fellowship to prepare herself for a position in teaching, supervision or administration.[2]

ANA's International Unit.   The International Unit is an educational program for exchange students. The International Council of Nurses organized this program to facilitate the exchange of ideas and to create better international understanding. As a member nation of the ICN the American Nurses' Association actively participates in this Exchange of Privileges Program.

As a professional organization the ANA also cooperates with the International Educational Exchange Service of the Department of State. The Exchange Visitor Program was set up by Congress in 1948 and two years later the ANA was officially designated a sponsor for nurse-exchange visitors under this program. The ANA has combined these two programs to organize its own exchange plan. It sponsors nurses from ICN countries who wish to further their nursing experience in the United States.

The ANA Exchange Program makes arrangements for nurses of the United States to have nursing experience abroad. The program is described in the *American Journal of Nursing,* June, 1953: "Nurses on the Two Way Street." For further information the nurse should write for the publication "Your Cap Is Your Passport," ANA Exchange Program, 10 Columbus Circle, New York 19, N. Y.

---

[2] "Federal Traineeships: Where to Apply." *American Journal of Nursing,* 59:1759 (Dec.) 1959.

RESEARCH IN NURSING

Research is assuming its rightful importance in nursing education, not only as a professional requirement but as a necessary tool in making decisions of policy regarding nursing service and nursing education. Research in nursing functions are urgent because of the greatly increased nursing load, and research in education is necessary to know what kind of professional education is best for nursing service.

Research Defined. Research may be defined as a critical and exhaustive investigation of and experimentation with some particular subject, clearly presented and free from bias, which, when finished should furnish valid information upon its stated objective.

In 1848, John Stuart Mill laid down well-defined rules for scientific research which still form the basis for our modern research. Modern investigators employ a number of methods, all of which require scientific thought, work, experimentation, and evaluation.

Research Workers. Research requires trained workers. Several people may be working on the same project, but there must be some one trained in research technics to direct and classify the findings. This director must have a sound educational background and an understanding of the principles of research, the technics and methods to be used, and the concepts of statistics. All this is necessary to obtain, compile, and classify information and to be able to draw constructive conclusions from the material.

Research always is tedious and time-consuming, but nursing can no longer base its claims upon opinions and guesswork. Research groups are at work in all parts of the country on all types of projects but always with their attention centered on better care for the patient.

The American Nurses' Foundation. As a means of coordinating and strengthening research activities the ANA established the American Nurses' Foundation in 1955 for organized research in nursing and in patient care.

The present objective in research of the ANF embraces four areas of study:

1. To promote or conduct studies, surveys and demonstrations in patient care, to seek ways to provide greater comfort and safety for patients, and to improve relations with patients and families for health teaching and rehabilitation.

2. To study the change of nursing care as the result of new drugs, equipment, techniques, and new philosophies of nursing care.

3. To determine the effects on patient care of administrative organization in hospitals, clinics, public health agencies, industries, nursing homes, and physicians' offices.

4. To study the nursing needs in different categories of illness with special emphasis directed toward the chronically ill and long-term patients in their homes and in hospitals.

To achieve this goal the American Nurses' Foundation is seeking support from nurses, industry, foundations, and individuals who are deeply concerned with health care for all.

The cost of the present program of research is a minimum of $1,000,000. In order to make the future of this research program secure, the Foundation is seeking an additional $1,000,000 as an endowment fund.[3]

CLASS EXERCISE

Prepare a list of available funds for graduate study. The class may be divided into three groups to investigate scholarships, fellowships, and educational loan funds.

Each group will obtain information along the following lines: experience required after graduation; state board performance; amount of loan funds available; interest rates; time permitted for repayment; list of universities receiving grants for the Federal Traineeship Program; list of memorial scholarships; scholarships offered by industries; scholarships provided by district and state associations; scholarships provided by the alumnae association of the school.

This should be set up as a continuous project from class to class. The material should be accessioned in the school library and revised by each class, with new items added as the funds are established·

REFERENCES

AMES, MARIE, and POTTS, PATRICIA J.: Teaching fellowships. *Nurs. Outlook* 4:584 (Oct.) 1956.

"Continuing education for the graduate nurse." University of Illinois College of Nursing, Chicago, 1960.

"Educational funds for graduate nurses." *Amer. J. Nurs.* 56:1018 (Aug.) 1956.

"Educational preparation for nursing—1960." *Nurs. Outlook* 9:551, (Sept.) 1961.

"Exchange for education: The story of the ANA's exchange visitor program." *Amer. J. Nurs.* 59:1666 (Dec.) 1959.

GELINAS, AGNES: We need research in many areas. *Amer. J. Nurs.* 50:443 (July) 1950.

"Give or Get $5." *Amer. J. Nurs.* 60:495 (Apr.) 1960.

HASSENPLUG, LULU WOLF (as told to Patricia D. Horgan): Finding your way to a college degree. *R.N.* 24:56 (July) 1961.

---

[3] Subscriptions to the ANF, Inc., are tax deductable within the limits prescribed by the Internal Revenue Code.

HENLE, ROBERT J.: Liberal education: A basis for nursing. *Nurs. Outlook* 9:161 (Mar.) 1961.

KLINGELHOFER, ANN: ANA approaches to research. *Amer. J. Nurs.* 60:56 (Jan.) 1960.

LECKIE, IRENE, and BAWES, ALBERTA A.: Shall I take a fellowship? *Amer. J. Nurs.* 57:1007 (Aug.) 1957.

LEGGE, VIVIAN L.: Degree nurses gain new status. *R.N.* 22:61 (Dec.) 1959.

LOBBAN, MARJORIE: The value of postgraduate study abroad. *Nurs. Mirror* No. 2646 (Jan. 13) 1956.

LOGSDON, HAROLD: The mainstay of nursing education. *Nurs. World* 129:8 (Feb.) 1955.

McGREGOR, ESTHER M.: Field instruction in graduate nursing programs. *Nurs. World* 131:7 (July) 1957.

MERTON, ROBERT K.: Search for professional status. *Amer. J. Nurs.* 60:662 (May) 1960.

NAHM, HELEN: A decade of change. *Amer. J. Nurs.* 59:1588 (Nov.) 1959.

"Nurses on the two way street." *Amer. J. Nurs.* 53:683 (June) 1953.

OSHIN, EDITH S.: How to get help for your education: Many programs are now available to give you financial aid. Here's what they are and when, where and how to apply. *R.N.* 24:43 (Nov.) 1961.

"Post-masters education in nursing." *Nurs. Outlook* 9:554 (Sept.) 1961.

"Principles of legislation relating to public funds for collegiate nursing education." *Amer. J. Nurs.* 59:820 (June) 1959.

SCHLOTFELD, ROZELLA M.: Reflections on nursing research. *Amer. J. Nurs.* 60:492 (Apr.) 1960.

SMITH, PURCELLE P.: The Mary M. Roberts Fellowship in Journalism for Nurses. *Amer. J. Nurs.* 55:1079 (Sept.) 1955.

SPALDING, EUGENIA K.: Current problems of nurse educators. *Teachers College Record* 57:38 (Oct.) 1955.

WHITNEY, FREDERICK L.: *The Elements of Research.* Prentice-Hall, Inc., New York, 1950.

UNIT IV

Organizations: National and International

CHAPTER 24

Organization

Organizations are almost as old as the human race. Primitive man realized that his chances for survival were better as a member of a group than when hunting and fighting alone. To live in groups required some sort of organization, leadership, and assignment of duties for the common good. The modern organization pattern has become elaborate, even complex, but the fundamental principle is still "United we stand; divided we fall."

Organization has been the nurse's strongest incentive for professional advancement. The early nurse knew the needs of nurses and nursing, but she realized that no one nurse could wield enough influence to bring about necessary changes and improvements. If the student will review her history of nursing, she will be amazed at the changes during even half a century. None of these advancements were brought about by any nurse working alone, but always through organization. The modern nurse owes her trusted and respected status in the community to the women who gave their time to develop better working conditions, more formal education, and better compensation.

Self-protection is a fundamental instinct, and through organization the nurse does protect her right to practice nursing with dignity and respect. Nurse-practice laws grew out of the state nurse associations.

The real nurse is activated by a spirit of service that puts service above

262

self. Few nurses know the number of bills annually introduced in the state legislatures that have no regard for the patients' interests. Through the legislative committees of organized nursing, most of these selfish bills die in committee. Through standing together in their district and state association, nurses render a spirit of service that protects the community and benefits the nurse.

No nurse can fully appreciate the strength of her organization until she has read "January 6, 1945."[1] It is a cardinal date in the history of American nursing. Janet M. Geister[2] has said "when we want things *together* mountains can be moved," but in the feverish days that followed January 6, 1945, a whole smoking volcano was moved!

CONSTITUTION AND BYLAWS

Each nurse is given a copy of the constitution and bylaws as she becomes a member of her alumnae and district association. Bylaws which follow a commonly accepted plan present the objectives and policies in a formal manner. It is each new member's duty to read this constitution and have a clear idea of the bylaws. In this way she has an intelligent understanding of the purpose of her association.

Constitutional changes are necessary from time to time. Some of the original purposes may have been accomplished; new ones may be needed and, due to language changes, sections may sound quaint or ambiguous. It is time then for a clarification of sections or terms.[3]

NOMINATING COMMITTEE

This is the most important standing committee of the organization. Usually the people selected by the nominating committee are the ones elected. Those who are elected control the function of the association. The following points should be considered by the committee: What experience have applicants had? Are they persons fitted for the office? Are they conservative, radical, or neither? Do they know the philosophy and science of organization as well as parliamentary procedure? Have they had any committee experience in this association? Is the district or state having geographic representation? Are all branches of nursing being represented?

Only some of the officers should be changed annually. This gives some experienced members responsibility for carrying on until new ones become accustomed to procedures.

---

[1] *American Journal of Nursing*, Vol. 45 (Feb. 1945), p. 85.

[2] Editorial, "United We Stand," *Trained Nurse and Hospital Review*, Vol. 112 (Apr. 1944), p. 285. (This journal is now called *Nursing World*.)

[3] The Landrum-Griffith Act which was signed into law in 1960 will make decided changes in the constitution and bylaws of the National Student Nurses' Association and the American Nurses' Association.

EXPERIENCE

Committee work is the best way to gain experience in association work. Executives select and appoint to committees those members who show interest. The nurse should accept a committee appointment willingly because it will give her insight into policies and an acquaintance with the members of the organization.

Every organization needs young members. They are likely to be a little radical and want to try new ideas. The older members are always a bit conservative because of experience. This makes for a good balance of power. As the younger members gain experience and prove their worth, they will be given more responsibility with the wise guidance of the older members.

MEMBERSHIP

Each registered nurse should feel responsible *individually* for the present as well as the future status of nursing, and to compare nursing as an occupation (a way to make a living) with nursing as professional practice.

The fundamental reason to belong to a professional organization is the *need to belong,* to be accepted, to be a part of the group; this is of deep psychological importance. This need is particularly important to the truly professional nurse, for she cannot afford not to be identified with the group.

How does the public see the professional nurse? Since World War II the image of the nurse has taken on special stature and significance. For the first time in recorded history the public is willing to grant professional status to the registered nurse but the public expects the nurse to fulfill the individual and group responsibilities that go along with this privilege and prestige.

SUMMARY

The chapters following in this unit are concerned with nursing associations and allied organizations. The student should remember that it is the individual interest shown by each member that makes these organizations function effectively and for her actual benefit.

REFERENCES

BUKER, HELENE: Membership is like friendship. *Public Health Nursing* 37:1 (Jan.) 1945.

DENSFORD, KATHERINE J., and JERNSTROM, ELAINE: Student participation in professional organizations. *Amer. J. Nurs.* 48:536 (Aug.) 1948.

''Does it matter what you think?'' *Amer. J. Nurs.* 49:349 (June) 1949.

Editorial: Elect strong nurse leaders. *Trained Nurse and Hosp. Rev.* 108:276 (Apr.) 1942.

Editorial: Professional associations. *Amer. J. Nurs.* 43:881 (Oct.) 1943.

GEISTER, JANET M.: The new look in nursing. *R.N.* 12:28 (Apr.) 1949.

''Get life into your association meetings.'' *R.N.* 12:75 (Nov.) 1948.

''Januray 6, 1945.'' *Amer. J. Nurs.* 45:85 (Feb.) 1945.

MASTORGI, ALBA A.: Are so many meetings necessary. *Nurs. Outlook* 8:628 (Nov.) 1960.

McGRATH, BETHEL: Getting nurses out to meetings. *Amer. J. Nurs.* 50:524 (Sept.) 1950.

''Nursing—and its organizations.'' *Amer. J. Nurs.* 49:197 (Apr.) 1949.

PHILLIPS, ELIZABETH C.: Professional organization activities. *Amer. J. Nurs.* 52:73 (Jan.) 1952.

STEADWICK, DOROTHY A.: Behind the scenes with a successful membership committee. *Amer. J. Nurs.* 48:586 (Sept.) 1948.

CHAPTER 25

National Student Nurses' Association

Near the midcentury student nurses in several large cities had formed student nurse associations. Chicago was the first on record. Later state student nurses were organized. In 1953 the national organization was formed. The membership was composed of all the state associations; the state associations were composed of all the district associations. This followed the traditional pattern of the American Nurses' Association.

A year before the NSNA was formed, the six national nursing organizations had combined into two national associations: the American Nurses' Association and the National League for Nursing. These two bodies had developed a Coordinating Council to prevent duplication of effort and to coordinate interests to the best advantage for nursing. This council assumed sponsorship for the student organization. The students soon demonstrated leadership ability that truly amazed the leaders in both parent organizations.

Purposes. Before the organization of student nurse associations young graduates were overwhelmed by the seemingly complex machinery by which professional nurses tried to foster high ideals of nursing practice and to promote the welfare of nurses in order that all people may have better nursing care.

The early district and state associations were formed in order to give students an understanding of district, state, and national organizations while they were students and while they could be given guidance and counsel.

Also, student organizations formed a bond of interest between schools in the same district and in the same state. These meetings became the means of understanding the interests and problems of the various schools: they were no longer isolated groups. Schools developed common interests on a district and on a state level. After 1953 national interests were developed.

Objectives and Interests. The original objectives—"training" for participation in professional nurses' organizations and as a channel of communications with other schools of nursing—are still important objectives. In keeping with the times other objectives have been added, such as recruitment, uniform bylaws, and training for disaster and national defense.[1]

The student participates in her district and state associations and through these activities becomes acquainted with the organization and objective of the ANA and NLN. It was hoped that this organizational experience would carry over to the ANA and NLN after state board examinations and registration. A recent survey shows that nurses who are registered but who are not members are in the youngest age group.

Interest in professional organizations should begin with the school admission. The student should be impressed with the fact that she is preparing to enter a profession. She should be aware that certain things are expected of a mature, professional person that are not expected of a person who holds a so-called nonprofessional job.

Representation. Representation to state and national meetings is by delegates. The quota of delegates is based on the number of paid-up members. These delegates have voting privileges at state and national meetings. They come well informed on state and national issues and return to their schools and district associations prepared to make a detailed report of the meeting attended.

There is a national convention each year to which the association sends delegates. In the even-numbered years (such as 1960, 1962, etc.) the NSNA meets with the biennial convention of the ANA; on the odd-numbered years the student association meets in convention with the NLN. During the three, four, or five years of the school program, the student has time and opportunity to become acquainted with both organizations of registered, professional nurses.

Dues. The district or state dues range from $1.25 to $2 a year. Dues to the national association are fifty cents; this money is used to finance national meetings, the expense of a representative to the International Council of Nurses, for the official publication called the *Newsletter,* for printing and postage to state and district associations, and for the maintenance of a headquarters and a staff.

---

[1] The purposes of the association are stated in the association bylaws. These purposes are also listed in *Facts About Nursing.*

Headquarters. National headquarters of the ASNA has the same mailing address as the offices of the ANA and the NLN—10 Columbus Circle, New York 19, New York.

CLASS EXERCISE

Review the constitution of the district and state student nurses' association.
What officers are elected each year?
How are these elections conducted?
List the standing committees of the district and state associations.
How much of the annual dues remains in the district treasury and how much in the state treasury?
How is the delegate quota decided?
Are these delegates appointed or elected?

REFERENCES

CANTWELL, PHYLLIS, and HEELEY, PATRICIA: Over a thousand arrived! *Amer. J. Nurs.* 54:208 (Feb.) 1954.

CORCORAN, JANET: NSNA's first six years. *Amer. J. Nurs.* 59:695 (May) 1959.

DERBY, PATRICIA ANN: *Amer. J. Nurs.* 58:563 (Apr.) 1958.

GILHOOLEY, MARY A.: and ELLIOTT, FLORENCE E.: The status of organization in schools of nursing. *Amer. J. Nurs.* 58:703 (May) 1958.

MAGUIRE, MARY J.: Mr. Robert please. (Parliamentary Law) *Nurs. Outlook* 3:194 (Apr.) 1955.

"Student organization round up." *Amer. J. Nurs.* 59:1444 (Oct.) 1959.

"The 1959 convention of the National Student Nurses' Association." (Program and Candidates) *Amer. J. Nurs.* 59:385 (Mar.) 1959.

Tomorrow's Nurse, published bimonthly at 51 Melcher St., Boston, Mass. It has a student nurse editorial board, selected from widely separated areas of the United States.

CHAPTER 26

American Nurses' Association and Its Divisions

THE AMERICAN NURSES' ASSOCIATION

The young nurse of today, enjoying the leisure that results from the eight-hour working day, accepts it as the "Divine right of kings," seldom taking thought of the effort put forth by her organization that she might have the same working privileges as those in other professions.

Because the national association works without "blowing of horns or sounding of trumpets," the nurse is not aware that the numerous opportunities for her educational advancement have been a direct result of the work and planning of organized nursing. The school attended by the modern student is a long trek from the apprentice type of school attended by the older nurses. This improvement has been accomplished through the legislative committee and the educational committee of the state association in striving for higher standards for its schools.

It is because of the united efforts of nurses as a group that the individual nurse is accorded professional status by society as a whole and by the federal government.

Membership. The membership of the American Nurses' Association is made up of the nurse associations of the 50 states, the District of Columbia, Puerto

Rico, Virgin Islands, and the Canal Zone. The present total membership is 171,000. *Facts About Nursing* gives the classification of ANA members of all states and territories each year in the chapter: "Distribution of Professional Nurses."

Purposes. The stated purposes of the ANA are to: "foster high standards of nursing practice, promote the professional and educational advancement of nurses, and to promote the welfare of nurses to the end that all people may have better nursing care."

At the biennial meeting of the ANA a platform is adopted by the House of Delegates which outlines the objectives of the association for the next two years. These objectives change considerably from biennium to biennium, but the welfare of the nurse and the care of the patient always remain as the primary purposes.

Organization. The supporting framework of the ANA consists of the Board of Directors, the House of Delegates, the Advisory Council, the sections, and the committees.

Board of Directors. This board consists of a president; first, second, and third vice-presidents; a secretary; treasurer; and eight directors. These fourteen officers, together with the chairmen of the eight national sections, make up the Board of Directors.

House of Delegates. The House of Delegates is the policy-making body of the national association. These delegates represent all states and territories. Each section of a state nurses' association shall be entitled to one delegate for every 200 members or fractional part thereof, and each state association shall be entitled to three delegates-at-large. All delegates shall be elected by secret ballot in order to conform to the requirements of the Landrum-Griffith Act of 1960.

Advisory Council. This council is composed of two representatives from each state association, the Board of Directors of the national association, the President of the NLN, and the editors of the American Journal of Nursing.

This body has only advisory capacity to the ANA Board of Directors, but it serves an important function in helping the board to make decisions which are not required to be presented to the House of Delegates.

Sections. The House of Delegates at the biennial meeting in Atlantic City, June, 1952, voted to form two national organizations to be known as the *American Nurses' Association* and the *National League for Nursing*. These associations carry the same names on state and district levels.

This reorganization meant a change of sections and of functions of sections in order to best further the interests of the individual nurse. Some sections were dissolved, and new sections were formed; the same procedure was followed in the state and district associations. At present there are eight distinct sections. In some states where the nurse population is low, some of these sections have not been developed because definite quotas are required before a section may be formed. These eight sections are as follows: Counselors, Executive Secretaries, and Registrars; Educational Administrators, Consultants and Teachers; General Duty Nurses with a Head Nurses branch; Nursing Service Administrators; Occupational Health Nurses; Office Nurses; Private Duty Nurses; and Public Health Nurses with a School Nurses branch. Sections promote high standards of nursing practice and advance the economic and professional interests of their members.

The name and address of each of these section chairmen are listed in the Official Directory of the American Journal of Nursing each January and July.

Meetings. Conventions of the American Nurses' Association are held biennially. The officers of the organization make their reports, elections are held, and subjects of general professional interest are discussed. Any registered nurse in good standing may attend these meetings upon presentation of her district membership card which will state the section to which she belongs. Voting at the biennial convention is by delegates from each section of the state nurses associations and three delegates-at-large from each state. Each state section is entitled to one delegate for every 200 members or fraction thereof.

Official Magazine. *The American Journal of Nursing,* first published in 1900, is the official magazine of the American Nurses' Association. The editorial and business office address is 10 Columbus Circle, New York 19, N. Y.

Headquarters. Nurses always are welcome at the headquarters of the ANA, 10 Columbus Circle, New York. The professional interests of nearly 200,000 nurses are handled here by a staff of more than a hundred people. Nurses may visit at any time throughout the year from 9:00 A.M. to 5:00 P.M., except on holidays.

THE STATE NURSES ASSOCIATION

State rights are recognized in professional nursing as well as in affairs of government. Although closely affiliated and working harmoniously with the national organization, each state maintains its individuality by having an organization that functions best for its particular locality, problems, and interests; therefore, the nurse interested in the state nursing organization will also be well informed about national policies and developments in nursing.

The nurses association is to the nurse what the medical association is to the doctor, what the bar association is to the attorney. The public recognizes it as the official organization that speaks for the nurse and protects her interests.

The state association is a grouping of all the district organizations. Here, through conferences of state legislators and the state association officials, laws are secured governing registration and nursing practice; in this way ethical and educational standards are made possible. Here, too, state-wide studies of nurses' professional problems are initiated and coordinated.

The collective membership of the district associations composes the state association. Thus, if a state is composed of nine districts with a total membership of 1842, then the state membership is 1842.

Organization. The state organization consists of the state officers and the board of directors.

State officers are elected for a two-year term by the state delegates from the district associations. Voting is conducted by secret ballot.

The name and address of the president, secretary, and executive secretary of the state associations are listed in the January and July "Official Directory" of the *American Journal of Nursing*.

Activities. It is the duty of the state association to carry out the projects voted by the House of Delegates. These differ in individual states, but usually consist of the following:

1. A state office of the Professional Counseling and Placement Service provides efficient counseling and job satisfaction without cost to the member.
2. A state bulletin is edited, published, and distributed to all members.
3. An office of Economic Security is provided in order to assist groups and individual nurses in negotiations that have established constructive group relations between nurses and employers resulting in better salaries and working conditions.
4. The state legislative committee plans and promotes state legislation to advance nursing and to protect the public.

The nurse, in paying her district dues, should be aware of the activities of her state association and should feel that the money she invests annually is returning ample dividends by constantly improving her professional status.

Executive Secretary. Many of the states have large memberships which involve a tremendous amount of work. This extra work is too much for the state officers, who are already busy in their own positions. In these states an executive secretary is employed as a paid administrator for the state association. Some twenty-five state associations now have full-time executive secretaries, and a few have part-time secretaries. The office at headquarters acts as a clearinghouse for the entire state association. Membership transfers between states and between districts within the state are made here; state dues are received; state conventions and institutes are arranged for and managed; legislative action is considered, and, if necessary, a lobbyist is provided; visits to district and alumnae organizations are arranged. The state loan funds are administered here, as is also the state relief fund.

Along with these duties, the executive secretary acts as an "information bureau" for the nurses of the state. The privilege of writing to this bureau should not be abused by nurses when the information may be readily available in their own hospital library or public health headquarters.[1]

The state nurses association should not be confused with the department that administers the nurse-practice act for that state. These offices have entirely different functions.

---

[1] The annual indexes and the cumulative index of the *American Journal of Nursing* are sources of information on almost any subject.

Pointers for State Meetings. Delegates are elected on a quota basis by secret ballot from the district association. They are issued a delegate card which will entitle the nurse to voting privileges in the House of Delegates.

The nurse-delegate should plan to arrive at convention headquarters in plenty of time for registration. At the desk she should present her district card and her delegate card. The nurse will be issued a delegate badge which must be shown in order to be admitted to the House of Delegates.

Microphones will be located in convenient places in the House of Delegates. When the nurse wishes to discuss a subject or make a motion, she should go to the microphone nearest her and state her name and the district she represents. If she wishes to make a motion, she should also submit it in writing. This will help the record and the stenotypist.

THE DISTRICT ASSOCIATION

The first organization to include *all* graduate nurses was *The Nurses Associated Alumnae of the United States and Canada,* organized in 1896.[2] In 1912 the name of the organization was changed to the American Nurses' Association.

The files of the *American Journal of Nursing* for 1913-1916 show that much work was done by a special committee on revision of the American Nurses' Association, and that at the 1916 biennial convention, held in New Orleans, the committee on revision of the ANA recommended, and the delegates at the convention approved, the constitution and bylaws for alumnae, district, state, and national associations.

The forming of district associations gave a great impetus to increasing the membership throughout each state. Long before this, small organizations had been formed within the states, sometimes comprising two or three counties, or one large city. In such cases, these were reorganized as districts of the state associations.

The nurse should not depend upon her national association to carry all the load. The division of responsibility begins with the district association. It is there that the individual nurse pays her debt to the advancement of nursing by giving her time, interest, and financial support.

Membership. The district association consists of all the nurses living in that area; this may be one large city or several counties. The membership of the district association forms the basis of the state association.

It is necessary to pay dues only once each year. If the nurse pays her dues in one district and moves to another district or another state, she should ask for a membership transfer.

Care should be taken to see that the district association has the correct address after a member has married or changed her residence. If the district has it correctly, it will be forwarded correctly to the state and national associations. Old addresses never die, they just cause confusion. For example:

---

[2] In 1907 this alliance was severed, Canada forming her Dominion organization known as the Canadian Nurses' Association.

Marie F. Woodward, 621 Buckingham Place, Chicago 13, is found to be Captain Marie F. Woodward, R.N., U. S. Army Hospital, Camp Atterbury, Indiana.

When a nurse becomes a member of the district, she will be presented with a copy of the constitution and bylaws. She should read every page of this booklet. It is her right as a member to know the rules and regulations of the organization; furthermore, it may save her genuine embarrassment later.

Advantages. As soon as the nurse has obtained her certificate of registration, she should apply for membership in the district association, thus allying herself with her professional organization. As an active member, she will continue to learn and keep herself informed on subjects of interest in her work.

The district association is the most important part of the nurse's organization. Here are her most intimate contacts with the national organization. It is here that her individual influence is felt most. If her alumnae and the district are in the same locality, her interest will be divided to some extent. Often the alma mater is in a distant state, and the nurse's interest in her alumnae is only that of a nonresident member; hence her district comes to be her major professional interest. Perhaps nowhere in the American Nurses' Association is the organization so strongly and intimately united as in the district association.

Dues. Dues are paid annually at the district level but the amount paid includes dues for the state association, the national association, and the International Council of Nurses.

Suppose that the district dues are $45. The nurse pays this amount to the district treasurer. Here begins a process of substraction. If the district dues are $15 for each member, this amount is subtracted and remains in the district treasury. The remaining $30 for each member is sent to the state association. The state dues are $22.50. Again, the state treasurer subtracts $22.50 for each member and forwards $7.50 to the national association.[3] From this the treasurer of the ANA will forward the dues for the International Council of Nurses.

This method of paying dues to all four associations is a convenient arrangement which the nurse appreciates when she considers the annoyance of paying each separately.

All state associations have a certain date, usually March 1, for "closing the books." This means that nurses whose dues are not paid by that date are dropped from membership. Therefore dues should be paid to the district treasurer not less than two weeks before this expiration date, in order that they may reach state headquarters in time to be entered in the state books.

Meetings. The nurse should feel that it is her professional duty to take an active part in the district meetings. It is not enough just to attend. "No, I don't go to the district meetings; I never get anything out of them." "How

---

[3] The present actual dues of the national association are $7.50.

much do you put into them?'' ''Well, I pay my dues.'' Have you helped on any committees? Have you tried to interest anyone else in attending meetings? If not, you have failed to live up to both your duty and your privilege.

Experience has shown that the meetings which are best attended are those with programs that are given by the nurses themselves. So often notices for the next district meeting say: ''A lecture on Dialysis of the Kidney will be given by Doctor B— at 8:00 P.M. All nurses are urged to attend.'' To most of the members it means ''another doctor's lecture'' to sit through, and few come.

An excellent program may be arranged by selecting a subject of general interest and presenting several aspects of it, nurses and doctors cooperating with other workers interested in the same subject, as in the following:

A Symposium on Multiple Sclerosis

Mortality and Morbidity in Multiple Sclerosis
Pathology of Multiple Sclerosis
Medical Treatment of Multiple Sclerosis
Feeding the Patient with Multiple Sclerosis
Nursing Care of the Patient with Multiple Sclerosis
Rehabilitation and Social Aspects of Multiple Sclerosis

The same idea may be carried out, making use of such general subjects as the ANA Economic Security Program, civil defense, and rehabilitation in nursing homes.

In districts where in-service education is difficult to plan, a district program on nursing, prepared by nurses and members of allied services, could be used to good advantage.

CLASS EXERCISE

This class project is planned to include all divisions which make up the American Nurses' Association and the International Council of Nurses. Information for this project can be secured from the treasurer of the district association, from the bulletin of the state association, and from *Facts About Nursing* published by the ANA.

Prepare a graph to show the district association as the basis of the state association, the state association as the basis of the national association, and the national association as a member organization of the International Council of Nurses. On this graph indicate the following: amount of dues for each organization; dates on which these dues are payable; number of members in the district, state, national and international associations. Indicate the increase in membership of each over last year.

Put this graph on display in the library; it will be of interest to all nurses.

REFERENCES

AMERICAN NURSES' ASSOCIATION: *Facts About Nursing* (an annual statistical publication). Published by the association in New York.

"American Nurses' Association and the National League for Nursing" (complete review of functions and organizational chart). *Amer. J. Nurs.* 56:69 (Jan.) 1956.

"ANA membership cards." *Amer. J. Nurs.* 54:49 (Jan.) 1954.

ASHIN, EDITH S.: How does the ANA stack up as a professional organization? *R.N.* 25:39 (Feb.) 1962.

BROWN, ESTHER LUCILE: *Nursing for the Future.* Russell Sage Foundation, New York, 1948.

"How the ANA was formed." *Trained Nurse and Hosp. Rev.* 100:687 (June) 1938.

JUHRE, ELSA M.: Clothes don't make a convention. *Amer. J. Nurs.* 54:840 (July) 1954.

' Nominations are in order." *Amer. J. Nurs.* 49:382 (June) 1949.

"Registered where you work?" *Amer. J. Nurs.* 49:382 (June) 1949.

"Representation at biennials." *Amer. J. Nurs.* 52:963 (Aug.) 1952.

The State Nurses' Association:

GEISTER, JANET M.: Organic unity of professional solidarity. *Nurs. Outlook* 6:215 (Apr.) 1954.

GRIFFITH, LILLIAN: Establishing a state office. *Nurs. Outlook* 3:28 (Jan.) 1955.

"How does your state association orient new officers and committee members?" *Amer. J. Nurs.* 56:620 (May) 1956.

HUGHES, EVERETT C., MacGILL, HELEN, and DEUTSCHER, ERWIN: *Twenty Thousand Nurses Tell Their Story.* American Nurses' Association, New York, 1958.

MERTON, ROBERT K.: The functions of the professional association. *Amer. J. Nurs.* 58:50 (Jan.) 1958.

PURDY, FRANCES: So you're going to have a convention. *Nurs. Outlook* 3:211 (Apr.) 1955.

The District Association:

BAKKEN, HELEN: An open letter to section members. *Amer. J. Nurs.* 54:1372 (Nov.) 1954.

ELDER, FRANCES: Needed—A change of climate. *R.N.* 18:34 (Sept.) 1955.

LEWIS, EDNA: We streamlined it. (Help for annual meetings) *Amer. J. Nurs.* 52:1083 (Sept.) 1952.

MAGUIRE, MARY J.: Mr. Robert, please. (Parliamentary law) *Nurs. Outlook* 3:194 (Apr.) 1955.

McGRATH, BETHEL: Getting nurses out to meetings. *Amer. J. Nurs.* 50:524 (Sept.) 1950.

"Programs for district meetings (Minnesota and Oklahoma)." *Amer. J. Nurs.* 52:714 (June) 1952.

SCHEWER, MATHILDA: To nurses everywhere. *Amer. J. Nurs.* 61:75 (Apr.) 1961.

STROM, EDITH E.: County fair. (proceeds used to send members to conventions and finance student projects) *Amer. J. Nurs.* 52:1521 (Dec.) 1952.

WALKER, VIRGINIA H.: An open letter to section members. *Amer. J. Nurs.* 55:432 (Apr.) 1955.

"Working with a committee." *Amer. J. Nurs.* 52:1082 (Sept.) 1952.

CHAPTER 27

The Alumnae Association

The first permanent societies of nurses were alumnae associations. Organized in 1888, the first of these was the Woman's Hospital School of Nursing, Philadelphia. These societies were organized principally to help the nurse work for her own school and to preserve her contacts with classmates and friends. Such organizations preserved ties that were sincere and precious.

Objectives. The alumnae association of each school of nursing decides upon its own objectives. These vary from school to school and objectives of diploma schools differ from those of collegiate schools. The main interest generally is to improve the school along modern lines, to keep informed of the school's activities, to keep alive school friendships, and to build up a reserve fund for the future needs of its members.

Activities. The association plans its own activities, and although it has no administrative function in the school, an excellent opportunity is provided for the school and the association to work together. The director of the school and the president of the alumnae association have much in common and they soon will find their objectives are much the same. The alumnae is an influential factor in recruitment, as it is also in public relations. The association can be helpful in the financial support of the school.

Most alumnae associations offer a scholarship to its members for advanced education. These are eagerly sought by graduates to be used for degree completion or for tuition while working full or part time.

The association can be influential in the selection of the type of student who may wish to enter the school. Graduates of the school are potential members of the association. Are the standards for the school in keeping with the type of members which the alumnae will welcome after registration?

The alumna will wish to keep in touch with the school. This can be done best by meeting the students. The students may be invited to share a meeting or program of interest to both alumnae and students. Alumnae association members would enjoy attending some of the concerts, exhibits, and theatricals given by students.

Maintaining Friendships. The newsletter or alumnae bulletin is the connecting link from class to class and from generation to generation. This method is in general use and ranges from a formal printed periodical to mimeographed sheets. It is "the tie that binds" and it is a good use of the association's funds.

Reunions. Class reunions should be one of the objectives of the alumnae. The university schools plan these reunions by classes in the individual colleges. The alumnae associations of the diploma schools do not have the reunion machinery available, but the association and the school plan together for a one- or two-day reunion every three to five years. The present students gladly act as guides. They appreciate their blessings a little more as they point out the improvements in the dining room, modern equipment, and living conditions.

Long-Range Objectives. Some alumnae associations establish a hospital fund to provide for hospital care for its members when needed. A pension fund could be a worthy project for the next quarter of a century. Nurses have been eligible for Social Security only since 1950 and still not all hospitals offer Social Security coverage. Many nurses, still living, were nearing the end of their nursing career when Social Security was made available. Nothing is as cold as public charity; a small monthly pension would be a reward for alumnae dues paid over the years.

One of the objectives of every alumnae association is genuine concern for its members. The student should be made aware of this during the nursing course. Dues to the association are a form of professional insurance. For the younger nurse it may mean advanced education; for the older nurse it may mean much-needed hospital care.

Fund Raising. In order for the alumnae association to build up a reserve to provide scholarships, hospital care, and pensions it must look beyond the annual alumnae dues. Various fund raising devices must be used in order to build up an adequate reserve. The following suggestions have been used successfully:

1. Greeting card sales show a good profit. Arrangements can be made with card manufacturing companies. These sales should include cards, gift wrap-

ings, and stationery. Plans should be made with inactive members to staff the sales booth, preferably in the nurses' residence. These sales can be conducted every two or three weeks from October to May.

2. A sale of parcel post packages is an interesting means of raising funds. A note is sent to every member to send a package to the association to be sold *wrapped* on Alumnae Day. The note should state the value of the contents to be enclosed as $1 or $2. There is a mysterious anticipation about such a sale.

3. There often are patients and friends of nurses who would be glad to make a contribution to the association if they were made aware of it. "The nurses were wonderful to my father. I wish there was something I could do for them." This could be an on-going project but it would mean that every member and the present student body be well informed about the purpose of the project.

4. An "every graduate" campaign yields surprising results. Letters should be sent to the members and non-members with an explanation of the drive for funds and ask for a contribution. For non-members an application form for membership should be enclosed with the campaign letter.

In large schools of nursing such an undertaking could be quite a chore for a small group of members. An agent or representative from each class could be appointed. She and her committee would be responsible for writing to each classmate. If the project included the last twenty classes, these twenty representatives would constitute a committee to formulate the letter, revise the address list, and arrange for mailing.

SUMMARY

The young healthy graduate nurse may feel that she can solve life's problems independently but she loses contact with her school friends. The alumnae association continues to function without her participation and support, but much later she may find that she needs the association more than the association needs her.

CLASS EXERCISE

Plan programs for one year for an alumnae association. These programs should be planned with the idea of helping members to keep up with new developments in nursing and to stress the place of the nurse in community affairs.

1. Invite a class of seniors to discuss and demonstrate new developments in medicine and surgery.

2. Invite an authority to present an illustrated lecture on civil defense, Conelrad stations, or other means for national survival.

3. Plan something of a social nature, such as a picnic, bazaar, or hobby show.

4. Plan a discussion of the World Health Organization. Maps should be used to indicate where health needs are greatest and what diseases are most prevalent. Explain how American nurses are participating in the World Health Organization.

5. The local Red Cross Nursing Service will welcome an opportunity to describe the present activities in the community.

6. The alumnae association will be interested to know of the activities of the city board of health and the board chairman will be pleased to have the opportunity to explain these functions to an understanding audience.

REFERENCES

CHARLOTTE, SISTER M., and JONATHAN, SISTER M.: Calling all alumnae. *Nurs. Outlook* 5:535 (Sept.) 1957.

"Check list for program planners." *Amer. J. Nurs.* 52:1090 (Sept.) 1952.

CONRAD, MARGARET E.: Alumnae funds. *Amer. J. Nurs.* 59:685 (May) 1959.

Editorial: Our alumnae associations. *Amer. J. Nurs.* 46:79 (Feb.) 1946.

GLADWIN, MARY E.: Alumnae associations, their opportunities and obligations. *Amer. J. Nurs.* 21:9 (Oct.) 1921.

KALTENBACK, WINIFRED, and CAVELL, CECILE: What are our alumnae doing? *Amer. J. Nurs.* 55:75 (Jan.) 1955.

MORRIS, MARY L.: Alumnae home coming. *Amer. J. Nurs.* 53:1101 (Sept.) 1953.

POWELL, FRANCES L. A.: For alumnae associations: These three purposes. *Amer. J. Nurs.* 40:1102 (Oct.) 1940.

CHAPTER 28

National League for Nursing

The National League for Nursing (NLN) is an organization of nurses and non-nurses established in 1952 through the amalgamation of seven national agencies. Many of these agencies had both nurse and non-nurse members.

PURPOSE AND PHILOSOPHY

The purpose of the NLN, stated in the Certificate of Incorporation of 1952 is "to foster the development and improvement of hospital, industrial, public health, and other organized nursing service and of nursing education through the co-ordinated action of nurses, allied professional groups, citizens, agencies, and schools to the end that the nursing needs of the people will be met."

The philosophy of the NLN is based on the eligibility of its members. Members include both nurses and non-nurses because the NLN believes that individuals and groups in all communities are interested in and are capable of making a worth-while contribution to the health and welfare of their community and indirectly to the state and nation.

ORGANIZATION

There is the NLN membership body of nurse and lay members made up of the state associations. The state associations are composed of local leagues for nursing. In states that do not have local leagues the nurse may join as an individual member.

As stated in the Certificate of Incorporation the NLN is concerned with nursing education and nursing service; therefore, there is a Division of Nursing Service and a Division of Nursing Education. The Division of Nursing Service is made up of the Department of Hospital Nursing and the Department of Public Health Nursing. The Division of Nursing Education has a Department of Diploma and Associate Degree Programs and a Department of Baccalaureate and Higher Degree Programs. Each of these four departments has a council of member agencies.

ACTIVITIES

The NLN has many activities directly concerned with nursing education and nursing service.

Fact Finding and Research. *Nurses for a Growing Nation* was a project of the League to get an estimate of the number of nurses needed by 1970 in the United States during time of peace. This report was published as a recruitment goal. The annual report prepared by the NLN in *Facts About Nursing* gives information on how the necessary number of nurses is being provided.

Testing Services. Most schools of nursing use a testing service to evaluate applicants. The NLN Testing Service offers tests, prepared by experts, for applicants to pre-service programs in professional nursing, for applicants to schools of practical nursing, and for the graduate nurse who wishes to enter a college or university for advanced nursing education.

This service provides also achievement tests in nursing subjects. These tests serve two purposes: the student can measure her potential in the coming state examinations, and the teacher can compare the performance of her students with that of students in similar programs in other schools of nursing.

The testing service also makes and scores the examinations of the State Board Test Pool, described in the chapter on Registration and Interstate Licensure.

Accreditation. Most schools of higher learning are subject to an accrediting body which sets standards by which its institutions are periodically evaluated. The National Commission on Accreditation appoints the agencies which investigate and accredit the program offered by the school.[1] In 1939 the National League of Nursing was designated as the accrediting agency for schools of nursing.

This is a voluntary program and it is not a legal requirement of the state examining board. However, accreditation of the NLN carries considerable

---

[1] "In 1909-1911, Abraham Flexner, at the insistence of the Carnegie Foundation for the advancement of Teaching, made two close and comprehensive studies of the status of medical education at home and abroad, and his strictures on American conditions excited a storm of comment and criticism . . . . ." From *History of Medicine* by Fielding H. Garrison.

prestige and acts as a measuring device for high school counselors. The list of fully accredited schools of nursing are listed in *Nursing Outlook* each February.

OFFICIAL PUBLICATION

In 1952 there was an amalgamation of several national organizations, chief of which were the National League of Nursing Education, the National Organization for Public Health Nursing, and the Association for Collegiate Schools of Nursing. The new organization, known as the National League for Nursing, established *Nursing Outlook* as its official publication. The magazine embraces the interests of public health nurses and teachers in diploma and collegiate schools of nursing. Editorial offices are located at 10 Columbus Circle, New York 19, N. Y.

HEADQUARTERS

The national headquarters of the NLN is located at 10 Columbus Circle, New York 19, N. Y. This organization maintains a staff of 200 persons to carry on an over-all program of nursing service for hospitals, public health, and nursing education on the diploma and higher education levels.

CLASS EXERCISE

From the state league for nursing obtain a list of the functions and services of the National League for Nursing. Follow through these activities and list all those that have directly affected the student experience of the nurse.

REFERENCES

Editorial: How was the vote? *Nurs. Outlook* 4:75 (Feb.) 1956.

ELLIOTT, FLORENCE, and SMITH, DOROTHY: National accreditation. *Amer. J. Nurs.* 55:456 (Apr.) 1955.

FILLMORE, ANNE: Our first five years. *Nurs. Outlook* 6:14 (Jan.) 1958.

FILLMORE, ANNE, SHEEAHAN, MARION W., and MILLER, JULIA M.: The NLN is everybody's business. *Nurs. Outlook* 1:22 (Dec.) 1953.

HOYT, ROBERT S.: Agency membership in the National League for Nursing. *Nurs. Outlook* 1:83 (Feb.) 1953.

''Let's look in at the league.'' (Detailed account of the activities of the National League for Nursing) *Amer. J. Nurs.* 49:246 (June) 1949.

MUNSON, HELEN W., and STEVENS, KATHERINE: *The Story of the National League of Nursing Education.* W. B. Saunders Company, Philadelphia, 1934.

NATIONAL LEAGUE FOR NURSING: *Criteria for the Evaluation of the Educational Programs in Nursing Leading to a Diploma.* Published by the League, New York, 1958.

''What NLN membership can do for you.'' *Nurs. Outlook* 1:78 (Feb.) 1953.

''Your vote in the NLN election.'' *Nurs. Outlook* 1:193 (Apr.) 1953.

CHAPTER 29

Other National Nursing Organizations

AMERICAN ASSOCIATION OF INDUSTRIAL NURSES (AAIN)

This association was organized in 1942 as a group of professional registered nurses working in industry. More than half of the membership comes from the highly industrialized states of California, New York, Ohio, Pennsylvania, Illinois, and Michigan.

Functions. The primary functions of the AAIN are:

"To formulate and develop principles and standards of industrial nursing practice in order that the nurse in industry may utilize more fully her professional knowledge and training in her service to workers and management—and to the community.

"To promote, by means of publications, conferences, workshops and symposia, both formal and informal programs of education designed specifically for the nurse in industry.

"To identify the rightful place of nursing in the industrial health program and to encourage cooperation among all groups engaged in protecting the health and welfare of the worker.

"To impress upon management, physicians, and allied groups the importance

286

of integrating into the activities of industry the services to be rendered by the industrial nurse."[1]

The national association is composed of local and state organizations. This association includes two important constituent groups: The Medical Advisory Council and the Management Advisory Council. These councils act in an advisory capacity to the local, state, and national groups. This makes for effective cooperation of nurses, physicians, and management, in "integrating into the activities of industry the services to be rendered by the industrial nurse."

Official Publication. The official magazine of the AAIN is the *American Association of Industrial Nurses Journal,* published monthly as a service to all members. It carries technical articles concerning industrial nursing and industrial medicine, reports of educational activities, and news of industrial interest on the local, state, and national level.

AMERICAN ASSOCIATION OF NURSE ANESTHETISTS (AANA)

The Doctors Mayo of Rochester, Minnesota, were probably the first to employ nurse anesthetists. The systematic training of nurses in administration of anesthesia began about 1910. Hospitals were beginning to demand skilled anesthetists, and there were not enough doctors interested in this form of medical practice.

The American Association of Nurse Anesthetists was organized in Cleveland in 1931. The major purpose of this organization was to improve educational standards for the nurse anesthetist. This objective was accomplished by requiring a national qualifying examination and by requiring full accreditation of schoo!s of anesthesia.

Requirements. The applicant who applies for registration at a school of anesthesia must be currently validly registered as a graduate professional nurse. The duration of the course must be eighteen months. The number of cases of clinical experience must be 450 totalling 500 hours of clinical instruction. The course requires 250 hours of formal classroom instruction.

The nurse anesthetist must have well-trained ears to *hear* any changes that may occur in the patient, well-trained eyes to *see* any changes, and well-trained touch to *feel* any changes in pulse and in muscle tone. She must be able to think quickly, and with good judgment, and to enjoy an atmosphere of intense activity. Equally important is her ability to calm the fear that always is present, whether manifested by the patient or a member of the surgical team. A capable anesthetist must be a good student of human nature—first, last, and always.

Legal Implications.[2]   There are more opportunities for the nurse anesthetist to become involved in legal suits than there are for the staff nurse or head

---

[1] *Facts About Nursing,* 1959, p. 233.

[2] These legal implications are clearly indicated in *Notes on Legal Aspects of Anesthesia by Nurses* by Clarene A. Carmichael.

nurse. For this reason all anesthetists carry professional liability insurance.

The anesthetist is personally liable for her own negligence, irrespective of whether or not the surgeon may be jointly or primarily liable. Although the court may consider the nurse an agent of the hospital, this does not relieve her of responsibility for her own carelessness. *But she is not responsible for the carelessness of the surgeon, his assistants, and the operating-room nurses.*

Nurse Anesthetists. Physicians who are specialists in the administration of anesthetics are known as *anesthesiologists.* Large medical centers may have several anesthesiologists. These in turn are supplemented by *nurse anesthetists.* In some of the smaller hospitals, one member of the medical staff has had special training in anesthesia and acts in a supervisory capacity to the nurse anesthetist.

Headquarters. The headquarters of the AANA is Prudential Plaza, Chicago 1, Illinois. Nurses who wish to consider a course in anesthesia may write AANA headquarters for an outline of the course.

The Guide Issue (published each August) of *Hospitals,* the journal of the American Hospital Association, lists the currently accredited schools of anesthesia.

GUILD OF SAINT BARNABAS

This is an international organization of nurses, which had its beginning in the Episcopal Church in England in 1876. The American organization was founded in Boston in 1886. Professional nursing was new in 1886; nurses were few, there were no nursing organizations, and both students and graduates had to adjust themselves to new environments. Social opportunities were lacking. Opportunities for attending church services either did not exist or were poorly planned. The Guild of Saint Barnabas (so named because it was organized on St. Barnabas Day, June 11th) came into existence to supply these spiritual and social needs of the nurse, and these are still its fundamental purposes.

The guild has a threefold program: spiritual, social, and cultural activities. Through its nationwide organization, it is able to exert a sisterly influence upon those who go from place to place. It promotes friendliness among all nurses, and it makes definite provision for contacts with women outside the nursing profession in its policy of including associate members who are non-nurses. These associate members cooperate with nurses in achieving the objectives of the guild, both local and national in scope, by effecting a useful, constructive, and altogether commendable society.

Some of the activities carried out by local branches include monthly guild meetings followed by social activities; an annual picnic; recognition of the Feast of St. Barnabas; inspirational addresses by speakers of note; discussions on fields of nursing; sick benefits and visiting of sick nurses; acquiring and management of apartment houses for nurses; providing rooms for committee meetings of nurses; holding supper, teas, picnics, and other forms of entertainment.

Headquarters of the Guild of St. Barnabas are in Quincy, Massachusetts. The organization's official magazine, *The News-Letter,* is published quarterly at the Guild's headquarters.

Membership. The membership of the Guild is interdenominational. Every professional nurse and every student nurse in an accredited school of nursing is eligible to be an active member. Clergymen, physicians, and women who are not nurses may be associate members. Each branch has a clergyman as chaplain. Officers and committee members are elected annually.

THE NATIONAL COUNCIL OF CATHOLIC NURSES OF THE UNITED STATES (NCCN)

The council was organized in June, 1940, "to encourage and advance the spiritual and professional welfare of the Catholic nurse." The present objectives of this organization are:

(1) To protect, encourage and advance the spiritual, professional and material welfare and social contacts of Catholic nurses; (2) To foster among all nurses the spirit of charity in the care of the sick by emphasizing spiritual and social values and opportunities in the exercise of the profession of nursing; (3) To provide an agency through which Catholic nurses will be able to speak corporately in matters of common interest to their profession; (4) To promote under the control of affiliated associations a program whereby Catholic nurses may dedicate a portion of each year to the voluntary care of the indigent sick.

The official magazine, *The Catholic Nurse,* is published quarterly, with editorial offices at 120 Boylston Street, Boston, Massachusetts.

This organization is composed of local units, diocesan unity, and the national association. Headquarters are at 1312 Massachusetts Avenue, N.W., Washington, D. C.

Membership. Any Roman Catholic professional registered nurse is eligible for membership. The applicant need not be actively engaged in nursing. Student nurses are given associate membership.

REFERENCES

American Association of Industrial Nurses

American Assoc. of Industrial Nurses, Inc.: Guide for the Use of the Daily Log. The Association, New York, 1957.

American Assoc. of Industrial Nurses and the National League for Nursing: Guide for Evaluating and Teaching Occupational Nursing Concepts. The National League for Nursing, New York, 1956, League Exchange No. 24.

BARSCHAK, ERNA: Working grandmothers and the occupational health nurse. *Amer. J. Nurs.* 57:481 (Apr.) 1957.

CONTA, LIONNE: What happens at the bargaining table? *Amer. J. Nurs.* 59:1436 (Oct.) 1959.

DEMPSEY, CATHERINE R.: The American Association of Industrial Nurses: How, and when it came into being. *Trained Nurse and Hosp. Rev.* 112:448 (June) 1944.

American Nurses' Association: Facts About Nursing. The Association, New York, Annually.

Management Advisory Council, AAIN: Principles of Management-Nurse Relationship in Industry. The association, New York, 1957.

Nurse Anesthetists

BARBEE, GRACE C.: Changing nursing patterns produce changing professional liability patterns. Part I. *Hosp. Manage.* 86:110 (Aug.) 1958; Part II, 86:108 (Sept.) 1958.

CARMICHAEL, CLARENE A.: Notes on Legal Aspects of Anesthesia by Nurses. American Association of Nurse Anesthetists, Chicago, 1959.

CREIGHTON, HELEN: *Law Every Nurse Should Know.* W. B. Saunders Company, Philadelphia, 1957.

LETOURNEAU, CHARLES U.: What is the present status of the nurse anesthetists? *Hosp. Manage.* 83:45 (June) 1957.

RAPER, HOWARD RILEY: *Man Against Pain.* Prentice-Hall, Inc., New York, 1945.

RATCLIFF, J. D.: The anesthesiologist. *Today's Health* 34:22 and 42 (July) 1956.

ROBINSON, VICTOR: *Victory Over Pain: A History of Anesthesia.* Henry Schuman, New York, 1946.

THATCHER, VIRGINIA: *History of Anesthesia.* J. B. Lippincott Company, Philadelphia, 1953.

Guild of St. Barnabas

HAM, MARGUERITE: Person to Person as One Nurse Speaks to Her Fellow Nurses. Guild of St. Barnabas, Quincy, Mass., pamphlet.

''Occasional paper—July, 1890.'' The News-Letter, Quincy, Mass., 1960.

Osborne, Edward: Origin in Boston of the Guild of St. Barnabas. The News-Letter, Quincy, Mass., 1917.

''Report of each chapter.'' The News-Letter, Quincy, Mass., 1960.

SPALDING, EUGENIA K.: *Professional Nursing: Trends, Responsibilities, Relationships.* 6th ed. J. B. Lippincott Company, Philadelphia, 1959.

National Council of Catholic Nurses

''Board of NCCN announces.'' The Catholic Nurse 9:56 (Dec.) 1960.

CONNELL, FRANCES J.: The Catholic Nurse in a Non-Catholic Hospital. The National Council of Catholic Nurses in the United States, Washington, D. C.

' History of the National Council of Catholic Nurses.'' *The Catholic Nurse* 1:35 (Dec.) 1952.

LYNCH, JOHN J.: Human experiments in medicine—moral aspects. *The Catholic Nurse* 9:18 (Dec.) 1960.

SISTER KATHLEEN MARY: Nursing education: Promotion of the Christian concepts of nursing. *The Catholic Nurse* 9:37 (Dec.) 1960.

CHAPTER 30

International Nursing

INTERNATIONAL COUNCIL OF NURSES (ICN)

This organization was founded in 1899. (See p. 119, Chapter 11, for a detailed account of the early history.) The association was established with the thought that unity of nurses from representative nations of the world would result in improved nursing care and conditions for health throughout the world, and in advancement of the profession of nursing itself.

The aims of the International Council of Nurses as stated in its Constitution and By-laws[1] are as follows:

The International Council of Nurses stands for self-government by nurses in their associations for the purpose of raising the standards of professional education and practice, as well as those governing the ethical conduct and public usefulness of nurses.

The International Council of Nurses stands for that full development of the human being and citizen in every nurse, which shall best enable her to bring her professional knowledge and skill to the many-sided service that society demands of her.

---

[1] International Council of Nurses: Constitution and By-laws As Amended, May, 1957.

The Council aims to provide a means of communication between nurses of various nationalities, to create opportunities for them to confer upon questions relating to the prevention, curative, and social aspects of nursing and the advancement of nursing and to afford facilities for the promotion of international understanding and the interchange of international hospitality.

The Council will undertake the management of any foundation or trust whose objectives comprise or are conductive to the education or advancement of nurses or nursing work.

The official organ of the International Council of Nurses is the *International Nursing Review*, published six times a year at council headquarters, 1 Dean Trench Street, Westminster, London S.W. 1, England.

Membership and Meetings. The national nurses associations from member countries and associate representative countries are considered to be the members of the ICN. In 1961 there were fifty-nine member countries and seven countries having associate representatives.[2]

Application for membership in the ICN is considered both by the membership committee and by the Grand Council. Countries that now have full membership in the International Council of Nurses are:

Australia	*Haiti*	*Northern Rhodesia*
Austria	*Iceland*	*Norway*
Barbados	*India*	*Pakistan*
Belgium	*Iran*	*Panama*
Brazil	*Ireland*	*Philippines*
British Guinea	*Israel*	*Poland*
Burma	*Italy*	*Republic of China*
Canada	*Jamaica*	*Singapore*
Ceylon	*Japan*	*South Africa*
Colombia	*Jordan*	*Southern Rhodesia*
Cuba	*Kenya*	*Sweden*
Denmark	*Korea*	*Switzerland*
Egypt	*Lebanon*	*Thailand*
Ethiopia	*Liberia*	*Trinidad and Tobago*
Finland	*Luxembourg*	*Turkey*
France	*Malaya*	*United States of*
Germany	*Mexico*	*America*
Ghana	*Netherlands*	*Uruguay*
Great Britain	*New Zealand*	*Venezuela*
Greece	*Nigeria*	*Yugoslavia*

Countries having associate representatives are:

Argentina	*Peru*	*Spain*
El Salvador	*Portugal*	*Syria*
Indonesia		

[2] Each year *Facts About Nursing* publishes a complete list of member nations and associate member nations.

Most of the work of the organization has been carried on through congresses which meet every four years. No nurse can think of herself as being a much-traveled person unless she has attended this most colorful of all meetings. Our country has been hostess to this great conclave three times and will be again, world conditions permitting.

Florence Nightingale International Foundation. This organization was established in 1934 as a permanent international memorial to Florence Nightingale in the form of an endowed trust for graduate nursing education on an international basis. Although the foundation is a legal part of the International Council of Nurses, it retains its own articles of incorporation and trust funds. The principal objectives of the foundation are "to promote research, to create a center of information on educational facilities, to establish and stimulate the award of scholarships, and to develop a section of the library dedicated to Florence Nightingale . . . assume responsibility for the 'long-term' educational activities of the ICN and in so doing will endeavor to benefit not only these countries which are affiliated with the ICN, but also those which are not yet members." (American Journal of Nursing, 50:9, Jan., 1950.)

The foundation is financed by earnings from the invested endowment, by grants for special research projects, and by monies contributed by national nurses associations.

Applications to the Foundation. Nurses desiring scholarships or fellowships from the foundation should apply to the Chairman, Florence Nightingale International Foundation, 10 Columbus Circle, New York 19, N. Y. Applications are considered and awards made to those "who are best qualified to help bring back a recognition of nursing as a world service."

Since not more than twenty students are admitted each year, only nurses already having an academic degree should consider forwarding their application to the foundation committee. European universities do not use the credit system in higher education; hence, work done at the foundation school could not be used as earned credits toward a degree in the United States. The level of instruction given presupposes both a basic nursing course and at least a baccalaureate degree.

Each country that is a member of the International Council of Nurses is asked to form a national committee. This committee will be represented on the grand council by two delegates and will be responsible in their respective countries for the selection of suitable candidates for the courses, and for the collection and awarding of scholarships.

Summary. The *American Journal of Nursing, Nursing Outlook,* and *International Nursing Review* frequently print articles and new notes concerning the activity of the International Council of Nurses which every nurse, who considers herself a professional woman, should read with interest. This organization is the "United Nations" for nurses.

Many times nurses, struggling for professional recognition by uninformed government officials, have used the prestige of the ICN to obtain sanction and approval for nursing education and legislation.

The International idea itself is so vast, so far-reaching, that, quite uncon-sciously, it impresses those persons who, ever so little, come in contact with it; we who have felt its powerful inspiration are responsible for its realization.

Singly, we are capable of doing infinitely little, but collectively, through the ICN, we should be able to make a great contribution worthy of the idea itself.[3]

CLASS EXERCISE

From current references develop a class discussion on the *International Council of Nurses with Which Is Associated the Florence Nightingale International Foundation* as an important factor in promoting world peace.

WORLD HEALTH ORGANIZATION

The World Health Organization (WHO) is a specialized agency of the United Nations and represents the culmination of efforts to establish a single international government health agency. The World Health Organization inherited the Health Organization of the League of Nations and the Health Division of the United Nations Relief and Rehabilitation Administration (UNRRA). It had its origin at the United Nations Conference in San Francisco in 1945, but was not founded as a permanent organization until September, 1948.

The purpose of WHO is "to achieve the highest possible level of health for all people." This is being done by assisting local authorities to build training programs for health and to improve the social and economic status of the nurses of that country.

Field work in WHO is done by teams, each composed of a doctor, a nurse, and a sanitary engineer. They recruit a large group of the inhabitants and demonstrate and carry out health measures. Their teaching is picked up and carried to near-by villages to be put into practice. In some countries where conditions are overwhelmingly difficult, WHO nurses have given actual basic training in nursing and sanitation to "dressers" for fundamental nursing care.

Four regional offices have been set up on a global basis, with a nurse in each. These offices are in Alexandria, Egypt; New Delhi, India; Bangkok, Siam; and Washington, D. C., where the office functions for both the Americas.

Besides the field work of WHO, the organization studies, on an international basis, major health problems affecting people in all parts of the world. These projects relate to malaria, tuberculosis, venereal diseases, maternal and child health, and sanitation. The World Health Organization is also continuing

---

[3] Margrethe Krause, Our International Fellowship, *American Journal of Nursing*, Vol. 48 (June, 1948), p. 375.

work begun earlier on biological standardization, addiction-producing drugs, health statistics, and international sanitary regulations.

Although the World Health Organization is only one of many councils within the framework of the United Nations, it touches the most common meeting ground of all—the desire of people to live in health and to provide health for their children.

Two publications of WHO are of special interest to nurses: *Chronicle of the World Health Organization* and *World Health*. Both of these are published in English at Palais des Nations, Geneva, Switzerland.

Qualifications. The World Health Organization is constantly in need of nurses for its many health programs around the world. Nurses are needed most in teaching and in public health.[4]

For some assignments special language skills are needed. In some countries the nurse teaches in English to English-speaking students, while in others an interpreter translates into the language of the students. Americans are sadly monolinguistic; perhaps international nursing will motivate nurses to become skillful in the use of at least one language other than that of the United States.

The Field Service Division of WHO has a fellowship program for study and research to enable nurses on these fellowships to study nursing-education methods, public health nursing, social welfare, midwifery, mental hygiene, and child guidance.

Nurses who are interested in this adventurous and fascinating work, as a two-year or more assignment may write to the Personnel Section, World Health Organization, Geneva, Switzerland.

EXCHANGE VISITOR PROGRAM

The American Nurses' Association, as a member of the International Council of Nurses, has been designated as a sponsor of the Exchange Visitor Program of the United States Department of State.

This program has been described in Chapter VI: *Graduate Study.* Nurses who seriously wish to participate in this international program should have their credentials compiled by the state office of the Professional Counseling and Placement Service or by the national office of the same organization. When this biography is assembled the nurse should request that a copy be sent to the International Unit of the American Nurses' Association.

Qualifications. The nurse must be a member of the ANA and have at least two years of experience as a registered nurse. A working knowledge of at least one language beside English is required for assignment to most countries. It is possible to work through an interpreter but it is inconvenient. Many language courses are offered in colleges, junior colleges, YMCA and YWCA, and by tutors. The nurse should plan on at least one year of concentrated language study in order to make her foreign experience valuable.

---

[4] Elizabeth Hill, Nursing in the World Health Organization. *American Journal of Nursing,* Vol. 58 (Apr. 1958), p. 528.

Cost and Expenses. The International Unit of the American Nurses' Association will give the nurse an estimate of the cost for a period of study or observation. The nurse should plan for a considerable amount beyond this estimate. She should go as a *traveler*—not as a *tourist*. Therefore, the nurse will need extra money to be able to investigate and appreciate the cultural, historic, and scenic interests of the country to which she is assigned.

There are opportunities for work experience for which a salary will be paid, but extra money will be needed for trips and a generous margin for emergencies.

CLASS EXERCISE

Prepare a map of the Eastern Hemisphere large enough to permit considerable detail. Fasten this map to poster board. Then from references published during the past two years, indicate the following:

1. Countries that have full membership in the ICN and those that have associate membership.
2. Countries in which nurses are working under assignment of WHO.
3. Countries to which American nurses have gone for work or observation under the Exchange Visitor Program.

REFERENCES

International Council of Nurses

BEST, ELLA: The International Council of Nurses. *Nurs. Outlook* 5:547 (Aug.) 1947.

BRIDGES, DAISY C.: Nursing—an international service. *Amer. J. Nurs.* 56:1273 (Oct.) 1956.

BRIDGES, DAISY C., and BROE, ELLEN J.: Nursing's one world. *Amer. J. Nurs.* 61:76 (Jan.) 1961.

BROE, ELLEN J.: The Florence Nightingale International Foundation. *Amer. J. Nurs.* 53:1345 (Nov.) 1953.

"Gift to ICN." *Amer. J. Nurs.* 58:1707 (Dec.) 1958.

GLAMAGERAN, ALICE: The western group. *Amer. J. Nurs.* 55:53 (Jan.) 1955.

"Grand Council of the ICN." *Amer. J. Nurs.* 47:361 (June) 1947.

"ICN—FNIF" (two international organizations unite). *Amer. J. Nurs.* 50:89 (Jan.) 1950.

"No matter how you say it." *Amer. J. Nurs.* 49:361 (June) 1949.

"Nurses complete study under FNIF." *Amer. J. Nurs.* 48:606 (Sept.) 1948.

Editorial: Nurses and the UN. *Amer. J. Nurs.* 50:515 (Sept.) 1950.

ODIER, LUCIE: The Geneva conventions. *Amer. J. Nurs.* 51:19 (Jan.) 1951.

"The Florence Nightingale International Foundation." *Trained Nurse and Hosp. Rev.* 100:660 (June) 1948.

"The ICN as a home owner." *Amer. J. Nurs.* 57:340 (Mar.) 1957.

"The ICN, the ANA, and the U.N." *Amer. J. Nurs.* 59:83 (Jan.) 1959.

"The professional press and the ICN." *Amer. J. Nurs.* 57:997 (Aug.) 1957.

"The ICN latchstring is out." *Amer. J. Nurs.* 44:594 (June) 1944.

"The ICN and nursing education." *Amer. J. Nurs.* 50:385 (July) 1950.

"The story of ICN House." *Internat. Nurs. Rev.* 3:2 (May) 1956.

TAYLOR, EFFIE J.: The International Council of Nurses. *Amer. J. Nurs.* 50:89 (Jan.) 1950.

TURNER, VIRGINIA A.: The eleventh quadrennial congress of the ICN. *Nurs. World* 131:7 (Aug.) 1957.

"What the International Council of Nurses does." *Amer. J. Nurs.* 49:131 (Mar.) 1949.

"With the ICN in Australia." *Amer. J. Nurs.* 61:60 (July) 1961.

World Health Organization

CHAGAS, AGNES W.: The WHO nursing consultant. *Amer. J. Nurs.* 55:1199 (Oct.) 1955.

CREELMAN, LYLE, and others: WHO and professional nursing. *Amer. J. Nurs.* 54:448 (Apr.) 1954.

DERBY, PATRICIA A.: My international experience. *Amer. J. Nurs.* 58:563 (Apr.) 1958.

HILL, ELIZABETH: Nursing in the World Health Organization. *Amer. J. Nurs.* 58:528 (Apr.) 1958.

KELLY, DOROTHEA N.: On the international scene. *Catholic Nurse* 9:44 (Dec.) 1960.

"Nurses' U.N.: Nursing knows no national boundaries." *Amer. J. Nurs.* 52:1209 (Oct.) 1952.

RIPLEY, IONE L.: The nurses' contribution to world health. *Nurs. World* 130:11 (Oct.) 1956.

Exchange Visitor Program

"ANA international unit activities increase." *Amer. J. Nurs.* 57:1182 (Sept.) 1957.

"ANA international unit reports." *Amer. J. Nurs.* 57:190 (Feb.) 1957.

ANA international unit's exchange service expands." *Amer. J. Nurs.* 59:1608 (Nov.) 1959.

BUSTELLI, MOYA: An exchange student's experience. *Amer. J. Nurs.* 58:1670 (Dec.) 1958.

MARTIN, RUTH M., and HUNT, ELIZABETH: The ANA's point of view. *Amer. J. Nurs.* 58:1666 (Dec.) 1958.

UNIT V

Professional Relationships

CHAPTER 31

Nursing Legislation

Nurses and nursing organizations need to be more alert and concerned with laws affecting themselves and their services. Legislation is every nurse's business. Nurses must accept and recognize their responsibility to study and discuss the social issues of the day and the legal means of controlling these issues. As lawmaking becomes more complex, the lawmakers depend increasingly on organized groups both to recommend and to support or oppose proposed legislation. Nurses constitute one of these groups. As nurses become more concerned and informed in legislative affairs, not only will nursing practice be improved and professional and employment standards be defined, but nurses themselves will become more aware of their greater responsibilities as citizens.

SPECIFIC LEGISLATION

In viewing the past half century of the accomplishments of organized nursing, nursing has become intimately interwoven with legislation. In fact, the chief motive for the organization of the state nurses' associations was the need for group action through which licensure laws, to protect both the public and the nurse, were promoted. The problem of state licensure is still with us and at the moment is a prominent legislative activity. At this time less than half of our states have laws which make illegal the *actual practice* of professional nursing by those not qualified, and other states' laws merely protect the title, "Registered Nurse."

Some recently enacted laws, or amendments to old laws, have direct or indirect effect on nurses' employment standards and practices. These include the Social Security Act, Unemployment Insurance Act, and the National Labor Management Act. Also, recent legislation has affected the structure, functions, and election procedures of the American Nurses' Association and its constituent state associations. The Landrum-Griffin Act of 1959 made necessary the revision of the bylaws of the American Nurses' Association and state and district associations to comply with the structural and functional changes required in the passage of this bill.

LEGISLATIVE ORGANIZATION

American Nurses' Association. The legislative program of the national association is conducted by two separate committees: a federal committee and a committee for assistance with state legislation.

Legislation of federal importance is studied and conducted through the Women's Joint Congressional Committee and the American Nurses' Association Special Committee on Federal Legislation.

The Women's Joint Congressional Committee was organized in 1920 as a clearinghouse for Congressional legislative work of national organizations of women, such as American Federation of Teachers, National Council of Jewish Women, American Nurses' Association, and American Association of University Women.[1] Each member organization is entitled to one delegate on this committee.

The American Nurses' Association Special Committee on Federal Legislation is the national association's own committee on federal legislation which works with the delegate of the Women's Joint Congressional Committee. The chairmen of these two committees make reports and recommendations concerning federal legislation to the board of the national association.

In January, 1945, the President of the United States urged that provision be made for drafting nurses. This proposal aroused every individual nurse as nothing else has done since modern nursing began. It is the nurse's privilege to read the exciting, dramatic action of the federal legislative committees and the Board of Directors of the ANA in the days and weeks that followed. Detailed reports and description of activities were carried in the American Journal of Nursing.[2] This is a concrete example of legislative machinery in a democratic society.

---

[1] For a complete list of these organizations, see *Brief Historical Review and Information about Current Activities of the American Nurses' Association including Certain Facts Relative to the National League of Nursing Education,* (American Nurses' Association, New York, 1940), pp. 38-39.

[2] See "January 6, 1945," *American Journal of Nursing,* Vol. 45 (Feb. 1945) p. 85; "The proposed draft of nurses," *American Journal of Nursing,* Vol. 45 (Feb. 1945), p. 87; "All the way—as volunteers?" *American Journal of Nursing,* Vol. 45 (Apr. 1945), p. 253; "Nurses draft bill passed by the house," *American Journal of Nursing,* Vol. 45 (Apr. 1945), p. 255.

The American Nurses' Association Special Committee on Legislation is a committee whose chief functions are the study and evaluation of nurse practice acts and assisting the individual states in their legislative programs.

All states now have "nurse practice laws," but they are far from uniform, and changes are made from time to time to advance and maintain professional standards. It is then that this committee may act as consultant in fundamental legislative principles by working with the state legislative committee.

State Associations. Each state nurses' association has a legislative committee which works closely with the board of directors. Both the legislative committee and the board watch closely to ascertain if any bills are presented at the state legislature that would affect nurses, nursing, or health. The state committee on legislation may also initiate legislation that would be beneficial to nurses, nursing, or health.

Members of the state committee on legislation should be representative of all fields of nursing and of geographic sections of the state.

The duties of the state committee are to watch proceedings of the state legislature and to initiate necessary legislation for the benefit of the state association.

District Committees. Each district has a legislative committee as a part of its organization. The American Nurses' Association Special Committee on Legislation has recommended to the Board of Directors of the American Nurses' Association that the district legislative committee be composed of a member from each Senate district and each House of Representatives district within the district nurses' association.[3] Such a committee would make it possible to disseminate information quickly and to reach legislators easily when action on impending bills is urgent.

The state committee will try to keep the district committee informed on current legislation by immediate notification when new bills are introduced affecting nurses. It then becomes the duty of the district committee to make personal contact with individuals and groups, and to ask them to express their approval or disapproval of the measure then before the House of Representatives or the Senate.

How Bills Are Prepared. The procedure in the preparation, submission, and enactment of all laws is much the same. One or more nurses feel that something should be done about some phase of professional work in which they are interested. They talk to other nurses about it and agree to present the idea at the next district meeting. There it is discussed and, if it is approved, is referred to the district legislative committee for development. When the district legislative committee is satisfied with its work, it may report back to the district or send its material to the state headquarters for consideration by the state legislative committee and by the board of the state association.

---

[3] See "Organizing a Legislative Program," *American Journal of Nursing,* Vol. 42 (Mar. 1942), p. 275.

Or, the first step may be taken by the state legislative committee itself in response to a state-convention resolution which resulted from agitation by delegates, or the state legislative committee may initiate the legislation as a result of its own deliberations.

The convention-resolution method is the best because it provides the greatest amount of the best type of educational publicity in the shortest time at the least expense. To attain maximum results from this method, the sponsors of the proposed legislation should prepare a skillfully worded resolution to the effect that, because of such-and-such conditions, the body assembled instructs the state legislative committee to prepare a bill for presentation to the law-making bodies, which bill is to contain such-and-such provisions. The preamble to the resolution should describe the conditions which make the proposed legislation necessary.

It is important that all material, records, press clippings, and letters upon which the statements in the resolution are based should be preserved in a "preparatory file" for later reference.

When the resolution is adopted and made a part of the convention record, the foundation for the necessary publicity is complete. The delegates will carry the news when they report to their districts, and the complete resolution will be published in the official report of the convention proceedings.

After the resolution has been adopted, the state legislative committee takes over the work. An attorney is employed, preferably one who has had experience as a legislator and, in any event, one who has had experience in drafting legislation and has an understanding of the place of the nurse in the social pattern. The attorney should be supplied with the following:

1. A copy of the resolution which contains the complete outline of the situation and its requirements

2. The "preparatory file" of resolution material which provides the background of the proposition

3. Copies of any existing laws which have a bearing on the proposed laws; these would assist the attorney in avoiding conflicts and duplications

4. Opportunities to confer with the state legislative committee when necessary

Under these conditions a properly qualified attorney should be able to prepare a bill so explicit and comprehensive that there need be no misinterpretation, no opportunities for opponents to attack it successfully, no question as to its benefits to society, and no loopholes to permit evasion of its provisions.

LEGISLATIVE ACTION

Any person or group may prepare a bill, but it must be introduced by a member of the legislature who will see it through.[4] This sponsor should be in full sympathy with the purposes of the bill, which can be explained fully to

---

[4] The success of Dorothea Lynde Dix, in her struggle for state hospitals for the mentally ill, was largely due to her unerring judgment in selecting the right legislator to introduce the bill for the appropriation of funds.

him during the preparation period. Here again, the preparatory file provides complete information. In committee, or on the "floor," he "knows all the answers"—nothing pleases a legislator more than to have all the answers at his instant command.

Copies of the bill should be sent to the district legislative committee so that the entire state membership may become familiar with its provisions and begin to create public support for the measure.

The bill is sent to the speaker's desk and given a number, title, and the name of the legislator introducing it. It is read by number, title, and name, and referred to the appropriate committees for study and investigation. Then follow anxious days, for many things can happen to a bill "in committee." It may be "killed," or it may "survive." When the bill is out of committee it will be scheduled for action on the floor in the form of debates and recommendations, and made a part of the legislative calendar. It is now ready for the legislators to express their approval or disapproval by means of the vote.

If the bill is passed on the final vote it is signed by the presiding officer of that house and sent to the other house for action which is much like the procedure in the first house.

If the bill has been passed by both houses it is sent to the governor for his signature. The bill may become a law without the governor's signature, or it may be passed over his veto.

It is only after the above action that a bill ceases to be a bill and becomes a law.

Critical Stages. When the state legislative committee sends out word that the bill is "in committee," the members of the district legislative committee should each send a brief letter to that legislative committee containing a statement as to why the bill would be beneficial, and the number of beneficiaries. Even if the bill is in committee for a week or two, no time should be lost in forwarding these letters. Do not use form letters. Personal letters carry the individual touch of the writers and more than repay for the extra effort involved.

The individual message may read: "I would appreciate your support of the nurses' bill"; or "The nurses' bill deserves to be passed, please vote for it"; or "The nurses' bill is a good bill, and you should vote for it." No set form of wording is necessary as long as the recipient will understand that the writer wants the legislator to vote for the bill. Spontaneity will carry more weight than formality.

The messages from the nursing groups may read: "Our association of members is vitally interested in (here insert the identifying name and number of the bill) Bill for the advancement of nursing, and the furtherance of the public welfare. Your vote and active advocacy of the bill will be appreciated." The inclusion of the number of members is essential; each member is a voter.

As in messages from individuals, it is best not to use a set form for all the groups; uniformity of wording creates a rubber-stamp atmosphere. The idea is to let the legislators know that an influential group of voters—influential in both members and prestige—is keeping an eye on the progress of the bill and expects it to be passed.

The same procedure is carried out when federal legislation is being considered. The federal committees notify the state legislative committees who, in turn, notify the district committees. Messages are sent to the state's representatives then convened in Washington. In this manner, every citizen is actually represented.

Lobbyist. A lobbyist is a legislative representative of a group or organization. When bills are introduced into the legislature that affect nurses favorably or adversely, a lobbyist should be retained to pave the way for the enactment or defeat of the bill. The chairman of the committee is the logical appointee as lobbyist. If the chairman cannot give the time, a similarly qualified person should be appointed.

As a lobbyist, she will be required to register at the state capitol, giving the name and business of her employer, and the reason for her current employment.

The lobbyist's first duty is to secure the names and addresses of the chairmen of all committees of the legislature, with special attention given to those committees to which bills affecting nurses, nursing, or health would be referred, such as the committees on public health, education, registration and licensing, etc. At the same time each district legislative committee would be supplied with a list of the names and addresses of the legislators from that district.

The lobbyist will establish contacts with the legislators, especially those who, because of their personalities or party positions, are recognized as "key" members. Through such contacts she may be able to secure the passage or defeat of a bill.

Coincident with her work on the nurses' bill, the lobbyist will keep watch for other bills that may affect nursing unfavorably. This is done by examining prospective bills in the legislative library. If an unfavorable bill is discovered, she will report the fact at once so that an attempt may be made to defeat that bill, or at least have its objectionable features eliminated.

Publicity. There can be no assurance of successful passage of a piece of legislation, regardless of the benefits it may provide, unless it is well publicized. A legislative committee which drafts a bill after the legislature has convened is likely to be disappointed. The groundwork of deliberations, study, expert opinions, and district cooperation should be laid before the legislative assembly.

Cooperation of all district and alumnae associations is most important, since these organizations are composed of individual members who will interpret the bill directly to the voting public. The legislative committee may realize the necessity of such a law and see the advantages of it for both the general public and the nurse, but in their eagerness, the committee may be likely to underestimate the necessity of educating the voters.

This education may be done best by first presenting it in detail to the alumnae and district associations, the National League for Nursing, the medical association, and the hospital association. These organizations are powerful factors in the dissemination of information to the laity, who regard the opinion of the organizations as authoritative. Emily Hicks, in describing how New York's nurse-practice act was won, says:[5]

Another word of caution is the result of another hard-won lesson. A state-wide educational program must reach the public as well as the State Association membership before the introduction of any bill into the legislature. Support for any measure whose story has not been presented in an adequate and convincing manner cannot be relied upon. No group can expect the public to get behind it unless it has first gotten before the public.

The lawmaking procedure as described may seem very complicated. It really is no more so than that followed in one of the many cases that daily pass through an operating room. It is merely a matter of teamwork, with each member of the staff knowing what to do, and when, and how.

POLITICAL INFLUENCE AND PERSONAL RESPONSIBILITIES OF THE NURSE

Some statements need to be made to emphasize the nurse's role in the promotion of legislation, especially legislation affecting nursing services and employment standards. It is generally agreed that one important measure of a profession is the degree to which it is socially oriented. More and more our way of life is tempered by federal, state and local laws. Nursing, one of the largest occupational and professional groups, is becoming affected more each year by specific and implied legislative action.

Let's ask, "How does the individual nurse fulfill her responsibility in promoting better legislation?" First, she might attend district, state, and national meetings and help set up the broad legislative programs and recommendations of the professional organization. The next step is to keep informed on what is happening in the state and federal legislatures. One way is by serving as a member of the legislative committees of her professional organizations. Another way is by reading professional literature which summarizes legislative activities affecting nurses and nursing. The third step in fulfilling her responsibility is to interpret the needs and interests of the nursing profession to the legislators and the public. It must be remembered that the legislators usually make their decisions on the basis of what their constituents inform them or advise them to do. In this way, every nurse as a citizen is entitled to promote the interests and welfare of nursing. The public, the legislator and the nursing profession expect the nurse to encourage and recommend legislation that promises better nursing and better health care of the nation.

A skilled lobbyist with a reputation for sincerity can render a valuable service, but only when it is known that she represents a politically powerful group can she do her best work. Nurses themselves constitute such a group. In each district their votes may be the deciding factor in a close election. Add to these votes the votes of those persons whom nurses can influence, and the

---

[5] Emily A. Hicks, A Crusade for Safer Nursing (How New York's New Nurse Practice Act Was Won), *American Journal of Nursing*, Vol. 38 (May 1938), p. 563.

potential political power of nurses becomes unquestionable. With confidence born of this knowledge every nurse should respond wholeheartedly to every request of her district or state legislative committee when a bill affecting nurses or nursing is before the legislature.

There need be nothing apologetic about requests for support from politicians and the public. Practically any bill sponsored by nurses is beneficial to the public welfare. Even the nurse-registration law, which seemingly benefits nurses only, protects the public from impractical, incompetent nurses at the same time that it protects the professional standing of the nurse.

When a bill is first presented, all nurses should begin at once to publicize its purpose. The district legislative committee supplies the need for this work. The private duty nurse, through her close contacts with the patient and his relatives, may tell them why the proposed legislation is good. The public health nurse may educate her patients likewise, and may do much to interest the lay members of her board who usually are persons of prestige in the community and whose influence may be relied upon to influence many others. Institutional nurses, in fact all nurses who meet lay people, should use every opportunity to publicize the bill.

If the nurse has any friends who are members of the legislature, she should get in touch with them at once; a friend at court is a valuable ally. Perhaps a nurse may have cared for a wife, husband, or parents of a legislator. Here is an excellent channel of influence. Send the former patient a copy of the bill with a request for support, or make a personal call and explain the purpose of the bill.

The cooperation of the medical profession and the state hospital association is important. Nursing legislation usually affects physicians and hospital administrators. Their interest and support can do much toward the successful passage of a bill.

In every community there are men and women who seldom hold political offices, yet who possess great power in anything pertaining to legislation. In many instances few persons in their respective communities know anything about these quiet workers. The job of identifying these leaders and establishing friendly contact with them should be part of the duties of the legislative committees. Access to such persons is best gained by cultivating the county chairman and other leaders of your political parties. The support of the leaders and the "men behind" is not difficult to develop after they are convinced that the nurses have no purely personal axes to grind. Once the contacts are established, it is best merely to let it be known what the nurses want and how many of them want it. The leaders will take the obvious necessary action.

With this complete organization picture in mind, each nurse will see the importance of the individual nurse during the progress of a bill.

CLASS EXERCISE

Outline the procedure necessary for the legislation of the following bill if it were proposed by the state nurses' association of your state:

THE BILL

Only professional, registered nurses with graduate work in psychiatric nursing shall be employed as supervisors in the state hospitals for the mentally ill in the state of ....

REFERENCES

American Journal of Nursing:

''Do public health nurses take more interest in political activities than institutional nurses?'' 49:133 (Mar.) 1949.

''Federal legislation'' (editorial). 50:685 (Nov.) 1950.

''How a bill becomes a law.'' 45:11 (Jan.) 1945; 45:85 (Feb.) 1945; (Illus.) 51:696 (Dec.) 1951.

''Look to your laws.'' (editorial). 61:51 (Feb.) 1961.

''Nurse practice acts.'' 49:197 (Apr.) 1949.

''Nurses as legislators in Sweden, Finland, and Japan.'' 51:104 (Feb.) 1951.

''Nursing legislation in the states.'' 51:692 (Dec.) 1951.

''Organizing a legislative program.'' 42:275 (Mar.) 1942.

''Ten tips on writing your congressmen.'' 56:459 (Apr.) 1956.

''White caps on Capitol Hill.'' 55:1204 (Oct.) 1955.

BALLARD, BERTON J.: The nurse's staunchest friend could be the public. *Amer. J. Nurs.* 56:586 (Sept.) 1956.

BECKER, RALPH E.: Lobbying and the nursing profession. *R.N.* 12:36 (Apr.) 1949.

DOCK, LAVINIA L.: What we may expect from the law. *Amer. J. Nurs.* 50:599 (Oct.) 1950.

GERDS, G., CONNORS, H. V., and THOMPSON, J. C.: Every nurse a lobbyist. *Amer. J. Nurs.* 60:1242 (Sept.) 1960.

Illinois Nurses Association: How new law (Landrum-Griffin Act) applies to INA members. Chart (Chicago) 67:22 (Apr.) 1960.

Illinois Nurses Association: Why we comply with Taft-Hartley Act (National Labor-Management Relations Act, 1947). Chart (Chicago) 56:10 (Oct.) 1960.

JAVITS, JACOB K.: Dear Congressman. *Amer. J. Nurs.* 53:554 (May) 1953.

JUDD, WALTER H.: Concerning letters to congressmen. Congressional Record, March 25, 1948. Reprinted in *Amer. J. Nurs.* 49:173 (Mar.) 1949.

WEISS, ETHEL V.: State labor legislation. *Amer. J. Nurs.* 50:719 (Nov.) 1950.

CHAPTER 32

Legal Problems

To hold a nurse legally responsible for her errors is a fairly new development in the law and should be the concern of every practicing nurse. This tendency on the part of the public to bring suit against the nurse, and also the hospital, has grown out of three concepts: (1) nurses are professional people and must accept professional responsibility for their acts; (2) there is an increase in social consciousness that makes individuals aware of responsibilities to other people; (3) damage suits against nurses and hospitals may be used as an easy method to obtain money and publicity out of all proportion to the damage involved. These concepts are bringing nurses, in greater numbers than ever before, into courts for legal liability. The charges range from failure to use bed rails for a confused patient to giving wrong medications.

Charitable hospitals no longer have the immunity they once held when courts felt that to pay damage claims would deplete the hospital funds used for charitable purposes. But the tendency to obtain easy money has prompted many damage suits and, besides, some hospitals have not taken the precautions necessary to diminish liability risks, such as providing fireproof stairways, fire escapes and exits, adequate bed rails, window locks, and first-aid equipment. Some hospitals have not even used "due care" in the selection of personnel.

For very practical reasons this chapter will be confined to a few representative nursing situations in which there are legal aspects to be discussed. Such a clarification is, of necessity, very general because state laws or interpretations of the common law are diverse. Even the digest of state laws relating to the practice of nursing as published by the American Nurses' Association makes no attempt to define the acts which are constructed by the statutes of the several states as evidence of the practice of nursing. For example, in some states nurses are placed in two classifications: those who are registered on the basis of their professional preparation, and those who are classified as "practical nurses." In other states there are various classifications mentioned by name in the law, such as registered nurses, trained attendants, trained nurses, practical nurses, without any attempt to define the duties or limitations imposed under any of these classifications.

ETHICS AND THE LAW

Doctors may give, and have given, nurses orders of every conceivable kind with an unhesitating expectation that the nurse will carry out these instructions to the letter. This has been an expectation rooted in the professional tradition that the doctor's orders are to be followed without question. But the nurse now has the background of a professional education; there no longer is a master-servant relationship between the doctor and the nurse. The nurse has every right to question an unusual order by the doctor. The court holds that the nurse is first a *citizen,* and second a *nurse.*

NEGLIGENCE

Negligence is the failure to do what a person of ordinary prudence would do. Here again, the education and experience of the nurse give her added responsibilities because she knows the accepted standards of care and treatment. True, the nurse does not prescribe treatment but she is responsible for carrying out the doctor's orders. If intravenous fluids have been started by the physician and the fluid infiltrates into the surrounding tissues and if the nurse does nothing about it the court may decide that she was negligent. (A person of ordinary prudence would have noticed the swelling.) Other examples of negligence may be failure to restrain a patient or to put on side rails, leaving an electric heating pad with a drowsy patient, leaving medicine at the bedside of a patient instead of administering the medicine, leaving a rectal thermometer in the anus of an unconscious patient. In the eyes of the court, all of these acts would not be done by persons of ordinary prudence.

The following are some of the cases where liability has been successfully asserted against the nurse:

Baby crawled to radiator and was burned. Nurse left baby alone.

Patient's hand mangled by bed-raising mechanism. Nurse failed to warn patient.

Missing surgical sponge or needle.

Paralysis caused by feet being strapped too tightly to operating table.

Burns caused by heating pads or lamps.

Patient scalded by tea left too near patient by nurse.

Patient falling from bed when nurse failed to answer light.

Wrong medication, solution, or blood.

Jumping (attempting to commit suicide), as a result of inadequate supervision.

Pneumonia caused by exposure to drafts.

Infection caused by nonsterile needle.

Baby smothering after surgery.

Breaking needle during injection.

Use of defective equipment.

FIRST AID

In most states, certain acts, when performed under emergency conditions, are exempt from operations of law governing the practice of medicine. A nurse may do anything in case of an emergency, even though in circumstances other than an emergency her act would clearly constitute the practice of medicine. No matter what the combination of circumstances may suddenly present, the nurse, because she is a nurse, should keep cool enough to remember two essentials: (1) to do only such things as are essential for the safety of the patient; and (2) the circumstances surrounding the situation. For example, a child is badly injured by an attack from a vicious dog. The child's home is in the city, only a few minutes from a physician and a hospital, yet a nurse living next door cares for the accident and dresses the wound. Compare these circumstances with the same kind of accident occurring on an isolated ranch in the southwest, 40 miles from the nearest physician, who, when he is reached by messenger, is away on a difficult confinement case and cannot come before the next day. In the latter case, the nurse cares for the accident as a first-aid measure, while the first nurse was clearly practicing medicine. To know when an emergency is an emergency calls for the fine judgment and discrimination known as common sense.

NARCOTICS AND BARBITURATES

The Harrison Antinarcotic Act is a federal law operative in all the states, and it is continuously and rigorously enforced through the various agencies previously mentioned. Under this law a nurse may have legal possession of narcotics only under the following conditions:

When she is registered under this law, as a druggist.

When she has obtained them as a patient, on the prescription of a physician holding a narcotic license.

When they are prescribed by a physician, holding a narcotic license, to be administered by her to a patient only during such time as that physician is connected with that patient's case.

When they are supplied to her by an institution, or an industrial concern, which has a narcotic license, for legal use in the course of her duties as an employee of such a concern, or institution.

Narcotics otherwise obtained, if found in her possession, will be confiscated and her possession of them will be accepted as factual evidence of her violation of the Harrison Law.[1]

Barbituric acid is the active principle from which many useful sedatives, such as Tuinal, Seconal, Butisol, have been prepared. The barbiturates exert a sedative action to induce sleep by depressing the motor cortex. The sale of these compounds as ''sleeping tablets'' has become enormous, and toxicologists and some psychiatrists feel that these medications should be included in the federal narcotic law. Most states have passed laws prohibiting the sale of barbiturates except by prescription.

POISONS

Poisons are second only to narcotics in the legal restrictions relating to their sale and use. They must be dispensed by, or under the supervision of, a registered pharmacist who is required to record every such sale. Such record consists of the name of the preparation, quantity delivered to the purchaser, alleged use of the preparation, date of delivery, name and address of the purchaser, and the signature of the dispenser. Nurses are not exempt from the rule requiring this record when they purchase poisons.

VENIPUNCTURES

''Shall nurses be permitted to do venipunctures?'' is only a new title to an old controversy: When is a medical procedure not a nursing procedure? As medical practice has become more complex, nurses have taken on more of the technical procedures. In 1900 only a qualified physician could give hypodermics! Many nurses now practicing can recall when blood pressures could be taken only by the physician; now the practical nurse is taught blood-pressure reading.

Nurses are as dexterous and capable of doing venipunctures as are physicians and technicians, but this procedure has not been made a part of the curriculum for formal teaching and supervision. With intravenous therapy a major part of medical practice, this is one more procedure which the busy physician is glad to yield to the skillful nurse.

The civil defense program assumes that all nurses are prepared, and in case of a national emergency will be expected, to do venipunctures. Doing venipunctures, however, is considered a part of the practice of medicine, and the nurse who does this procedure is disobeying the law and has no legal protection.

The laws of the state medical boards are being studied and revised in order that the courts and the nurse may know what procedures may legally be performed by the nurse. Until this subject is no longer controversial, it is wise to inquire of the hospital authorities before giving medicine by this route.

[1] See Carl Scheffel and Eleanor MacGarvah, *Jurisprudence for Nurses* (New York, Lakeside Publishing Co., 1938), p. 139.

ANESTHETICS

A registered nurse may administer an anesthetic to a patient *in the presence of* and in accordance with the directions of the surgeon in charge. Under these conditions the court holds that the administration of anesthesia by a registered nurse is a duty incident to the practice of medicine. Such circumstances as these occur most frequently in office practice where only a short anesthesia is necessary.

For the administration of anesthesia in hospitals, most states require that anesthetics be given only by anesthesiologists or nurse anesthetists who have completed a course in anesthesia and who have successfully passed the National Qualifying Examination.   .

GIVING MEDICAL AID TO CRIMINALS

While sympathy and service in the relief of human suffering are the basic ideals of nursing, the nurse should not allow sympathy to make her a lawbreaker by giving aid to criminals. In the once-popular gangster movies, the romantic figure in white who so tenderly ministered to the handsome wounded gangster was rewarded by a ''God bless you, lady,'' from the presumably heart-thrilling bad man. Those pictures were incomplete. None of the films showed that the nurse, who concealed from the police the fact that she had aided or harbored a suspected or convicted fugitive from the law, was a lawbreaker herself and that she usually paid a penalty through imprisonment, followed by professional and social ostracism.

One may not be too emphatic in advising the nurse to notify the nearest police station or the sheriff's office as soon as possible after having given aid to persons who might be construed as being fugitives from the law. Even though the nurse acted under threat of injury or death if aid was refused, she is not relieved of the legal responsibility of promptly reporting the facts to the proper authorities.

RESTRAINTS

The nurse as a professional person has the right to decide if a patient needs some form of restraint; it is not necessary to have a doctor's order to take this precaution. The use of side rails on the beds of postoperative patients, elderly patients at night, or patients with both eyes patched is a common procedure in hospitals. In fact, the only requisite is that the nurse be aware that restraint, such as bed rails or ankle and wrist restraint, should be applied; not to do so constitutes negligence.

Chemical restraint, in the form of tranquilizers, has greatly reduced the need for mechanical restraints, such as restraining sheets and wrist and ankle cuffs. These new tranquilizing drugs have greatly changed the nursing care of patients in mental hospitals.

From her classes, experience, and observation, the nurse should be able to detect signs of abnormal behavior in her patient and should take immediate measures to avoid an accident. Absence of the nurse from the room for even five minutes may mean the death of the patient, and for this the nurse can be held liable on grounds of negligence.

If complete restraint is ordered by the physician, the patient should be watched carefully to see that pressure sores do not develop or that the circulation does not become impaired. The restraint may have seemed loose enough at the time it was applied, but if the patient struggles he may cause the restraint to tighten and thus obstruct circulation. No complete restraint should be applied for more than one hour without releasing one arm or one leg for a short time while the nurse is close by.

When restraining a patient, the windows should be locked. Any patient who is disturbed enough to need to be restrained should also have the windows locked. Any nurse with considerable experience knows of some tragedy in which this precaution was not taken.

AID IN MAKING WILLS

The ever-present imminence of death renders aiding in the making of a will, and witnessing of wills, a not-unusual part of a nurse's experience. Her ability to be helpful under such circumstances depends upon her knowledge of such procedures, especially upon her conception of what constitutes a valid will, which is the legal declaration of a person's intentions which he WILLS to be performed after his death.

Primarily, the validity or nonvalidity of a will is established in the light of these questions: Does it truly represent the last wishes of the testator as to the disposition of his property after death? Does it indicate such disposition of his property as he would make when capable of sound judgment and free from undue influence? Are the bequests in accordance with the laws of inheritance and the laws governing the disposition of property by will?

The nurse should keep in mind these three requisites for the making of a will: It must be dated, signed at the end, and witnessed.

The nurse should not assume the responsibility of helping a patient make a will except under conditions in which an attorney cannot be secured. When such a procedure becomes necessary, the nurse should assure herself that the patient has testamentary capacity, but a nurse, whose knowledge of law is meager, may wonder what constitutes testamentary capacity. In Niemes v. Niemes, *et al.*, 97 O. S. (Ohio) 145, a leading case in Ohio on this subject which probably represents broadly the view in other states, the court said:

Testamentary capacity exists when the testator has sufficient mind and memory:

First, to understand the nature of the business in which he is engaged;

Second, to comprehend generally the nature and extent of his property;

Third, to hold in his mind the names and identity of those who have natural claims upon his bounty;

Fourth, to be able to appreciate his relation to the members of his family.

The attestation clause is one of the most important parts of the will when it is probated. If there is any doubt in the nurse's mind that the testator does not have testamentary capacity, she should not sign the attestation clause which states that the testator has such capacity.

If the patient is too ill, too weak, or too handicapped by a severe wound of the arm or by an amputation to sign his name, then his name may be written by the nurse and the testator makes his mark thus:

His (x) mark signature of Charles Brown.

Student Nurses and Wills. If it is necessary for the patient to make a will, the student should not act as a witness to the will. The reasons for this advice are:

1. The student may not be of legal age.
2. When the will is probated it may be difficult to arrange class schedules for the student to appear in court or to return from an affiliation in another school of nursing.
3. The patient may recover and the student may have graduated and be living in a distant state or country and her address may not be known. If the later probation of the will involves litigation it causes difficulties for all concerned.

THE NURSE AS A WITNESS IN LEGAL PROCEEDINGS

The prospect of a day in a law court as a witness means either a day of horror, or just another day, depending upon the nurse's attitude toward the law and the extent of the rights and obligations of a witness.

When called as a witness, she should remind herself that the standard legal procedure is being followed, that she had little or no part in the development of that procedure, that there is nothing she can do to change it at the moment, that the sensible thing is to obey the court summons if she is physically and ethically able to do so, and that she has only to tell what she believes to be the truth, which should not be so terrifying a prospect for anyone who has a clear conscience and who knows that our courts have an excellent system of laws and rules designed to protect the honest and competent witness from embarrassment.

If the nurse feels that she is being treated unjustly in being called as a witness, she has, under certain conditions, a legal right to refuse to obey the summons. Her refusal is justified only when the summons, technically known as a subpoena, has not been served legally. If the service has been legal, her refusal may result in her arrest for contempt of court.

If the service has been legal, the nurse must obey the summons unless she is actually prevented from doing so by sickness, in which case she must protect herself by having a licensed physician certify in writing that she is unable to respond to the summons because of sickness, and by notifying the judge of such inability to attend.

The witness can avoid most of such troubles if she will keep the following points in mind:

1. Go slowly; be deliberate. Police find that in the "third degree" they can seldom tangle a man until he gets to talking faster than he thinks.

2. Understand the question before you attempt to answer. The witness has

the privilege of asking to have the question repeated, or of asking that the court stenographer read it.

3. Answer only what you are asked and stop unless the answer needs explanation.

4. Watch for two questions in one.

Kinds of Testimony. Testimony as presented in court is of two kinds—fact and expert. Nurses are seldom called for expert testimony but may be called for fact testimony, which is just what the word implies: that which she knows to be a fact, such as things she actually saw, or heard, or perhaps felt, or did. As an example: The nurse might state that she saw the patient admitted to the emergency room with a badly bleeding leg; that she saw the bone protruding from the wound. This is classed as fact testimony. But suppose at this point the attorney should ask the nurse if she thought the patient would be able to walk all right? This is expert testimony, and the nurse should refuse to answer, appealing to the judge if necessary. Also, testimony is of economic value: for fact testimony, she may collect the regular fee allowed by law, but in giving expert testimony she may set her own price.

PRIVILEGED COMMUNICATIONS

In some states nurses are included with clergymen, doctors, and lawyers, as persons who cannot be compelled to disclose certain kinds of information when such information has come to them as privileged communications. For instance, in Arkansas a statute covering this point reads:

No person authorized to practice physic or surgery, and no trained nurse, shall be compelled to disclose any information which he may have acquired from his patient while attending him in a professional character, and which information was necessary to enable him to prescribe as a physician, or to act for him as a surgeon or trained nurse.

Nurses are similarly privileged in New York but not in Ohio. In practically all cases such privileges are qualified by expecting certain types of information, such as that obtained from criminals, applicants for insurance, claimants under workmen's compensation laws, or persons having communicable diseases.

The nurse should ascertain if the statutes of her state specifically grant the nurse rights under the doctrine of privileged communications. In the absence of such statutory rights the nurse will find that the common law prevails, whereby no information obtained from the patient is regarded as privileged communications.

CLINICAL RECORDS

Few nurses realize the importance of details and accuracy in keeping clinical records. There is no better way to emphasize this than to attend a case in court, in which the patient's record is presented as evidence. There is often a complete lack of things that would make a record legally useful: erasures have been made, and the opposing attorney claims that these are an attempt to falsify the record; the same physician's name appears on each page, although he was out of the city for two weeks and a colleague looked after his practice. A man who sustained a brain injury claims he suddenly developed diabetes as a result of the accident. The man's record is requisitioned, but it makes no mention of liquid intake. Every record should be kept in such manner that it would furnish facts for testimony months or even years afterward.

The most important rule to follow in keeping a reliable record is to record services, observations, and events as soon as possible. Daily, in hospitals all over the land, nurses depend upon memory to carry important details through the breathless routine of several hours. Perhaps in the morning care of four or five patients several points of legal importance were involved: a newly admitted patient had a small burn on the right foot; another declared that life was not worth the pain of getting well, and why bother; in a vague way the nurse had noted that the woman in Room 22 had pin-point pupils after a friend had visited her, but in the haste to care for the next patient the observation was forgotten; and near noon when the nurse is ready to do her charting, she records only, "Sponge both," for each.

Nurse's Signature. A legal signature is the manner in which the person identifies himself in writing. This is commonly done by using the first and last name. A shorter form may be used, but not initials, since more than one nurse may have the same initials. In signing bedside notes on the patient's medical record, the nurse must be clearly identifiable by her signature and she must sign in the same manner on each and every occasion in which her signature is required.

CONTRACTS AND EMPLOYMENT[2]

In addition to the technical and ethical phases of a nurse's work, there are other matters involving the law: compensation for her services, the identity of those persons responsible for the compensation, the conditions under which she is to perform her duties, the possibilities of injury or illness resulting from her employment, and the concurrent item of the obligations assumed by her when she accepts employment, all subject to contract whether the contract is written or oral or merely implied by the actions or statements of the parties to the contract. In these matters it is well for the nurse to realize that, because of her professional status, she is affected by legal tenets which do not apply to nonmembers of her profession.

If the nurse has reason to believe that the patient is psychopathic, a minor, a married woman not living with her husband, or a woman who is undergoing a legal separation or divorce, the nurse should be careful to learn the facts so that she may know whom to hold responsible for her compensation, and, where necessary, she should make definite arrangements for payment with responsible persons.

[2] Condensed from pages 46-60 of *Jurisprudence for Nurses* by Carl Scheffel and Eleanor MacGarvah (New York, Lakeside Publishing Co., 1938).

Once a nurse has begun her duties on a case she cannot leave the patient without notifying the patient, a responsible person, or the hospital executives that she intends to leave the case. After such a notice is given she must remain on the case sufficiently long to give those acting on the patient's behalf a reasonable time to secure another nurse. This applies equally to those nurses doing part-time or hourly nursing.

WORKMEN'S COMPENSATION

Most states have compensation acts which amount virtually to a health and accident insurance. This state compensation is meant to take care of the so-called hazardous occupations, such as coal mining, steel erection, building. The cost of insurance in companies usually writing health and accident policies is very high for these occupations. Consequently, the individual states have set up laws to compensate or care for these workmen or their dependents.

Nurses ask if they are entitled to workmen's compensation. This form of insurance is set up for the occupations and not for the professions. Therefore the nurse must prove that her employer's business was an occupation and that she was injured in the course of her employment. Most hospitals carry workmen's compensation insurance for their employees and, in most states, are permitted to include the nurses employed in that institution. This does not include the private duty nurse who is in the hospital. Private duty nurses are independent contractors and as such are not eligible for compensation.

CRIMINAL RESPONSIBILITY

As individuals, nurses are noticeably law abiding. As a class, because of the nature of their duties, they are constantly in danger of committing involuntary crimes—crimes in which there may not be even a suspicion of criminal intent, yet the result is such that an offense is committed against an individual or society or both. Practically all such crimes result either from ignorance of the law or from the commission of some grossly negligent act.

For instance, if a nurse leaves a case without giving sufficient notice of her intention to leave that another nurse can be secured to take her place and if the patient suffers injury because of the resulting lack of nursing service, the offending nurse can be held liable not only for breach of contract or negligence or both, but also for criminal negligence.

Another example: A registered nurse became an involuntary criminal under the Medical Practice Act of Ohio, and under the Harrison Antinarcotic Law. She had been giving hypodermic injections of morphine to a patient, the morphine having been obtained on a prescription written by the patient's doctor. The doctor left the case. The nurse had an unused portion of the morphine and continued to administer the hypodermic injections as prescribed for the patient. When the doctor left the case, the nurse ceased to be under his direction, and under the Harrison Antinarcotic Act, she ceased to be his agent. She would have had no further right to administer narcotics even though the narcotics had been lawfully owned by the patient.

There are many other phases of a nurse's obligations. Few nurses know all of these obligations, and fewer still are aware of the criminal responsibility incurred by failure to observe them. For instance, among the many little-known duties imposed on nurses by some civic ordinances and state laws is that of reporting births, deaths, and communicable diseases. Still another instance involving nurses in litigation is the restraint of patients; the nurse doing private duty will do well to be informed on this particular statute of her state.

As stated in the opening paragraphs of this chapter, the nature and scope of the subject matter renders it impossible to cover more than a few of the situations peculiar to a nurse's duties, a limitation which applies particularly to the criminal responsibility of the nurse. The author has purposely included only those situations which are most likely to be encountered by the nurse in her everyday experience. Each year when court convenes, the nurse should watch the court calendar for suits involving nurses and doctors and should make a special effort to attend the court sessions as part of her general education in nursing.

MALPRACTICE INSURANCE

Malpractice is the term used to distinguish negligence when it applies to professional persons. While the nurse always has been held liable for negligence, her professional status is one of higher responsibility, and courts are more and more charging her with the results of her errors. In case of the nonprofit hospitals, courts have even gone so far as to hold the nurse solely liable for injuries to patients even though they occurred on the premises of the hospital.

To provide against such contingencies, the American Nurses' Association, with its usual concern for the individual nurse, has provided a master liability policy with a reliable insurance company for members of the association to protect themselves against alleged malpractice. Members of the association may obtain insurance coverage up to $5,000 at the annual rate of $10.[3] Nurses may be insured for larger amounts at higher annual premiums. The company concerned will also provide legal counsel without limitation until the case is terminated. Such an insurance policy will do much to give peace of mind to nurses whose duties bring them into actual contact with patients.

CLASS EXERCISE

Confer with the attorney for the hospital to obtain specific information concerning legal points in your state.

1. Does your hospital carry workmen's compensation for student nurses as well as for other employees?

---

[3] This rate is higher in Texas, where the minimum rate for annual premiums is set by law at $20.

2. Does your state grant privileged communications to nurses?
3. What is your state law concerning the custody and adoption of children?
4. In your state, what diseases are listed as "reportable" to the health authorities?
5. In your state, what restrictions are placed on the giving of anesthetics by professional nurses?
6. What penalty does your state provide for imposters who practice nursing without a license?
7. Is it legal to employ nurses from other countries?
8. Is it legal for the practical nurse and the nurse's aide to do procedures considered to be in the realm of professional nursing?
9. Is it legal for the student nurse to work for hire as a nurse?
10. What is the legal status of the graduate nurse who is an Exchange Visitor?

REFERENCES

BARBEE, GRACE C.: Legal problems of office nurse. *Amer. J. Nurs.* 51:168 (Mar.) 1951.

BARBEE, GRACE C.: When is the nurse held liable. *Amer. J. Nurs.* 54:1343 (Nov.) 1954.

BARBEE, GRACE C.: The nurse, the nursing home, and the law. *Amer. J. Nurs.* (Aug.) 1961.

BARTSCH, JOSEPHINE: Handling orders that violate ethics. *RN* 24:46 (Apr.) 1961.

BRENNER, ROBERT L.: Operate on the wrong patient? *RN* 23:33 and 23:78 (June) 1960.

BRYANT, EUGENE: Legal aspects of industrial nursing as applied to the Workmen's Compensation Law. *Nurs. World* 129:24 (Sept.) 1955.

CANTLIN, VERNITA L., and CANTLIN, EDWARD F.: Legal facts for proper practice. *Nurs. World* 133:17 (Sept.) 1959.

COOPER, SIGNE S.: Drug administration and the law. *RN* 24:59 (Jan.) 1961.

CREIGHTON, HELEN: *Law Every Nurse Should Know.* W. B. Saunders Company, Philadelphia, 1957.

CREIGHTON, HELEN: Your liability in off-duty first aid. *RN* 22:36 (May) 1959.

"Damage suit highlights hospital liability problems." *Modern Hosp.* 79:65 (Sept.) 1952.

DRIPPS, ROBERT D., LINDEN, MAURICE E., MORRIS, HAROLD, PHILLIPS, WILLIAM A.: Medical, social, and legal aspects of suicide. *J.A.M.A.* 171:523 (Oct. 3) 1959.

FREDERICKS, AMY: You can help them "lay down the law." *RN* 25:42 (Jan.) 1962.

GERHARDT, PAUL: You don't have to be wrong to be sued. *Amer. J. Nurs.* 61:68 (Jan.) 1961.

GRIFFIN, WINIFRED H.: Court! Court! Court is in session and there is a nurse on the jury. *Amer. J. Nurs.* 58:1547 (Nov.) 1958.

HALL, GEORGE E.: The office nurse and the law. *RN* 23:36 (Mar.) 1960.

HAYT, EMANUEL, HAYT, LILLIAN R., GROESCHEL, AUGUST H., and McMULLAN, DOROTHY: *Law of Hospital and Nurse.* Hospital Textbook Company, 1958.

HERSHEY, NATHAN: The law and the nurse. *Amer. J. Nurs.* 62:75 (Feb.) 1962.

HERSHEY, NATHAN: The law and the nurse: Negligence. *Amer. J. Nurs.* 62:98 (Mar.) 1962.

HERSHEY, NATHAN: The law and the nurse: The doctrine of respondeat superior. *Amer. J. Nurs.* 62:78 (Apr.) 1962.

LAYCOCK, MIRIAM F. (DOROTHY WILSON, ed.): Changing status of nurses in civil liability actions in California, 1925-1949. *Nurs. Res.* 3:44 (June) 1954.

LESNIK, MILTON J.: Nursing functions with legal control. *Amer. J. Nurs* 53:1210 (Oct.) 1953.

LETOURNEAU, CHARLES U.: When the medical record is summoned to court. *Hosp. Manage.* 80:42 (Aug.) 1955.

LUDLAM, JAMES E.: Bedrails—up or down. *Amer. J. Nurs.* 57:1439 (Nov.) 1957.

O'CONNER, R. B.: Malpractice and standing orders. *RN Nurses* 14:26 (May) 1951.

PARKER, ALLEN J.: Let your will be done. *RN* 22:70 (Mar.) 1959.

PARKER, CHERRY: Lady, drop that wrench! *Nurs. Outlook* 9:548 (Sept.) 1961.

PASTORE, EVELYN: The nurse and malpractice. *Nurs. World* 126:45 (Oct.) 1952.

PHILLIPS, CLARE: Guide for buying malpractice insurance. *RN* 22:33 (Apr.) 1959.

REGAN, WILLIAM A.: Private duty relief. *RN* 23:53 (June) 1960.

REGAN, WILLIAM A.: Patients, press, police—and you. *RN* 23:57 (Oct.) 1960.

REGAN, WILLIAM A.: Legal pointers: Signatures. *RN* 23:37 (Dec.) 1960.

REGAN, WILLIAM A.: Is a nurse who has an occupational illness such as dermatitis or tuberculosis or radiation illness eligible to receive benefits under the Workmen's Compensation Act? *RN* 24:39 (May) 1961.

REGAN, WILLIAM A.: When is the private duty nurse legally liable? *R.N.* 24:62 (July) 1961.

REGAN, WILLIAM A.: You and the doctor shortage. *RN* 25:53 (Mar.) 1962.

SCOTT, WILLIAM C., and SMITH, DONALD W.: Employee—or independent contractor. *Amer. J. Nurs.* 49:143 (Mar.) 1949.

SCOTT, WILLIAM C., and SMITH, DONALD W.: Workmen's compensation and the nurse. *Amer. J. Nurs.* 50:136 (Mar.) 1950.

SCOTT, WILLIAM C., and SMITH, DONALD W.: Disclosure of professional information. *Amer. J. Nurs.* 55:1217 (Oct.) 1955.

SCOTT, WILLIAM C., and SMITH, DONALD W.: Legal aspects of nursing practice: Immunity of charitable hospitals. *Amer. J. Nurs.* 55:1279 (Dec.) 1955.

SCOTT, WILLIAM C., and SMITH, DONALD W.: Legal aspects of nursing practice: The Taft-Hartley Act and the professional employee. *Amer. J. Nurs.* 57:346 (Mar.) 1957.

SCOTT, WILLIAM C., DONALD W.: Changes in hospital liability. *Amer. J. Nurs.* 58:68 (Jan.) 1958.

STOKES, JOHN H.: The question of venipunctures. *Amer. J. Nurs.* 52:307 (Mar.) 1952.

TERENZIO, JOSEPH: Some legal aspects of evening and night duty supervision. *Nurs. Outlook* 4:609 (Nov.) 1956.

CHAPTER 33

Nursing Publications

The amount of discussion about graduate work and credits toward a degree indicates the effort that nurses are making to keep abreast of these fast-moving times. The purpose of this chapter it to tell the nurse how she may keep well informed while carrying on her regular activities. This *in-service* education is available to every nurse through current periodicals. The nurse who reads the nursing magazines is always well informed on current events in nursing. She may be twenty years away from her basic training and a hundred miles from any medical center yet be familiar with the latest treatments, apparatus, and medications. All this is made possible through systematic reading of a few well-chosen magazines.

The most progressive ideas are first made public through the magazines. Only authors and publishers realize the length of time required to write and publish a book. We read of new procedures and medical discoveries usually before they are put into books. Sometimes a series of magazine articles that have proved especially valuable are collected and published in book form.

Never in the history of mankind has there been such a vast amount of material written, published, and broadcast, particularly about subjects relating to health and disease. This is being done to meet the demands of higher education and of increased leisure for the general population. Much of this material may be classed as pseudoscientific. Also, much is being published for popular consumption which may be beneficial to the laity but is usually a waste of time for the nurse. Therefore, the nurse must cultivate early a sense of values in her selection of scientific literature.

Newspaper articles are seldom more than an indication of what is being done in research on various subjects. Since newspaper writers rarely have medical training, these articles usually are written as an interview with a medical authority.

The following questions will be found practical in learning to evaluate magazine articles:

1. *Who is the author?* What is his standing in his particular field? Is he qualified to write upon this particular subject?

2. *Where were the facts obtained?* Is this an original article? Is it merely a collection of facts assembled from the reading of a nonmedical writer?

3. *Who sponsored this author?* Is the magazine reliable? What is the objective of the publishing company? Is it interested in the education of those who read these articles, or is it concerned only with sensational articles for its own advancement?

These questions are surely to be followed by: "How are we to go about getting the answers?" Questions 1 and 2 may usually be answered in one of two ways: The author's position and type of work will be given under the title of the subject on a *contributors' page.* When investigating an unfamiliar magazine, look at the table of contents and the contributors' page if no information about the writer is given at the beginning of the article. In this way, the nurse will soon build up a literary acquaintance with some of the authorities of nursing and allied fields.

Nursing magazines may be divided into two classes: official and commercial.

An official magazine is one which is controlled and owned by the organization which sponsors it, and thus is known as the "official organ" of that organization.

Commercial magazines are those published for financial gain by a publishing company or private individual. There are several excellent commercial periodicals which the nurse will learn to know by applying the above rules. Among commercial magazines that contribute to nursing are Modern Hospital, Hospital Management, RN—A Journal for Nurses, and Nursing Survey.

When a magazine is published by a nursing organization, great care is taken to make its information reliable and authentic, uncolored by prejudice of personal feelings. Nurses give out information with satisfaction and assurance because they have read it in the official magazines. As nurses, they have come to accept these periodicals as a guarantee of factual information.

PERIODICALS OF THE ANA AND NLN

The American Journal of Nursing. This journal is now an established part of nursing, for both the student and the graduate. It is a necessary part of her professional equipment. How we came to have this official organ should be of interest to every nurse. In 1935, the *American Journal of Nursing* published the "Story of the American Journal of Nursing," which may be found in the school library.

"The nurses who planned the *Journal* in the beginning had in mind three functions which it would carry on for the members of their group: It would be a continuous record of nursing events; a means of communication between scattered groups of nurses; and one means of interpreting nursing to the public."[1]

The *Journal* has done all of these. It has been a most potent factor in securing nursing legislation and in keeping the nurse informed of her national and international organizations, government nursing, loan funds, Red Cross, nursing education, and recreation. Along with these it always has devoted a large portion of its space to the care of the patient at the bedside. This clinical information comes from excellent sources. The editors each month give the nurse an introduction to the author of each article, and she will be interested to find how people who hold extremely demanding positions give of their time and effort that all nurses may have the best in medical literature.

The *Journal* publishes an official directory in January and July of each year, listing names and addresses of officials of international, national, and state organizations as well as the chairmen of both standing and special committees. The addresses of the state board of examiners are given also in the official directory.

A number of schools offering graduate work are listed in the *Journal*. Since there are no groups or organizations regularly inspecting or accrediting graduate work at present, advertisements of these courses are approved by the editor following conference with the Executive Secretary of the National League for Nursing.

Both the student and the graduate nurse should personally subscribe to the *Journal*, which is $5.00 per year. Subscriptions should be sent directly to headquarters, 10 Columbus Circle, New York 19. An index is printed each year in April, and the nurse should always request her copy because it will give her assistance in looking up references to articles published during the previous year.

Nursing Outlook. With the reorganization of five national nursing associations in June, 1952, the National Organization for Public Health Nursing became one of the departments of the National League for Nursing. Its official publication *Public Health Nursing* became absorbed by the official publication of the League for Nursing—*Nursing Outlook*.

Nursing Outlook furnishes nurses with information on all nursing—public health nursing, hospital nursing service, industrial nursing, and education. It devotes its contents to problems of nursing service in hospitals and public health and presents new material especially planned for nursing-service administrators, public health consultants, and nurse educators. The nonmember of the National League for Nursing will read *Nursing Oulook* with interest because of its authentic information on national health committees, the World Health

---

[1] *Story of the American Journal of Nursing* (New York, American Journal of Nursing Company, 1935).

Organization, international exchange of nurses, and activities on a local level because of ideas that can be used in public health clinics and in colleges which have schools of nursing in order to attain better nursing service in the community.

The first issue of *Nursing Outlook* was published in January, 1953. It is published by the American Journal of Nursing Company at national headquarters of the ANA, New York.

Nursing Research. Abraham Flexner, in 1916, established certain criteria as fundamental functions of all professions. Nursing has been phenomenally successful in meeting all these requirements except that of research "and to require the members constantly to resort to the laboratory and seminar for a fresh supply of facts."[2]

For the most part, nurses have been so busy getting the job done that there has been no time for research, which requires contemplative thinking, experimenting, and evaluating. Also, to be of value, research must be done in a scientific manner. To do this the nurse must have had an education beyond her basic nursing course in order to know the technics of scientific research.

Nurses are in a unique position to see both sides of a research project, since they work with both the medical profession and the social scientists. Therefore any research project should be aimed toward improving the physical condition of the patient through nursing, furthering the rehabilitation of the patient, and furnishing an understanding of both mental and physical health needs. But nursing research should be the work of the university school, since instruction and research are already its chief aims, and tools, materials, and research technics are available.

Nurses are aware of the need for applied scientific research, not merely to qualify as a profession but as a major step in planning nursing for the future. Therefore, *Nursing Research* was published to serve two purposes: "... to inform members of the nursing profession and allied professions of the results of scientific studies in nursing, and to stimulate research in nursing."[3]

The National League for Nursing is the sponsor of *Nursing Research.* It is published by the American Journal of Nursing Company at 10 Columbus Circle, New York 19. The need for such a publication was apparent when the original subscription list had 5000 subscribers. The subscription price is $5.00; the magazine is published four times a year.

THE PERSONAL SUBSCRIPTION

The nurse should have her own subscription to those periodicals most useful to her particular line of work. She seldom has time to read them thoroughly if she depends upon the copies at headquarters or the hospital library; but if she owns a copy it always is available, and she can read and assimilate it at her leisure. Then, too, articles have a way of failing to catch our attention the

---

[2] "Is Social Work a Profession?" Proceedings of the National Conference of Charities and Corrections, Chicago, 1915, pp. 576-590.

[3] Editorial, *Nursing Research,* 1:5 (June) 1952.

first time we look over the list of articles. This is because our interest varies from day to day and from month to month. The nurse reads only the articles of interest at the time. If a child is brought to the outpatient department with a peculiar skin eruption on the buttocks and the mother timidly offers the information that "it gets bad like that after eating eggs," the nurse makes a mental note of possible food allery. When she again looks at her magazine, the article on allergy suddenly thrusts itself upon her attention. We see that in which we are most interested.

Also her personal subscription gives the nurse the privilege of clipping articles of special interest; or, better still, if she has her magazines bound in good buckram, they will become a most valuable part of her library.

BINDING

A magazine that is worth reading regularly is worth keeping permanently, and bound magazines are most usuable. All magazines related to health publish a yearly index which is a necessary part of every bound volume. Some of these are published separately, while others are included in the June and December numbers in a special section. If they are mailed separately, write for your copy early in July and January. By learning to use these indexes, you will be able to tap sources of information on any subject.

Consult the librarian at the local library for the name of a reliable bindery. You will have the privilege of selecting your own binding. The bindery will remove the covers and advertising sections, but the covers of most of our nursing magazines should not be removed since most of them are decorated with works of art that are of special interest. In writing your name on unbound copies of magazines, take care not to mar the picture.

In most states, the state association publishes a bulletin of special interest to nurses of that state. This contains current articles on nursing, organizational changes, district news, and official directory of the state, etc. This publication is the official organ of the state association and it is sent to each paid-up member as one of the services of the state association.

INDEXES

A great deal of good nursing literature is being produced in both official and nonofficial magazines, American and foreign, that contain articles of lasting value. These publications are not limited to schools of nursing but they are of interest to nurses in general.

There is need for a nursing index to cover these periodicals and books. At present we have two major indexes: *Index Medicus,* now published by the Library of Medicine and the *Hospital Literature Index*. These two indexes include only twelve nursing periodicals.

A *Nursing Index* would be of value to nurses in all fields as well as nursing schools, public libraries, research students, and social workers.

OTHER PERIODICALS

The following magazines will be found helpful in keeping the nurse informed and will greatly increase her in-service education. From this list, select those which appeal most to your work and interest and then select one or two that are general in scope, making any nurse better informed and interested in life:

1. *The American Journal of Public Health and the Nation's Health* is published by the American Public Health Association, 1790 Broadway, New York 19.

2. *The Canadian Nurse* is the official magazine of the Canadian Nurses' Association and is published at 1411 Crescent Street, Montreal, Quebec, Canada.

3. *Hospitals* is the official magazine of the American Hospital Association, published for hospital administrators, and is of interest to all hospital nurses. It is published at 840 N. Lake Shore Drive, Chicago 11, Illinois.

4. *Hospital Progress* is published by the Catholic Hospital Association, 1438 South Grand Boulevard, St. Louis 4, Missouri.

5. *Today's Health* is published by the American Medical Association for the laity, yet no registered nurse should regard it as beneath her intellectual level. The public health nurse will find it especially useful in helping her to answer questions asked by her patients.

6. *National Business Woman* is published by the National Federation of Business and Professional Women's Clubs, Inc., 2012 Massachusetts Ave., N. W., Wash. 6, D. C. Nurses are independent women and should know more about other independent women. This magazine which is available only to members of the Federation can do much to broaden the social and cultural, as well as the business background of the nurse.

7. *The International Nursing Review* is published at the headquarters of the International Council of Nurses, 1 Dean Trench St., Westminster, London S. W. 1, England. This magazine, issued quarterly, has two advantages: (1) It gives the nurse an international conception of nursing, which means a better understanding of other races and nationalities. (2) It is published in English, French, and Spanish. The nurse who has studied foreign languages will find it interesting to keep up her reading in another language.

8. *Mental Hygiene* is published by the National Committee for Mental Hygiene. Since this subject is assuming the importance that it merits, the nurse is enabled to keep in touch with its progress by including this magazine in her professional reading.

9. *Nursing Times,* which is the official organ of the College of Nursing, is published by Macmillan & Co., Ltd., St. Marin's Street, London, W. C. 2.

10. *The Star* is published by patients of the United States Public Health Service Hospital, Carville, Louisiana, "radiating the light of truth about Hansen's disease."

11. *The Nursing Survey* is devoted to nursing education especially, and is published six times a year by the F. A. Davis Company, 1914 Cherry Street, Philadelphia 3, Pennsylvania. The subscription price is $3.00 per year.

12. *RN* is published monthly by The Nightingale Press, Oradell, New Jersey. Cost of a subscription for one year is $3.00.

13. *Safety Education*, a magazine for teachers and administrators, is published by the National Safety Council, 425 North Michigan Avenue, Chicago 11, Illinois. Excellent for school nurses.

14. *Public Health Reports* is published by the United States Public Health Service at Bethesda, Maryland. It is an excellent magazine for both the student nurse and the practicing public health nurse.

15. *Modern Hospital* is published by the Modern Hospital Company, 919 North Michigan Avenue, Chicago 11, Illinois. This magazine has excellent articles on nurses and nursing as seen from the hospital administrator's viewpoint.

16. *World Health* is published by the World Health Organization, six times a year.

17. *Journal of Psychiatric Nursing* is published bimonthly by the F. A. Davis Company, 1914 Cherry Street, Philadelphia 3, Pennsylvania. Its subscription price is $3.00 per year.

CLASS EXERCISE

The class will make a careful study of nursing and allied periodicals. With this information decide upon five magazines that will be best for the hospital nurse, the public health nurse, and the office nurse.

REFERENCES

AFTAB, SHIRLEY H.: Sixty years of Trained Nurse. Trained Nurse and Hosp. Rev. 132:14 (Jan.) 1949.

BELIN, CONSTANCE R.: What's goin' on here? *Nurs. Outlook* 1:34 (Jan.) 1953.

"Binding your journals." *Amer. J. Nurs.* 49:76 (Feb.) 1949.

DEWITT, KATHERINE, and MUNSON, HELEN: The Journal's first fifty years. *Amer. J. Nurs.* 50:590 (Oct.) 1950.

DIETZ, LENA DIXON: Let's have a nursing index. *Davis Nurs. Survey* 24:112 (Aug.) 1960.

Editorial: A new magazine for nursing. *Amer. J. Nurs.* 52:1077 (Sept.) 1952.

Editorial: Needed: An index to nursing journals. *Nurs. Outlook* 7: 569 (Oct.) 1959.

"1962-The year of the written word." *Nurs. Outlook* 10:83 (Feb.) 1962.

"How the Journal began." *Amer. J. Nurs.* 49:331 (June) 1949.

"1962—The year of the written word." *Nurs. Outlook* 10:83 (Feb.) 1962.

"Order your indexes and bibliography cards now." *Amer. J. Nurs.* 44:163 (Jan.) 1944.

"Order your Journal index now!" *Amer. J. Nurs.* 54:149 (Feb.) 1945.

POLAND, F. W.: Writer's Cramp. *Canad. Nurse.* 55:523 (June) 1959.

ROBERTS, MARY M.: The Journal editors. *Amer. J. Nurs.* 49:330 (June) 1949.

SEIDL, GEORGE W.: Writing for publication. *Amer. J. Nurs.* 51:427 (July) 1951.

"The Journal as a business," and "How the money is spent." *Amer. J. Nurs.* 51:8 (Mar.) 1951.

TURNER, RUTH: We try our hand at journalism. *Amer. J. Nurs.* 50:449 (July) 1950.

"What are professional periodicals." *Amer. J. Nurs.* 37:1369 (Dec.) 1937.

"What happened to that article you wrote?" *Nurs. Outlook* 5:220 (Apr.) 1957.

YAST, HELEN: Library service. *Hospitals.* 34:92 (Apr. 16) 1960.

CHAPTER 34

Public Relations

Public relations, as it concerns nurses, is the promotion of good human relationships between the nurse and the public which she serves.

Every profession is geninely concerned about the relationships with its public. Public opinion is a powerful influence, and no one is in a better position to mold favorable public opinion than are nurses. The nurse has three areas of public relationships—the patient, the medical profession, and the citizens of the community. There is a great difference between good publicity and good human relationships. Nurses always make good publicity material, but modern nursing needs better human relations. The general public needs to know more about nursing, and the nurse needs to know more about people outside the institution in which she works. By and large, the public still regards nursing as a cloistered profession, and nurses have done very little to change this attitude.

Nursing, as a profession, needs the support of the public for schools of nursing, public health, economic security, and better care for the aged. The better the public knows nurses and the aims and needs of nurses, the more willing they will be to support these projects when they are introduced.

The following presentation of areas of public relations aims to make a nurse aware of herself in connection with an important part of everyday living.

THE PATIENT

A great deal of the nurse's good public relations with patients is done naturally and spontaneously as part of the job. The little old lady who hadn't been used to kindness exclaimed, ''When I get home, I'm going to tell every body in the village how wonderful you all were to me!'' The nurses who heard her remark looked at each other, wondering what they had done. Without being aware of it, they had been contributing to good public relations. The weary parents of a very ill child were advised by the nurse to leave their telephone number with her and go home for a short rest. Because of her attitude, they left with complete confidence. The nurse was unaware of public relations, yet her thoughtfulness had far-reaching results. Simple kindness and human understanding will do much to establish good public relations for the nursing profession.

THE PUBLIC HEALTH NURSE

The public health nurse has an excellent opportunity to improve public relations through the patient, the medical profession, and the community; in fact, the community is also her patient load. Public health nursing developed out of favorable public relations, and it has had the interest and cooperation of the community since its origin. The successful public health nurse is aware of the importance of maintaining friendly working conditions with other health agencies, community chests, religious groups, and her own non-nurse board members. Indeed, the high regard in which public health is now held is largely due to the thoughtfulness of public health nurses.

THE INSTITUTIONAL NURSE

Under this heading is included a wide range of nursing in general and specialized hospitals, government hospitals, and nursing education. These hospitals give employment to the largest number of nurses because they care for the greatest number of patients. Hospitals rank fifth in business enterprises and provide employment for thousands of people. All this is built around the patient, whether the hospital be large or small, private or tax-supported, endowed or supported by the community chest. In a country such as ours, every patient has his or her own area of influence, and it can have a powerful effect on public opinion. A large medical center in a vast, isolated area is dependent upon the state legislature to maintain the medical school, nursing school, dietetics school, occupational therapy school, etc. Everyone in every department, from the laundry foreman to the administrator, must be alert to the practice of good human relationships in order to keep the hospital filled with satisfied patients who provide clinical experience for members of the various schools. Good public relations is not only obeying the golden rule, but it has a very practical side.

THE NEIGHBOR

The nurse cannot easily escape the responsibility of neighborliness; R.N. means Real Neighbor as well as Registered Nurse. By virtue of her profession, she has become an important person in her neighborhood. As a neighbor she is subject to questioning and pleas for advice: "Doctor said to give Billy whooping cough serum. Do you think I should let the children go to school?"

When answering these questions, take time to give an adequate explanation, taking care that you give due respect to the intelligence of the questioner. Nurses know so much more about medical conditions than non-nurses that they sometimes forget that other people, too, have wide fields of information and interest.

As a neighbor, take care not to give the impression of practicing medicine; R.N. does not mean M.D., and favorable relationships with the medical profession in your community are necessary. Leave to the physician those things reserved for physicians.

THE CITIZEN

A criticism of nurses is their apparent lack of community interest, yet few people in a community are so well qualified to become useful citizens as are nurses. As a professional educated person, the nurse will be readily accepted by other civic-minded citizens. The relationship will be broadening for her, and she can make a real contribution to the community which will be personally satisfying to her creative self.

The nurse can develop an interest in the government of the city, county, and state. This is a democratic government; it deserves and demands the interest and support of worth-while citizens if it is to be preserved, and where can better people be found than in the professions? It is high time that some of the "best people" became interested in better government. The start can be made at the local level with much self-satisfaction; the League of Women Voters is an interesting organization in which to gain an idea of political machinery.

Outside of the institution or public health work, the nurse can join other civic leaders in meeting the problems of her community. She is in a position to know many of the health needs of the people. As the public health nurse, she knows the sanitation and housing needs; as the school nurse, she is an ideal person on the committee to prevent juvenile delinquency; as the outpatient nurse, she knows where most of the tuberculosis comes from. Because of her civic interest and personal contacts, she can and will be given support in remedying these conditions.

Nurses are in demand as public speakers, and they have much to contribute to such groups as women's clubs, Red Cross, parent-teachers' meetings, church groups, and future-nurses clubs. Here is an excellent opportunity to develop favorable public relations and at the same time to let your audience learn something of nursing and nurses. (Nurses need to talk more about nursing and less about patients.) Perhaps the subject requested by the group is heart disease. After the nurse has been presented by the chairman of the program committee, she can get acquainted with her audience by bringing in some pertinent current event in nursing: "This is off the subject of heart disease, but I know that you will be interested to learn that the state board of education has appropriated funds to develop a college of nursing in our state university. As a nurse, it gives me great satisfaction to know that nursing is being recognized on this basis." There will probably be a social hour after the talk, and here again is an opportunity to educate the audience.

In preparing a talk to a non-nurse audience keep in mind the probable background of the group. People are health conscious. Radio and television and popular books on health have done much toward providing a background on antibiotics, uses of blood, cancer, heart disease, and many other common ailments.

THE RADIO OR TELEVISION SPEECH

Being a success as a platform speaker does not necessarily mean that a nurse may be equally successful "on the air." Some excellent speakers, especially women, are utter failures from a radio standpoint because they lack radio personality, or, as is frequently the case, because of a radio consciousness so apparent to the listeners that the speaker's best efforts are spoiled.

Other things being favorable, a few rehearsals with the radio-station staff are likely to dispel radio consciousness, especially if the speaker's mind is really more concerned with her subject than with herself. Thereafter, as in any other form of public contact, her success will depend on the degree of her interest in what she has to say.

Preparation of a radio or television address requires more care than that given to a platform talk because of the rigid time schedule observed in broadcasting stations and because of the greater necessity for maximum interest content of the audience, since the dial knows no courtesy.

THE PRESS

The newspaper is an excellent media for informing the public about nursing activities. The nurse should make an effort to develop cooperative relationships with the local newspapers. Nurses and nursing always are news. A nurse was chairman of a committee to preserve a bird sanctuary in her community; the metropolitan daily ran a three-column spread with the nurse's picture. The graduate of a local school of nursing is leader in the development of group therapy treatment in one of the state mental hospitals. The newspaper presented a delightful human interest story. This was good public relations for both the mental hospital and the school of nursing.

Nursing organizations on the state or district level need the newspapers for meeting notices and other activities. In exchange for this courtesy the public relations committee of the organization can pass on an interesting story about nursing for the Sunday edition.

Most newspapers carry a "letter column." This can be used as an excellent means for a public expression of gratitude "for help in our recent fire disaster" or for "the toy contribution to children's department of our hospital."

THE LAW

Perhaps the most important hospital area relative to public relations is the emergency room, where speed, urgency, and tensions are magnified.

The head nurse in the emergency room makes many of her own public relations decisions. Most hospitals adopt certain policies to be followed in which the size of the town and the efforts to serve the community are considered.

Victims of shootings, fire, explosions, poisonings, and car accidents are, by law, entered on police records. This is public information. The nurse is free to give the press the name, address, age, sex, marital status, employer, and occupation of the patient, and nature of the accident. However, the hospital may withhold information from the press that would reflect discredit on a patient or his family, such as suicide, intoxication, drug addiction. Also, most hospitals, as a consideration to patients and their families, do not release the prognosis of a patient.

"Police cases" include lawbreakers and certain accident victims. Any patient who is not a police case has the same right-of-privacy that any other patient has. Although he may be a prominent politician, actor, or industrialist, or whatever makes one famous in the public eye, he may refuse to have pictures taken and may have his name withheld from the public if he wishes.

SUMMARY

In the final analysis of public relations, the thermometer stands at kindness and understanding, whether it concerns the nurse working in the venereal disease clinic or the nurse on the "team" of the World Health Organization in Ethiopia. Nurses can build good public relations only as they can appreciate the feelings of the people with whom they work. Nurses can sell nursing not by gay posters, radio and television announcements, and full-page advertisements, but by the individual nurse in her exhibition of kindness, right living, community participation, and social education.

CLASS EXERCISE

1. Name ten worth-while contributions that the married nurse living in an urban community may make toward the improvement of social and political conditions.

2. Name ten worth-while contributions that may be made by the married nurse living in a rural community.

REFERENCES

ALFANO, GENROSE: What rapport means to me. *Nurs. Outlook* 3:326 (June) 1955.

AMBERG, ROSE G.: A nurse looks at intergroup relations. *Amer. J. Nurs.* 59:1584 (Nov.) 1959.

BERNAYS, EDWARD L.: The nursing profession—a public relations viewpoint. *Amer. J. Nurs.* 45:351 (May) 1945.

BOYD, HARRY, and FREY, THOMAS E.: The press and the hospital. *Nurs. Outlook* 6:80 (Feb.) 1958.

BURLING, TEMPLE, LUNTZ, EDITH M., and WILSON, ROBERT W.: *The Give and Take in Hospitals.* G. P. Putnam's Sons, New York, 1956.

BURNS, FLORENCE S.: Future nurses clubs. *Amer. J. Nurs.* 53:84 (Jan.) 1953.

CABOT, HUGH, and KAHL, JOSEPH: *Human Relations.* Harvard University Press, Cambridge, Mass., 1953. (Especially interesting to nurses.)

CROOM, LOUISE: Classes in public relations. *Amer. J. Nurs.* 51:85 (Feb.) 1951.

Editorial: Brotherhood every day. *Amer. J. Nurs.* 53:161 (Feb.) 1953.

FAY, AUDREY B.: Public relations pays in pediatrics. *Amer. J. Nurs.* 52:1506 (Dec.) 1952.

FISHER, MARGUERITE J.: Professional women as effective citizens. *Amer. J. Nurs.* 49:757 (Dec.) 1949.

FLORES, FLORENCE: Visitors unlimited. *Amer. J. Nurs.* 53:1350 (Nov.) 1953.

GEISTER, JANET M.: Public relations begins at the bedside. *Amer. J. Nurs.* 50:463 (Aug.) 1950.

GRAF, LOUIS: How to handle press relations. *Hosp. Manage.* 80:50 (Aug.) 1955.

HANNA, MARK: Good public relations requires good public speakers. *Amer. J. Nurs.* 48:163 (Mar.) 1948.

HARLOW, REX F., and BLACK, MARVIN M.: *Practical Public Relations.* Harper & Brothers, New York, 1952.

HENDERSON, JEAN: Public relations in nursing. *Amer. J. Nurs.* 48:514 (Aug.) 1947.

HENNICK, HENRIETTA R.: The student's parents are your friends. *Nurs. Outlook* 3:284 (May) 1955.

HERWITZ, ADELE: An international look at employment problems. *Amer. J. Nurs.* 59:355 (Mar.) 1959.

HUDSON, MARCELLA: What housewife R. N.'s can do. *Nurs. World* 129:10 (Oct.) 1955.

JOHNSON, LUCIUS W.: Ah-er-uh-unaccustomed as they are. *Modern Hosp.* 80:60 (Jan.) 1953.

LINDSAY, ROBERT: Public relations can help you gain economic security. *Amer. J. Nurs.* 57:46 (Jan.) 1957.

McCABE, IRENE F., and CHRISTOPHER, WILLIAM I.: Public relations institute stresses the importance of the "little things" in the daily hospital routine. *Hospitals* 27:66 (Feb.) 1953.

MITCHELL, M.: Interpreting nursing to the community. *Nurs. Mirror* 112:1217 (June 30) 1961.

NOTTER, LUCILLE E.: Visitors are important people. *Nurs. Outlook* 3:372 (July) 1955.

PENNOCK, META R.: New ethics in publicity. *Trained Nurse and Hosp. Rev.* 87:753 (Dec.) 1931.

POWELL, ENOCH, "Human Relations in Hospital Service," *Nursing Mirror* 112:1125 (June 23) 1961.

POWERS, DAVID G.: *How to Say a Few Words.* Doubleday & Co., Inc., New York, 1953.

PROCK, VALENCIA: The nurse's role in a joint education program for the health professions. *Nurs. Outlook* 9:557 (Sept.) 1961.

"Public relations and you." *Amer. J. Nurs.* 51:667 (Oct.) 1951.

REAGER, RICHARD C.: Tell your story well. *Amer. J. Nurs.* 50:461 (Aug.) 1950.

REED, ELIZABETH: Don't read your speech. *Amer. J. Nurs.* 55:1212 (Oct.) 1955.

ST. GEORGES, MAUBERT: *Public Relations.* Alexander Hamilton Institute, New York, 1953.

SNYDER, DAVID U.: Pubic relations counseling in the nursing profession. *Amer. J. Nurs.* 56:860 (July) 1956.

SPEIGEL, MAE O.: Organizing community resources to meet health needs. *Nurs. Outlook* 4:272 (May) 1956.

"Telling our story." *Amer J. Nurs.* 56:23 (Jan.) 1956.

WEEKS, LEROY R.: Medical profession and clergy as community servants. J.A.M.A. 47:256 (July) 1955.

"What can an inactive nurse do to make her professional preparation and experience useful and effective in her community." *Amer. J. Nurs.* 55:1211 (Oct.) 1955.

WIENER, NORBERT: *The Human Use of Human Beings.* Houghton Mifflin Co., Boston, 1954.

WILSON, ELAINE: Try it on television. *Amer. J. Nurs.* 54:436 (Apr.) 1954.

CHAPTER 35

Personal Economics

Economists have said that no woman makes an honest effort to save before she is thirty. The element of romance was dominant previous to the Depression years beginning with 1930, but now women, and society as a whole, have become budget conscious. Thirty years ago few young graduates would have given a thought to the financial future. Today, many of them are investigating and investing in postal savings, life insurance, endowment policies, and deferred retirement annuities, while many for the first time are learning to budget their income. The modern woman has begun to think in terms of budgets if not of savings. She has begun to practice thrift.

The late David Francis Jordan, professor of finance and author, defines thrift as: . . . *a determination to live with a margin for future advancement; to earn a little more than one spends, or to spend a little less than one earns, getting meanwhile the value in strength, in satisfaction, or in other worth for the money one feels free to spend. The spirit of thrift is opposed to waste on the one hand, and to recklessness on the other. It does not involve stinginess, which is an abuse of thrift, nor does it require that each item of savings should be a financial investment. The money that is spent in the education of one's self or one's family, in travel, in music, in art, or in helpfulness to others, if*

340

it brings real return in personal development, or in better understanding of the world we live in, is in accordance with the spirit of thrift.

Nurses salaries have advanced considerably during the past decade but these, except in the higher administrative brackets, are not equal to salaries paid to women in other professions, such as teaching and social work.

The current salary range for nurses in each state and in the large metropolitan areas is listed in *Facts About Nursing,* published annually by the American Nurses' Association. This book is to be found in all nursing libraries. Information on nurses salaries is listed under "The Economic Status of the Nursing Profession," and includes all categories of nursing.

A TYPICAL SAVINGS PLAN

While the amount for each purpose may vary, a typical savings plan should include provision for (1) emergencies, (2) financial credit and convenience, (3) dependents, and (4) old age.

Emergencies. A nurse should have a small sum of money, equal at least to a month's salary, set aside as an emergency fund in case of illness, unemployment, unexpected traveling, or a sudden call home. This fund can be maintained as a savings account payable on demand and replenished as soon as possible after the emergency has been met.

Financial Credit and Convenience. For convenience and safety, a nurse should maintain a checking account. Paying everything by check means that she need keep very little cash on her person or in living quarters, and thus reduces the danger of theft or the inconvenience of a lost pocketbook; besides, canceled checks are receipts for which one is often grateful. When correctly filled in, the check stubs constitute a record to be used to verify expenses in the nurse's budget. A checking account is an excellent bank reference when asking for a charge account at a department store, gas station, or other place of business.

Dependents. By "dependents" is meant not only those who are dependent upon the nurse for the necessities of life, but also those for whom, through relationship or gratitude, the nurse has come to feel a certain responsibility. Sad and lonely indeed must be the nurse who has no one to care for but herself. Most persons feel a real pride in knowing that their loved ones are provided for. For this reason, every nurse should buy a life insurance policy with the first money earned after completing her nursing course. She can then buy an ordinary life policy for an annual premium of approximately $20 for each $1000 of insurance. Even so small a policy will give a satisfying measure of protection to her dependents in case of her death, and she may still have the pleasure of spending as she pleases some of the first money she has earned—a happy combination of circumstances which admittedly gives her a glorious feeling of independence. If she dies, her dependents receive the proceeds of the policy; if she survives the dependents, she has a valuable investment with various settlement options.

Old Age. There are three possible rewards for the work of the registered nurse: (1) satisfaction of the urge to serve humanity, (2) financial independence during her working life, and (3) financial security when she retires from active work.

THE ECONOMIC SECURITY PROGRAM

Because much of early nursing was private duty, both the nurse and the public thought of nurses as independent contractors. But as industry expanded, so did institutions employing nurses, and it became evident that it was necessary to increase salaries and provide better working conditions. The two needs had much in common. The labor inequalities during World War II convinced nursing leaders that something definite should be done to protect the economic security of nurses, and, as a result, economic security became one of the planks of the 1946 platform of the American Nurses' Association.

Out of this discussion developed the Economic Security Program, based on the belief *that all nurses are entitled to a salary commensurate with their professional qualifications and responsibilities.* This program not only benefits the nurse economically, but it increases her professional stature. The public will appreciate and respect a profession whose services are valued as are those of other professional workers of comparable educational qualifications.

The Economic Security Program should be important to the nurse-student. For the most part the student has been adequately provided for since infancy, which includes present living conditions. The monthly allowance, too, is adequate for cosmetics, recreation, and small charities. Because of twenty years of protection, the student has nothing in her experience for comparison. Her allowance compared with the salary of a staff nurse looks astronomical. Six months after graduation she finds her salary inadequate to meet living conditions. She looks for positions that offer higher salaries and begins a serious study of nursing economics.

The new graduate can make her best contribution to herself and to nursing by actively supporting the Economic Security Program in the state office headquarters.

Bargaining Agent. The state or district association acts as a bargaining agent for the association. Nothing could be more destructive to the high regard for nurses which the public now holds than coercive negotiating. Bargaining between nurses and their employers is done in a dignified, professional manner.

Each section of the state association sets minimum-wage standards and sends copies of these wage standards to all employers of nurses. The state association employs at headquarters a person whose duty it is to act as bargaining agent for nurses in groups or as individuals. The group decides what it desires in the way of salaries and improved working conditions and presents these stipulations to the bargaining agent for consideration and discussion. Then one or more representatives from the group, together with the bargaining agent, meet the employer for a negotiation conference. Since the problem is presented and discussed by both sides with sane, unemotional understanding, a reasonable adjustment is usually reached to the mutual satisfaction of nurses and employers.

INSURANCE

A life insurance policy is a promise to pay money either to an individual (called the insured), or to his estate, or to named beneficiaries in the event of his death. If the policy is payable at the end of a certain period to the insured while he is living, it is known as an endowment policy. If the policy is payable only in the event of death, then it is known as a life policy.

Life policies, or those payable only at the death of the insured, are given different names which are used to indicate the manner in which the insured pays the premiums. A *whole life* (also called *ordinary life*) policy is one for which the insured contracts to pay premiums during his entire life. If, on the other hand, the insured does not wish to pay premiums during his entire life, but wants to limit the payments to a term of years (such as 10, 20 etc.), it is then called a *limited life* policy.

An *annuity program* is one which, by systematic payments or one large payment to an insurance company, provides a guaranteed life income. The amount of the income and the age at which it is to commence is governed by the proportion of your earnings which can be set aside as savings, by the number of dependents, by the age at which you may wish to retire from active work or to begin drawing on your savings, and the like. A competent insurance salesman, trained to analyze these factors, can then recommend a suitable annuity program.

As a rule, life insurance agents suggest a whole life policy or limited life (usually twenty-payment) policy as best meeting the immediate requirements of the young graduate.

OTHER PLANS

Postal Savings. The postal savings system was instituted by an act of Congress, 1910, for the purpose of encouraging thrift and to provide a safe depository for the accumulation of savings.

A postal savings account may be opened in person or by mail at any local post office. Deposits of any amount of dollars but not less than $5 may be made until the total deposits reach $2500. The annual interest rate on deposits is 2 per cent. Deposits plus the accrued interest may be withdrawn at any time from the post office where the deposits were made.

United States Savings Bonds. Millions of Americans are buying government savings bonds systematically, as personal reserves and to add regularly to their funds for important lifetime purposes, such as buying a home or providing for retirement and travel.

United States savings bonds are designated by letters, such as Series E, Series H, and Series K. Consult your local bank for detailed information and advantages of the various series of bonds.

Pension Plans. Employees of some nonprofit hospitals, which also include employees of state hospitals, are eligible for old-age-security pensions. In order to provide for their employees, many nonprofit hospitals have set up their own pension plans. In such plans, both the hospital and the employee contribute a certain part; the plan is payable at a specified age, usually sixty-five years.

HEALTH AND ACCIDENT INSURANCE

When buying insurance of this type, be sure of two things: (1) that the policy contains the clause, "Illness disability paid for all diseases without restriction," since many companies refuse to pay for all "Illnesses peculiar to women"; (2) that the nurse thoroughly understands the wording covering the nature and frequency of medical attendance required in order to qualify for indemnity.

The number of subscribers for *hospital insurance* is increasing rapidly. Credit departments of voluntary hospitals find that more than half of their patients carry some form of hospital insurance, either group or individual, by commercial or nonprofit organizations. With the hospital bill already paid, people are less reluctant to go to the hospital. This means that minor illnesses are treated before they become serious or chronic. Hospital insurance is indirectly teaching preventive medicine to the general population.

More detailed and definite information on hospital insurance can usually be found in the hospital periodicals. Also, see the current annual index of the *American Journal of Nursing*.

RELIEF FUND

The American Nurses' Relief Fund was established in 1911 for the purpose of providing financial relief to sick nurses who were in need. This fund was national in scope, each state association and each district association having its relief fund committee. At the biennial convention in 1932 the house of delegates voted as follows:

That the residue of the Relief Fund, both legacies and gifts, after legitimate expenditures for administration and distribution have been deducted, be allocated to the membership at the time of the 1932 Biennial Convention together with the interest accruing thereafter in proportion until the date of distribution.

That while the allocation of the relief fund monies be on the basis of the April, 1932, membership, the Board of Directors of the American Nurses' Association delay the sale of the relief securities until such time as the Board may deem wise, taking into consideration the original cost, face value, and market value of the securities, and that upon the sale of the securities the sum of their selling price plus the accrued interest be allocated in accordance with the foregoing motion.

This vote of the house of delegates has been carried out; securities have been liquidated, and the funds have been distributed to the various states.

Since the relief fund has been taken over by the state associations, the plan in most states is as follows: The state organization decides to raise a stated amount for nurses' relief service. Each district or alumnae association investigates each case appealing for service. In many cases help may be given without any actual expenditure of money, which means much to the self respect of the member who is being helped. When money is really needed, the case is referred to the headquarters of the state nurses' association for official action. Many districts keep on hand a small fund for ambulance service, travel expense, and other emergency needs.

FEDERAL SOCIAL SECURITY

The Social Security Act of 1935 did not include nurses, but obtaining this benefit for nurses has been one of the activities of the American Nurses' Association. With the cooperation of other health agencies, the bill known as the Social Security Act Amendments became a law in August, 1950, and effective January 1, 1951. This law brings nurses under the coverage of the old-age survivors, and disability insurance benefits. The latest amendments to the Social Security Act became law in September, 1960.

Nurses in industry and in profit-sharing clinics have had Social Security, but that did not include the great group of nurses in religious, educational, charitable, and other nonprofit institutions. Federal Social Security provides benefits at the lowest possible costs; therefore, it is to the advantage of the nurse to seek employment in institutions covered by federal Social Security.

Provision is made for the private duty nurse to have Social Security coverage by classifying her as a self-employed person. She does not pay a monthly tax, but she keeps a record of all income from patients and pays her Social Security tax annually, as she does her income tax. If she has worked part of the year in some other capacity which has Social Security coverage, such as office nursing, industrial nursing, etc., she should deduct that amount from her private duty earnings.

Tax rates for the self-employed are slightly higher than the rates quoted above, but, even so, this plan furnishes a cheaper annuity than can be purchased in any other manner.

INCOME TAX

Nurses as well as other employed people are subject to federal income tax, and since there is a tightening up of the administrative machinery that regulates the collecting of this government tax, all nurses should pay close attention to the regulations governing it.

The *American Journal of Nursing,* with its usual interest in the personal economics of nurses, publishes annually an article on federal income tax to include revisions, withholdings, and deductions. Read this article each year before filling in the income-tax returns.[1]

---

[1] The cost of uniforms is deductible from income tax. This is true only if the nurse does not wear the uniform as street wear to and from work.

BUDGETS

Any budget must be based upon fixed charges to be met and over which one has no control, such as rent, electricity, and refrigeration, if an apartment or house is being maintained. Budget figures merely indicate the proper proportion of the total income which should be allotted for various expenditures. The number of persons being aided or supported by the wage earner is still another factor, as are individual differences.

Sample budget forms can be secured from most banks. Forms also may be secured from the Bureau of Home Economics in the United States Department of Agriculture and from the Institute of Life Insurance. No budget is of value unless it is followed. The few minutes necessary to enter the day's items constitute a small price to pay for the financial comfort yielded by an honestly kept budget.

A FORMAL WILL

A will should be a part of the financial plan of every nurse, whether married or unmarried. To the healthy young graduate this may seem morbid and unnecessary. "I have nothing to will." "My husband can have anything I have." "My parents can have mine." All this means nothing unless it is written down, signed and witnessed. It is people of modest means who have the most need of a will. It helps to prevent the expensive red-tape of the probate court.

The safe way is to have a will drawn by a competent lawyer. The fee is usually from $15 to $25. This document will state whom the nurse wishes to act as her executor—her husband, sister, or trusted friend. The cost of a will is a small price to pay for a great deal of peace of mind.

CLASS EXERCISE

The class estimates that the nurse can make an annual saving of $500. Members of the class assume responsibility for obtaining information on reliable sources of investments: government bonds, savings and loan companies, stocks and bonds, and other reliable securities. How can the nurse invest this amount annually to the best and safest advantage?

REFERENCES

American Journal of Nursing:
    ANA economic security program: What it is and why. 58:520 (Apr.) 1958.
    Economic security—your program. 52:1496 (Nov.) 1952.
    Individual, the section, and the state nurses' association in collective bargaining. 51:540
        (Sept.) 1951.
    New guide for improving employment conditions. 52:1522 (Dec.) 1952.
AMERICAN NURSES' ASSOCIATION: Manual for an Economic Security Program. The
    Association, New York, 1952.

BAKER, JOHN M.: I don't want my wife to nurse. *Amer. J. Nurs.* 57:1466 (Nov.) 1957.

BARUCH, BERNARD M.: Economic controls and the nurse. *Amer. J. Nurs.* 51:491 (Aug.) 1951.

CANTA, LIONNE A.: What happens at the bargaining table. *Amer. J. Nurs.* 59:1436 (Dec.) 1959.

COHEN, WILBUR J.: Health insurance under Social Security. *Amer. J. Nurs.* 4:502 (Apr.) 1960.

CREIGHTON, HELEN: Get those employment details in writing. *RN* 23:51 (Feb.) 1960. ''Developments in health insurance.'' *RN* 20:60 (May) 1957.

EARLE, HOWARD: How to save money on your health insurance. *Today's Health* 39:32 (Feb.) 1961.

ELDER, PETER: Income tax deductions. *Amer. J. Nurs.* 57:318 (Mar.) 1957.

FEINSINGER, NATHAN P.: Labor legislation, economic security, and individual freedom. *Amer. J. Nurs.* 52:426 (Apr.) 1952.

''For Us, for Nursing, for Patient Care.'' *Amer. J. Nurs.* 61:66 (June) 1961.

GERARD, MARGARET: Richer than you think. *Amer J. Nurs.* 61:89 (Mar.) 1961.

GLOVER, MILTON H.: Methods of providing income for old age. *Pub. Health Nurs.* 44:461 (Aug.) 1952.

GORBY, JOHN H.: Employee credit unions. *Mod. Hosp.* 79:55 (Aug.) 1952.

HAVIGHURST, ROBERT J., and SHANAS, ETHEL: Retirement and the professional worker. *J. Geront.* 8:81 (Jan.) 1953.

HOOD, EVELYN E.: Economic security in British Columbia. *Amer. J. Nurs.* 56:583 (May) 1956.

''How much nurses are paid.'' *Amer. J. Nurs.* 61:89 (May) 1961.

JORDAN, CLIFFORD H.: Where do nurse educators stand on the economic ladder? *Amer. J. Nurs.* 61:70 (Aug.) 1961.

JORDAN, DAVID F., and DOUGALL, HERBERT E.: *Investments. 7th ed.* Prentice Hall, Inc., Englewood Cliffs, N. J., 1960.

JORDAN, DAVID F., and WILLETT, EDWARD F.: *Managing Personal Finances.* 3rd ed. Prentice-Hall, Inc., Englewood Cliffs, N. J., 1951.

PORTER, SYLVIA: How to live on what you make. *Atlanta Journal and Constitution.* May 24, 1953. Condensed in Reader's Digest, September, 1953.

RODGERS, DONALD I.: Teach your wife to be a widow. *Collier's,* June 7, 1952.

SCOTT, WILLIAM C., and SMITH, DONALD W.: Travel expenses and your income tax. *Amer. J. Nurs.* 56:1003 (Aug.) 1956.

SHELDON, NOLA S.: The private duty nurse and her Social Security coverage. *Amer. J. Nurs.* 51:235 (Apr.) 1951.

SHEPPARD, HAROLD L., and SHEPPARD, AUDREY P.: Paternalism in employer-employee relationships. *Amer. J. Nurs.* 51:16 (Jan.) 1951.

TITUS, SHIRLEY, MUNIER, JOSEPH D., and MERMELSTEIN, THELMA: Economic facts of life for nurses. *Amer. J. Nurs.* 52:1109 (Sept.) 1952.

''Survey of salaries and personnel practices in effect October, 1960 for teachers and administrators in nursing educational programs.'' *Amer. J. Nurs.* 61:71 (Aug.) 1961.

WHITAKER, JUDITH G.: The changing role of the professional nurse in the hospital. *Amer. J. Nurs.* 62:65 (Feb.) 1962.

WHITMAN, HOWARD: Planning your own security. *Today's Health* 39:26 (May) 1961 (Part I); June, 1961 (Part II).

WINSLOW, JOHN: Protecting your Social Security credits. *RN* 23:41 (Feb.) 1959.

WINSLOW, JOHN: New helps in solving your money problems. *RN* 22:39 (Nov.) 1959.

WINSLOW, JOHN: Check your check knowledge against these pointers. *RN* 25:65 (Mar.) 1962.

CHAPTER 36

Graduate Problems

The graduate nurse is confronted with problems—ethical, social, and professional—that do not concern the student nurse. The graduate is "on her own," and she is expected to know and do the correct thing, although her state board examinations may be as recent as last week. In order to save the new graduate some of the difficulties and embarrassments from the hard school of experience, a few of these situations are discussed. Also, a rather lengthy reference list is appended, dealing with still more problems, as the titles will indicate.

GIVING ADVICE ON CHOICE OF DOCTORS

"What doctor shall I have? You are a nurse; you know who is best." Even as freshmen students this question is heard, and of graduates it is asked even oftener. Giving advice about a choice of doctors is a risk even in the nurse's own family. If the results are unfavorable, the nurse is blamed: "Miss R— said to call him." Sometimes the question may be phrased: "We have been having Doctor L— in our home for twenty years but he seems a bit old and we thought maybe we should have a younger doctor. Do you think Doctor L— is still pretty good?" Never try to advise people about discharging a longtime

348

family physician. If it is at all possible, urge them to retain his services. The faith that people have in a physician is as much a healing element as is the medical treatment.

HOW YOUR PATIENTS LIVE

A few nurses are prudishly concerned about the morals of their patients. This is indeed a narrow-minded view. The nurse may find that her patient sells liquor illegally; this is none of her concern. The physician sent her to care for the fractured leg, not the man's morals. She may disapprove of the moral delinquency, but she is acting as assistant to the physician and not to the clergyman. One is reminded of the nurse who refused to stay on a serious pneumonia case after she had learned that the man and woman in the house were not legally married. She said it was against her principles. Nurses should have less of such "principles" and more of the golden rule.

TALKING IN PUBLIC

Regardless of how interesting one's work may be, it should be an unfailing rule that when one leaves it, it must not be discussed in public. It is decidedly disconcerting to hear two nurses in a bus or restaurant discussing their work or their patients. True, a nurse need not be ashamed of her profession (many nurses, indeed, feel a bit superior to the laywoman), but nursing of any kind is a personal service which requires intimacies not intended for the public ear. The nurse should have interests so numerous and varied that she need not be limited to her work as a source of conversational material.

No lawyer talks all the time of law, no business man speaks only of his merchandise, no broker of only stocks, and no doctor just of life and death. Why should we talk only of patients and nursing? . . . There should be an unwritten law about talking shop and gossiping about other people's business.[1]

PRACTICING WITH IRREGULARS

Nurses often are concerned about what to do when working with so-called "irregulars." A professional nurse who accepts a call and finds a practical nurse in charge accomplishes little by assuming a superior air and being disagreeable. Such a situation is an opportunity to prove the advantages of her professional education. By virtue of her training, the nurse should prove herself even more adaptable than the practical nurse and should be able to give better nursing care; these obvious differences will be quickly recognized by the patient and the family. Furthermore, her training should enable a nurse to meet any crisis more efficiently and with better judgment than can the practical nurse. When a skilled nurse demonstrates that training has its

---

[1] Gladys E. Willet, ' The Truth Hurts,'' *American Journal of Nursing*, Vol. 38 (April 1938), p. 475.

advantages, the difference in price for service will count in favor of the registered nurse.

Whether or not the professional nurse teaches or demonstrates any nursing procedures for the practical nurse whom she may find on the case depends upon the circumstances.

As for medical irregulars, and those physicians outlawed by their own profession because of some unethical conduct, no nurse in good standing in her own profession can afford to jeopardize this standing by cooperating with an individual who does not have the endorsement of the medical profession. ''All professions grade down to something unprofessional in the lower fringes of their membership, and it is a duty to society and to the professions to cut this soiled fringe away'' by having no contact with it.

ADVERTISING AND PRODUCT ENDORSEMENTS

The graduate nurse may be approached by commercial firms with a request that she endorse one or more of its products, the endorsement to be used for advertising purposes. The giving of such endorsements is a practice frowned upon by the nursing profession and is one of the things that nurses in good standing ordinarily do not do. The proposals are made very attractive, and the compensation is adequate; the procedure, however, is pregnant with unethical possibilities, and no nurse should risk her professional standing by agreeing to it until after she has obtained unquestionable assurance of the accuracy of the verbal or printed statements she is asked to make. The nurse should use every precaution in investigating requests for her endorsements or for her professional services in other forms of publicity. For purely technical information she may refer to the laboratories of the American Medical Association, Chicago, Illinois. For advice concerning the ethics involved, she may consult the Committee on Ethical Standards of the American Nurses' Association.

WEARING THE UNIFORM—WHEN AND WHERE

For several years there has been an increasing discussion of the propriety of nurses wearing their uniforms in public places and on the street. There is no official ruling on the uniform, but an excellent precedent has been set in the fact that the use of the insigne of the Red Cross Nursing Service has been circumscribed by an act of Congress, and specific ruling made as to when, where, how, and by whom the insigne may be worn. Since only graduate nurses are accepted as Red Cross nurses, there can be nothing presumptuous in our professional nurse's uniform by definite rulings concerning its use.

The nurse may be guided by the following general statement: A professional atmosphere is created by a graduate nurse's uniform and cap wherever they are worn. Hence, professional ethics should govern one's decisions as to when and where the nurse may appear in professional garb. Since the rules of ethics of any profession represent the group opinion, the author may do no better than present some suggestions which embody the opinions of leaders in the nursing world, as expressed in conferences and correspondence during the past few years.

As members of one of the newest of the professions, nurses may be guided in general by the customs of the older professions. Military and naval officers wear their service uniforms only when on active duty. Judges wear their judicial robes only while on the bench or in their private chambers. Clergymen wear their vestments only while conducting or participating in a religious ceremony. Doctors wear their office smocks only in their offices. University and college executives and faculty members refrain from wearing their caps and gowns except when participating in some strictly institutional ceremony. Indiscriminate use of the distinguishing garments of any professional group causes even the laity to suspect that the wearer is a charlatan.

Applying these practices to various nursing situations, the following inferences may be drawn:

It is the considered opinion that a nurse may wear the uniform when employed by a medical firm to explain the use of its products at a convention if duties involved come within the practice of profession and if the uniform does not make her unduly conspicuous.

If employed in a department store, in the division of health service, she should wear a uniform.

If employed in an educational capacity in some department store, that is, in some work which engages her nursing education, she may wear a uniform.

Most nurses are agreed that if employed in a store primarily as a saleswoman she should not wear the uniform. In this case its use manifestly would mean that the uniform was being commercialized.

The world-wide popularity of movies in which doctors' and nurses' uniforms dominate the settings has been capitalized by the same type of promoters who dress theater doormen and ticket takers in rear admirals' uniforms. The author has seen restaurant and soda-fountain attendants in uniforms practically identical with those worn by nurses. This situation will become worse before it becomes better. It may be improved only when professional nurses, individually and through their organizations, discourage the use of the uniform for any purpose other than those indicated in the preceding paragraphs as being in accord with the spirit of the nursing profession.

The American Journal of Nursing, August, 1937, page 911, in publishing the digest of minutes of the meeting of the board of directors of the American Nurses' Association, says:

With regard to the matter of nurses appearing in uniform, it was the opinion of the members of the Board that the nurse in uniform should appear in public only when dressed in outdoor uniform such as that adopted by the Nursing Service of the American Red Cross, the United States Public Health Service, and the Public Health Nursing Associations.

TELEVISION CODE

In January, 1960, an amendment was made to the National Association of Broadcaster Television Code. "The amendment prohibits the portrayal of physicians, dentists,—and nurses by actors in television commercials. No props or setting may be used in a commercial which would give the impression that the individual is a member of the medical, dental, or nursing profession, when not.''

RED CROSS INSIGNE

Reference has previously been made to restrictions imposed on the use of the Red Cross insigne. Because of these references, a condensation of the Regulations for Wearing the Badge of the Red Cross Nursing Service approved by the National Committee of the Red Cross Nursing Service, as of December 8, 1931, is appended:

1. It may be worn by an enrolled Red Cross nurse only, and then as a badge and not as a pin.
2. When in uniform, the Red Cross nurse may wear her badge: (a) with an indoor Red Cross uniform to fasten the collar in front; (b) with an outdoor Red Cross uniform to fasten the collar; (c) it may be worn 2 inches below and 3 inches to the left of the lower left-hand point of the collar.
3. It may be worn at a Red Cross function with civilian clothes or with evening dress. When worn this way, it must not be worn as a pin but should be worn on the left, in relatively the same position as described in (c) above.
4. It must not be loaned to any person, even though she might be an enrolled Red Cross nurse. The badge should never leave the possession of the nurse to whom it has been issued. When the application for enrollment has been approved, the nurse will receive a numbered appointment card and badge, record of which will be kept on file by the local committee on Red Cross Nursing Service and by the nursing service at national headquarters. The badge and card will remain at all times the property of the American Red Cross.

SCHOOL PINS

The school pin should be worn only with the uniform. Again, it becomes the insigne of the nurse's school. Sometimes the recent graduate, in her happy pride of accomplishment, wears her pin with street clothes and with evening dress. Nurses generally are agreed that this is not in good taste, no matter how proud the owner may be to wear it.

COSMETICS

The woman of today has become so accustomed to the use of cosmetics that she uses it even when in uniform. To use it or not to use it has caused considerable discussion. Theodocia Crosse, the late author of Social Customs, and an authority on social usage, in answer to the author's query on the subject, made the following statement: ''Strictly speaking, no make-up should be worn by nurses in uniform. However, the modern young woman is so accustomed to wearing it that to forego it entirely when in uniform seems an uncalled-for extreme, particularly in view of the fact that a slight amount of lipstick, rouge, or powder may enhance the nurse's appearance and make it more pleasing to the patient. But only by a conservative use should it be endorsed. Perhaps a test as to whether too much is being used or not might be found in the question: Is it immediately obvious that I am wearing make-up? If it is obvious, then too much has been applied.

"Bright nail polish is not in good taste in the sickroom. It serves no purpose, and is not in keeping with the modesty and utilitarian character of the nurse's uniform. Furthermore, many people have a distinct aversion for brightly colored nail polish, and the use of it may be offensive to the patient."

THE USE OF "R.N."

The title, *Registered Nurse,* is purely professional and should not be confused with social affairs. The letters *R.N.* should be used only on professional cards, statements, and professional stationery, and always when a professional signature is required. The nurse should remember that this title does not indicate an academic degree; it indicates only that she has successfully passed her state board examinations and that, having done so, she is registered or licensed to practice nursing in that state.

Always use *R.N.* with the signature in writing for professional samples and scientific literature, as advertised in nursing periodicals. This is the advertiser's protection against "practicing medicine" by sending samples to lay people, thus encouraging self-medication. Some manufacturers also require the nurse's state registration number.

PROFESSIONAL COURTESY

Should the nurse expect a discount for service from her physician or dentist? A nation-wide cross-section survey of nurses was made on this question. Three out of four nurses answered in the negative.[2] The nurse, as an independent person, expects to pay her way.

A simple way of solving this problem without embarrassment to either the doctor or the nurse is through insurance. Many forms of income protection insurance which include physician's fees are available. When ill the nurse may present her insurance card to the physician with the remark: "If there are additional charges please have your secretary send me a statement."[3]

IF A STRIKE OCCURS

Unions of nonprofessional employees in hospitals are being organized in many cities and especially in large medical centers. The nurse is committed to give nursing care, but where does "nursing care" stop and "strike-breaking" begin?

[2] Martha Dudley, "How Nurses Choose Their Doctors," *RN* Vol. 23 (June 1960), p. 56.

[3] The nurse should retain this statement for income tax deductions.

The American Nurses' Association House of Delegates, in June, 1960, issued a complete statement of the "Nurses in Disputes Policy." The following quotation from this statement should be the nurse's guide in any hospital strike or threat of strike:

"The ANA believes that the best relations among management, nurses, other employees and the public will be maintained if management, the other employees and the public recognize that nurses by virtue of their professional obligations occupy a neutral position in management-labor disputes and continue to perform their distinctive nursing functions during such disputes solely in fulfillment of their professional duties to patient."

This policy of neutrality may be difficult to decide in the actual situation. The rule-of-thumb should be to separate non-nursing activities from nursing activities: nurses will not replace elevator operators, laundry, kitchen or housekeeping personnel.

Sometimes a conflict arises between doctors who wish "business as usual" and nurses who are committed to a policy of neutrality. The director of nursing service, who is a nurse, knows the nurses' position. She will give this information to the administrator who in turn will inform the doctors that nurses will provide only nursing care, and request that admissions be curtailed until conditions are again normal.[4]

CLASS EXERCISE

Describe one actual situation involving a question of ethics in the following: loyalty to the physician as a public health nurse; choice of physician; advertising; graduate uniform.

REFERENCES

ALCOTT, LOUISE, MOORE, MARY R., and CAMDEN, HONORE: Combining marriage and nursing. *Amer. J. Nurs.* 55:1344 (Nov.) 1955.

"Are we guilty of bad manners?" *Amer. J. Nurs.* 42:815 (July) 1942.

BARTSCH, JOSEPHINE: Handling orders that violate ethics. *RN* 24:46 (Apr.) 1961; 25:58 (Feb.) 1962.

BONNEY, Virginia: Directing students to programs appropriate for abilities and goals. New York State League for Nursing, *Primed for Progress*, Bulletin No. 1, 1960.

CROSSE, THEODOCIA: *Social Customs*. J. B. Lippincott Co., Philadelphia, 1938.

---

[4] The nurse's responsibility in hospital strikes is given in detail in "If a Hospital Strike Occurs," *American Journal of Nursing*, 60:344 (Mar.) 1960.

DEVERS, ALICE C.: Employment during pregnancy. *Nurs. World* 127:23 (Jan.) 1953.

DUDLEY, MARTHA: How nurses choose their doctors. *RN* 23:56 (June) 1960.

DUDLEY, MARTHA: Are hospitals meeting their nurses' health needs? *RN* 25:60 (Jan.) 1962.

Editorial: Industry and the professional. *Amer. J. Nurs.* 44:420 (May) 1944.

Editorial: "Jargonitis—a curable disease." (A plea for correct English) *RN* 20:48 (Sept.) 1957.

"For the patient who needs a flying ambulance." *RN* 24:35 (Aug.) 1961.

FRENCH, GAIL: Fashions and grooming. *Trained Nurse and Hosp. Rev.* 122:225 (May) 1949.

GAULT, DOROTHY PATTERSON: A hoop to hang your cap on. *RN* 24:63 (Sept.) 1961.

HEWES, LYDIA: Name pin introduce staff to patient. *Mod. Hosp.* 79:91 (Aug.) 1952.

"If a hospital strike occurs." *Amer. J. Nurs.* 60:344 (Mar.) 1960.

KRALOVICH, ANNE M.: The graduate nurse's uniform. *Amer. J. Nurs.* 49:148 (Mar.) 1949.

LEGGE, VIVIAN L.: Care for a relative with a terminal illness? *RN* 24:77 (Sept.) 1961.

MANOCK, JANE W.: Hospital strikes. *Amer. J. Nurs.* 59:1346 (Oct.) 1959.

NIGHTINGALE, FLORENCE: *Notes on Nursing.* Appleton-Century-Crofts, Inc., New York, 1917. Reprinted in 1946.

NORMAN, MABELCLAIRE: How to keep up with new medicines. *RN* 24:57 (June) 1961.

OSHIN, EDITH S.: You have a stake in hospital accreditation. *RN* 24:60 (Apr.) 1961.

OSHIN, EDITH S.: When your patient must travel by plane or train. *RN* 24:33 (Aug.) 1961.

PETERS, DOROTHY: The Kewanee story. *Amer. J. Nurs.* 61:74 (Oct.) 1961.

PHILLIPS, CLARE: Open hearing on tips. *RN* 20:38 and 20:78 (Dec.) 1957.

REICHERT, PHILLIP: The modern nurse and medical advertising. *Amer. J. Nurs.* 54:1092 (Sept.) 1954.

"Rx for visitor trouble." *RN* 24:11 (June) 1961.

STANDARD, SAMUEL, and HELMUTH, NATHAN (editors): Should the Patient Know the Truth? Springer Publishing Co., New York, 1955.

SWITAL, CHET L.: The nurse and her silhouette. *RN* 12:48 (Mar.) 1949.

VANDERBILT, AMY: *Complete Book of Etiquette.* Doubleday & Co., Inc., New York, 1953.

"What is my responsibility?" *Amer. J. Nurs.* 61:55 (Oct.) 1961.

"Will just being good women suffice?" *RN* 12:24 (Feb.) 1949.

WOLFF, ILSE S.: Should the patient know the truth. *Amer. J. Nurs.* 55:546 (May) 1955.

Index